W9-BLA-891

The Essential Guide TO

Healthy Healing Foods

by Victoria Shanta Retelny, R.D., L.D.N.
with Jovanka JoAnn Milivojevic

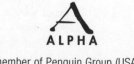

ALPHA

A member of Penguin Group (USA) Inc.

ALPHA BOOKS

Published by the Penguin Group

Penguin Group (USA) Inc., 375 Hudson Street, New York, New York 10014, USA

Penguin Group (Canada), 90 Eglinton Avenue East, Suite 700, Toronto, Ontario M4P 2Y3, Canada (a division of Pearson Penguin Canada Inc.)

Penguin Books Ltd., 80 Strand, London WC2R 0RL, England

Penguin Ireland, 25 St. Stephen's Green, Dublin 2, Ireland (a division of Penguin Books Ltd.)

Penguin Group (Australia), 250 Camberwell Road, Camberwell, Victoria 3124, Australia (a division of Pearson Australia Group Pty. Ltd.)

Penguin Books India Pvt. Ltd., 11 Community Centre, Panchsheel Park, New Delhi—110 017, India

Penguin Group (NZ), 67 Apollo Drive, Rosedale, North Shore, Auckland 1311, New Zealand (a division of Pearson New Zealand Ltd.)

Penguin Books (South Africa) (Pty.) Ltd., 24 Sturdee Avenue, Rosebank, Johannesburg 2196, South Africa

Penguin Books Ltd., Registered Offices: 80 Strand, London WC2R 0RL, England

Copyright © 2011 by Victoria Shanta Retelny

All rights reserved. No part of this book shall be reproduced, stored in a retrieval system, or transmitted by any means, electronic, mechanical, photocopying, recording, or otherwise, without written permission from the publisher. No patent liability is assumed with respect to the use of the information contained herein. Although every precaution has been taken in the preparation of this book, the publisher and author assume no responsibility for errors or omissions. Neither is any liability assumed for damages resulting from the use of information contained herein. For information, address Alpha Books, 800 East 96th Street, Indianapolis, IN 46240.

THE COMPLETE IDIOT'S GUIDE TO and Design are registered trademarks of Penguin Group (USA) Inc.

International Standard Book Number: 978-1-61564-108-6

Library of Congress Catalog Card Number: 2010919340

13 12 11   8 7 6 5 4 3 2 1

Interpretation of the printing code: The rightmost number of the first series of numbers is the year of the book's printing; the rightmost number of the second series of numbers is the number of the book's printing. For example, a printing code of 11-1 shows that the first printing occurred in 2011.

Printed in the United States of America

Note: This publication contains the opinions and ideas of its author. It is intended to provide helpful and informative material on the subject matter covered. It is sold with the understanding that the author and publisher are not engaged in rendering professional services in the book. If the reader requires personal assistance or advice, a competent professional should be consulted.

The author and publisher specifically disclaim any responsibility for any liability, loss, or risk, personal or otherwise, which is incurred as a consequence, directly or indirectly, of the use and application of any of the contents of this book.

Most Alpha books are available at special quantity discounts for bulk purchases for sales promotions, premiums, fund-raising, or educational use. Special books, or book excerpts, can also be created to fit specific needs.

For details, write: Special Markets, Alpha Books, 375 Hudson Street, New York, NY 10014.

Publisher: *Marie Butler-Knight*

Associate Publisher: *Mike Sanders*

Executive Managing Editor: *Billy Fields*

Acquisitions Editor: *Tom Stevens*

Development Editor: *Jennifer Moore*

Senior Production Editor: *Janette Lynn*

Copy Editor: *Catherine Schwenk*

Cover Designer: *Rebecca Batchelor*

Book Designers: *William Thomas, Rebecca Batchelor*

Indexer: *Julie Bess*

Layout: *Ayanna Lacey*

Senior Proofreader: *Laura Caddell*

Dedication

For my three loves: Scott, Grant, and Samantha—you make everything possible.

Contents

Part 2   Healthy Foods in Focus   73

Part 3   Drink to Your Good Health   187

Appendixes

Introduction

For me, there's no better topic than the wonderful world of food—especially food that keeps you healthy, happy, and productive for life! From the moment you are born, food is life, love, and nourishment for your growth and development. Food is also medicine; it heals your body, fends off chronic diseases and disorders, and keeps every cell in your body in tip-top shape. *The Essential Guide to Healthy Healing Foods* takes you into the landscape of nourishing foods. However, we go beyond talking about food to discussing your relationship with what you eat, why you eat, and when you eat. This book is a window into the world of healthy food choices. It is meant to arm you with the basic nutrition knowledge you need to become a mindful eater in a world where mindless eating runs rampant.

How to Navigate This Book

To give you a complete landscape of healthful eating, *The Essential Guide to Healthy Healing Foods* is divided into five parts. Each part delves into a different facet of food and eating.

Part 1, Eat Well to Live Well, explores how the wide range of nutrients work together to promote optimal health throughout life. From the fiber-filled carbohydrates, lean proteins, and healthy fats that your body needs in large quantities to the vitamins and minerals you need in smaller amounts, we help you understand why you should strive to eat a combination of all these nutrients. One food or meal does not make or break a healthy diet; rather, it's the way you eat over the course of time that matters. These chapters help you start substituting healthy foods for unhealthy foods and maintain a nutritious diet in the face of continuous temptation. You'll also discover how you and your family can make smarter choices at every age.

In **Part 2, Healthy Foods in Focus,** you get close and personal with the foods that contribute to your good health. From fruits and veggies to whole grains and fabulous fats, you'll learn what gives certain foods their healing and healthful properties, as well as what can sometimes make them dangerous. We also explore the world of food allergens—where they lurk, what the symptoms are, and how to work around allergies and still maintain a healthy diet. Also, we take a look at interesting ways to spice up your health and cooking by swapping salt with sodium-free, flavor-packed herbs and spices.

Part 3, Drink to Your Good Health, delves into the nature of liquid nutrition. The downside of drinking your calories rather than eating them is that they can quickly lead to weight gain. The upside is that water, tea, coffee, and even alcohol (when drunk in moderation), can play a major role in your health and wellness. It all comes down to balancing liquid with solid food calories, and we give you some tips on savvy drinking tactics.

Ever wonder what foods are good for revving up your metabolism? Or what you should eat to sleep better or boost your immunity? **Part 4, Real Food to the Rescue,** looks at overall wellness and how cutting-edge nutrition tips can help you stay healthy, fend off inflammation, and get more shut-eye.

Part 5, Foods to Fight Disease, explores the major role that food plays in fending off chronic diseases, such as diabetes, heart disease, cancer, and osteoporosis. With what you eat playing a primary role in whether or not disease creeps into your life, this part highlights foods that can help prevent and control major diseases. Armed with nutrition know-how, you can better tackle and defend against illnesses and live a longer, healthier life.

An important aspect of eating healthy, healing foods is cooking with them at home. To help you get comfortable using a wide variety of nutritious foods, we've included recipes throughout the chapters to showcase how to use some of these foods in your own kitchen.

On the Side

This book is peppered with tidbits of nutrition and food-related information. Here's how they break down:

Definition	Here you'll find definitions of uncommon terms associated with food, eating, and nutrition.
Healing Hints	These tips help you get the most out of foods' healing properties. Whether a new cooking method or selection strategy, these snippets are meant to help you maximize your foods' nutritional value.
Munch on This	These side notes give you background information on food, nutrition, and health. Think of them as food for thought.
Food wise	Here you'll find myth-busting facts and precautionary notes as you navigate the world of food and nutrition.

Acknowledgments

For me, there's no better book to write than one about healthy and healing foods! Food is my personal and professional passion. Many thanks to Marilyn Allen, my literary agent, for giving me the opportunity to express this fire in my belly. And to Tom Stevens, my go-to editor at Alpha, who helped turn my words into a cohesive book. This book would not have been possible without the editing finesse and expertise of JoAnn Milivojevic. Thank you, JoAnn, for the extra time, support, and for making the book-writing process much less daunting for me.

Much thanks goes to my nutrition colleagues and friends, who inspire me to be a better nutrition professional every day and contributed to this work more than they know—especially Kate Geagan, M.S., R.D.; Robin Plotkin, R.D., L.D.N.; Dawn Jackson Blatner, R.D., L.D.N.; Bethany Doerfler, M.S., R.D.; Judy Doherty, P.C. II; and Heidi McIndoo, M.S., R.D.—thanks so much for giving me the support to forge ahead with my dreams. And to my patients who inspire me with their hope, strength, and fortitude—I learn so much from you.

Much love and gratitude to Scott, my husband, love, and best friend—thank you for believing in me when I didn't and being my taste tester! And for my two precious gifts, Grant and Samantha, who always go with the flow and love me unconditionally, even when my time got tight and there wasn't much to give. But, there was always time for our bedtime prayer, "Dear God, thank you for this day, for a chance to live in a healthy way." May your love of healthy living never end.

As I walk on life's journey, there's no greater pleasure than saying thank you to my Mom and Dad who gave me the courage to stick with my passions and the love to know when to let go. And for Gram, thank you for feeding me well always—her delicious cooking and ease in the kitchen meant more to me than she ever knew. Last, but certainly not least, to my sisters, Viv and Gigi, may you always know that you were responsible for my passion for food and health (and you know what I mean!). For that, I am forever grateful …

Trademarks

All terms mentioned in this book that are known to be or are suspected of being trademarks or service marks have been appropriately capitalized. Alpha Books and Penguin Group (USA) Inc. cannot attest to the accuracy of this information. Use of a term in this book should not be regarded as affecting the validity of any trademark or service mark.

Part 1

Eat Well to Live Well

The chapters in this part explore how nutrients work together to promote optimal health throughout life. You'll find out about macronutrients, such as carbohydrates, proteins, and fats, and micronutrients, such as vitamins and minerals. Although your body needs different quantities of these nutrients, all are necessary for optimum health. You also learn how and why you should strive to eat a combination of all nutrients.

You gain insight into how to maintain a healthy, nutritious diet in the face of continuous temptation. America's seductive eating environment can lead to a number of eating disorders, which I explore and point out paths to overcome them. And equally important, you'll discover how you and your family can eat more mindfully, make better choices at the grocery store, and enjoy new foods.

chapter 1

Food for Life

Understanding how nutrients work together for optimal health

Getting the most from The Big Three nutrients

Making sense of organics

Deciphering nutrition labels

Ensuring good food quality

What you eat is directly related to your health. That's probably not an earth-shattering revelation to you. But consider this: according to the World Health Organization, 2.7 million die each year because they are not eating enough fruits and vegetables!

In ancient times certain foods were revered for their healing powers. Today, nutrition science validates the idea that good food leads to good health. So, as it turns out, an apple a day may just keep the doctor away. On the other hand, foods that lack nutrients not only pile on unnecessary calories, but they can cause a cascade of events that may lead to the onset of chronic diseases—and repeat visits to your doc.

In this chapter I help you be a better food detective. You'll learn to sleuth out the high-nutrition foods, gain a better understanding of what good nutrition really means, and, most important, find out how to get more of the good stuff into your daily diet.

The Complex Nature of Food

The beauty of healthy and healing food is the interplay of nutrients. Neither a single food nor a single nutrient acts alone. It's the *combination* of nutrients in foods that provides a biological defense against viruses, bacteria, and damage to cells, which can lead to illness and chronic diseases. That's why it's so important to include a wide variety of healthy foods in your diet.

Along with variety, balance and moderation are also important. Here are some quick tips on what to eat for health and for weight management:

- Consume a variety of nutrient-dense foods (see the next section).

- Meet recommended amounts of nutrients and calories by having a balanced eating plan. I help you with that in Chapter 2.

- To prevent weight gain as you age, eat less and exercise more, especially after age 30.

All About Nutrients

The goal of healthy eating is to maximize the amount of *nutrients* you can give your body at any one time. Fueling up with *nutrient-dense foods,* such as vegetables, fruits, and whole grains, helps your body heal and function at optimal levels. On the other hand, eating *empty-calorie foods* can threaten long-term health with weight gain and nutrient deficiencies.

Definition

A **nutrient** is a chemical substance in foods. Nutrients provide energy, growth, enable repair of cells, and regulate body processes. **Nutrient-dense foods** provide a lot of vitamins, minerals, and fiber with relatively few calories. **Empty-calorie foods** contain more calories than nutrients; examples include candy, cookies, white bread, fried foods, and alcoholic beverages.

Nutrients can be further broken down into macronutrients and micronutrients. Macronutrients are carbohydrates, proteins, and fats—these are what registered dietitians call "the big three" nutrients. We need to fortify our bodies with adequate supplies of these three key nutrients every day.

Your body also needs micronutrients, but in much smaller amounts. Micronutrients are minerals and vitamins. Minerals include iron, cobalt, chromium, copper, iodine, manganese, selenium, and zinc. Minerals are essential for supporting the chemical reactions in the body for proper functioning of organs, bones, and hormones. Likewise, small amounts of vitamins are essential for your health. For instance, the B-vitamins and vitamin C help your immune system and reproductive systems run smoothly and give your skin a healthy glow.

The Big Three Nutrients

As you'll soon see, "the big three" macronutrients (carbs, protein, and fats) all play unique roles in your body. Fiber is considered a macronutrient, too, but I will discuss it later in the chapter. Keep in mind, though, that one is not more important than the others. They work together to sustain the intricate matrix of health.

Carbohydrates

Carbohydrates, or carbs for short, are a vital nutrient as they supply energy in the form of glucose (sugar) to your brain and to every cell in your body. High-fiber carbs, such as whole grains, vegetables, and fruits, are best for your health as they help keep your blood sugar stable, fend off hunger longer, and fill you up faster with fewer calories.

The Institute of Medicine (IOM) recommends that the average person (not overly active) get at least 130 grams of carbohydrates per day. This means you should spread your carbs out throughout the day at meals and snacks, such as whole-grain bread, whole-grain pasta, brown rice, oatmeal, and whole fruits and/or vegetables. Remember, one serving of carbs equals 15 grams. (For more carb counting details, check out Chapter 21.)

Let's face it, carbs are controversial, and the most infamous nutrient thanks to a flurry of *fad diets* in recent years. Most people have a love-hate relationship with them. Your body needs carbs for energy. If you don't eat enough carbs your body will turn to stored glucose (glycogen) in your liver for energy. Once the liver's glycogen stores are depleted, the body begins to use fat for fuel. If this goes on for too long, the liver may get stressed, your workouts and physical conditioning may be compromised, and you may become dehydrated (not to mention your breath may begin to smell like the funky odor of nail polish remover). Not a good combination!

definition

Fad diets promise big weight loss in a short period of time with drastic measures like taking out a major nutrient or food group because it is perceived as fattening or harmful. Instead aim for a diet that is balanced with healthy carbs like whole grains, fruits, and vegetables.

Protein

Protein is not just for muscle-building bubbas at the gym. Our bodies rely on protein—or, more specifically, its building blocks, amino acids—for many essential functions. Proteins are powerful players in our cells, metabolism, and immune system. They also help us digest foods properly.

Eating a variety of protein-rich foods is important because your body cannot make all of the amino acids on its own. How can you get enough? By eating high-protein foods daily such as beans, legumes, tofu, skinless chicken breast, turkey breast, lean beef, and low-fat milk, yogurt, and/or cheese.

The general guideline provided by the *Dietary Guidelines for Americans* recommends 5 to 7 ounces of meat or meat alternatives per day. Like all nutrients, it's important to spread protein out throughout the day—research has shown that our bodies can only use 4 ounces at a time. There are 7 grams of protein in an ounce of meat, so that's 35 to 49 grams per day.

But how much protein do *you* really need? That depends on your age and body weight. For adults (19 + years), calculate this:

> $0.8 \times$ kilograms (kg) of body weight (kg = your weight in pounds divided by 2.2) For example: If you are 150 pounds, divide $150 \div 2.2 = 68$ kg
>
> $0.8 \times 68 = 54$ grams of protein per day

That's 7 to 8 ounces of protein-rich foods a day for average adults.

> **Munch on This**
>
> The typical American adult does not lack protein in his or her diet. According to research published in the *American Journal of Clinical Nutrition,* some American adults eat as much as 91 grams of protein per day! Discover your own personal protein consumption by using the calculation described in this section.

Fat

Fat is a necessary, vital nutrient for life and health. Fats, also known as lipids, make up every cell in your body! They regulate hormones, insulate your organs, facilitate the absorption of fat-soluble vitamins, and are good for hair and skin. Now isn't that enough to take fats more seriously? But wait, there's more. Much more.

Fat makes us feel satisfied and happy after eating it. From a culinary perspective, fat adds flavor and smoothness. Fat may actually be one of our taste senses, along with salty, sweet, sour, bitter, and savory, which explains why fatty foods taste so good.

Fat comes in two forms. There are *unsaturated fats* known as the "good" fats, and *saturated fats* known as the "bad" ones. For your health, the unsaturated fats from olive oil, canola oil, fish, and nuts are good for your heart. The not-so-good side of fat is that too much of the saturated and the so-called *trans fat* fats can lead to heart disease, stroke, and high cholesterol.

On the list of fatty foods to limit—*not* eliminate altogether—are whole milk, full-fat yogurt and/ or cheese, fatty cuts of meat (bacon, prime rib, etc.), and tropical oils (coconut, palm oils, etc.). However, feel free to banish those pesky trans fats, a.k.a. partially hydrogenated vegetable oils, altogether! I cover fats in greater detail in Chapter 10.

> **Definition**
>
> **Unsaturated fats** are heart-healthy fats, which help keep blood cholesterol levels in check and blood vessels clear. **Saturated fats,** if eaten in large quantities, can lead to high cholesterol and clogged arteries. **Trans fats** are vegetables oils that have been processed (hydrogenated) in order to make products last longer on grocery store shelves. They are detrimental to health and can lead to heart disease.

Remember that eating fat—in moderation—does *not* make you fat. It's overall calories that count. A mere 10 extra calories a day can cause you to gain a pound in a year! Keep in mind that carbs and protein have four calories per gram and fats have nine calories per gram. So watch the extra nibbles, bites, and sips!

Whole Foods

When we talk about whole foods the whole truly is greater than the sum of its parts. Whole foods are unprocessed and unrefined and typically do not contain added ingredients, such as sugar, salt, or fat. As a result, whole foods are typically higher in fiber, vitamins, minerals, and *antioxidants* than refined processed foods. Examples of whole foods include whole grains, whole fruits and vegetables, dry beans, peas, lentils, unprocessed meat, poultry, and fish. Whole foods can also contain polyphenols and flavonoids, two types of antioxidants, commonly found in fruits, vegetables, and tea leaves, especially green tea.

Whole foods contain a host of vital, healing compounds. Let's get acquainted with a few of them:

- **Antioxidants**   Nutrient components of foods, primarily found in vitamins A, C, and E and selenium ("ACES" for short). They fend off cell damage by free radicals, which can cause diseases. Free radicals are toxic molecules in the body that cause damage to the cells, premature aging, and chronic diseases.

- **Dietary fiber**   There are two types of dietary fiber: soluble and insoluble. Both types travel through the body undigested. Soluble fiber helps rid the body of excess cholesterol; it is found in oats and citrus fruits. Insoluble fiber helps with healthy function of the large intestine or colon; it's in the skin of fruits and vegetables, plus whole grains, and seeds.

A good example of a whole food is a whole grain. A whole grain maintains its triad of health: the bran, endosperm, and germ. Bran contains fiber, B-vitamins, and trace minerals. Endosperm provides energy in the form of carbohydrates and protein. (This is the only part left in a refined grain.) Germ contains antioxidants, vitamin E, and B-vitamins.

So get your whole foods in every day. At mealtime, eat whole grains in the form of whole-grain breads, whole-grain pasta, brown rice, and/or oatmeal. Get even more whole foods by piling your plate with a variety of fresh vegetables and snacking on whole, fresh fruits at least two to three times a day.

Food Quality Matters

Food quality is a primary consideration of healthy eating, and this requires making the right choices every day. But with an overabundance of options out there, navigating the grocery store aisles can be downright daunting. Do you pay the extra price for organic produce but buy conventionally produced milk and meat? What about wine with sulfites or not? Is it okay to buy Angus beef hot dogs if they are free of nitrites, an additive in cured meats that is linked to chronic diseases? Let's try to distill what you really want to eat to get the best bang for your health buck!

Organic vs. Conventionally Grown Foods

From a logical standpoint it makes sense to not want to ingest pesticides, fertilizers, and growth hormones. Organic foods don't have these. Cutting back on the use of these substances is not only better for you, but the health of the planet.

Food scientists debate whether or not organically grown produce actually contains more nutrients. Some studies have shown that they do, but in insignificant amounts. Nonetheless many people think organics are better for themselves and the planet, and it shows up at the cash register: dollar sales of organic produce grew more than 12 percent in 2009, reaching total sales of $9.5 billion!

Let's decipher some jargon commonly used by the health community:

- **Organic**   A designation used by the U.S. Department of Agriculture's National Organic Program to certify food that is produced without synthetic chemicals or fertilizers, genetic engineering, radiation, or sewage sludge.

- **Conventional foods**   May be produced with synthetic chemicals, irradiation, or in the presence of sludge or toxic waste.

- **Recombinant bovine somatotropin (rBST)**   An artificial growth hormone injected in dairy cows to increase milk production.

In the United States, organic foods are regulated by the Organic Foods Production Act (OFPA) of 1990. This act ensures that organic growers and handlers use only organic materials and are certified to sell products labeled "organic." In the United States products that contain at least 95 percent organic ingredients can display the USDA certified organic seal shown in the following figure.

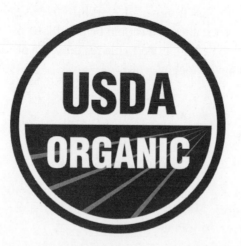

Look for this seal to identify organic food that's been certified by the USDA.

Organics Across the Food Spectrum

The USDA has standards for organic crops, livestock (including cows, hens, chickens, and pigs), and packaged goods, dairy, and seafood. With crops, strict guidelines ensure that land is free of pesticides and substances for at least three years prior to harvest. There must be buffer zones to protect fields from unwanted substances from neighboring farms. Livestock or animals must be fed organic food, permitted to roam outside and get sunlight daily, and cannot be fed hormones, antibiotics, or be overcrowded.

Packaged goods that are designated as organic cannot be packaged in any materials that have come in contact with synthetic fungicides, fumigants, or preservatives. In fact, 95 percent of organic packaged good's ingredients must be produced organically in order to get the USDA certified organic seal. Organic dairy products cannot contain antibiotics, synthetic growth hormones, or toxic pesticides.

The USDA standards for organic seafood are still being developed. Due to fish's highly publicized heart-health benefits, there is a shift toward sustainable marine life in order to keep the waters flowing with healthy species of fish. Responsible farming practices are leading to what is called a "sustainable blue revolution," which will ensure that the fish on your table is free of contaminants like mercury and PCBs, antibiotics, and hormones. (Read more on safe fish and seafood to eat in Chapter 10.)

Produce is probably the most popular organic product on the market. When it comes to your fruits and vegetables, there are three rules of thumb: eat a varied diet, rinse all produce, and buy organic whenever possible. The Environmental Working Group's *Shopper's Guide to Pesticides* publishes a list of fruits and vegetables that should be purchased organically ("The Dirty Dozen") as they were found to be high in pesticide residue. The products on the right ("The Clean 15") are safe to buy conventionally grown.

The Dirty Dozen	**The Clean 15**
(Buy These Organic)	(Lowest in Pesticides)
Apples	Asparagus
Bell peppers	Avocado
Blueberries	Cabbage
Cherries	Cantaloupe

The Dirty Dozen	**The Clean 15**
Celery	Eggplant
Grapes (imported)	Grapefruit
Kale/Collard greens	Honeydew Melon
Nectarines	Kiwi
Peaches	Mangoes
Potatoes	Onions
Spinach	Pineapple
Strawberries	Sweet corn
	Sweet peas
	Sweet potatoes
	Watermelon

Remember, eating any type of vegetables and fruits—whether conventional or organic—is better than not eating any! It's okay to buy conventional produce, but take precautions: wash with a scrub brush (used only for your produce) and cold water and/or peel the fruit or vegetable (this process takes away some vital nutrients, but it's a trade off!) to take away as much pesticide residue as possible. No need to use special produce soaps—the fewer chemicals you use, the better!

Nutrition Label Know-How

When it comes to choosing packaged foods, there is no better way to assess what you're about to put in your mouth than the Nutrition Facts Panel (NFP) on the box, bag, carton, or bottle.

munch on This

Anything packaged in a box, bag, carton, or bottle is required to have a Nutrition Facts Panel. Nutrition labeling for raw produce—fruits and vegetables—and fish is voluntary.

In an ideal world, we would eat only fresh, unprocessed foods, but that's not realistic. Because convenience is king in our fast-paced world, processed and packaged food is a fact of life—but it doesn't mean good nutrition has to be compromised. The NFP tells you at a glance what you need to know about any packaged food. Using it, you can limit certain nutrients and get more healthful ingredients. You want less saturated fat, sugar, and cholesterol, and more nutrients like omega-3 fats and dietary fiber. What should you look for on a food label?

Corn chips with new trans fat label

Nutrition Facts
Serving Size 1 oz (28g/29 chips)
Servings Per Container: 10

Amount per serving

Calories 150	Calories from Fat 90
	% Daily Value*
Total Fat 10g	15%
Saturated Fat 1.5g	6%
Trans Fat 0g	
Cholesterol 0mg	0%
Sodium 280mg	12%
Total Carbohydrate 16g	5%
Dietary Fiber 1g	
Sugars less than 1g	
Protein 2g	

Vitamin A 6%	•	Vitamin C 0%
Calcium 4%	•	Iron 2%
Vitamin E 6%	•	Vitamin B6 2%

*Percent Daily Values are based on a 2000 calorie diet. Your daily values may be higher or lower depending on your calorie needs.

Learning how to read the Nutrition Facts Panel on packaged food helps you make healthier food choices.

Reading a Nutrition Facts Panel is easy once you know what everything means. One of the most important things to look at is the serving size. If a serving is ½ cup and you eat 1½ cups, you are getting three times of all the nutrients listed on the label! Also, pay attention to the calories and fat per serving, as these will go up as your portion size increases.

For the rest of the nutrients on the NFP, pay attention to the percent daily values (DV) or the average amount of each nutrient in a product based on a 2,000 calorie daily diet. If you eat more or less than 2,000 calories a day, the DV for some nutrients may not equal 100 percent.

A good rule of thumb is this: for the nutrients that you want to limit, such as total fat, saturated fat, trans fat, cholesterol, and sodium, aim for less than 5 percent DV on the label; on the other hand, for nutrients that you want to increase like vitamins, minerals, and fiber, aim for above 20 percent DV.

Selection and Storage

Healing foods are easy to find because many of them do not come in packages, boxes, or bags. We're talking fresh fruits and veggies here. However, they still have to be kept fresh to maintain optimal quality. If not stored properly, fruits and veggies will quickly begin to lose their nutrient value. We'll explain how to store them properly so you can maintain freshness for as long a period of time as possible. Always remember before and after handling produce (and all foods) to clean hands and storage containers to eliminate the chance of contamination from bacteria.

Food quality depends on a variety of factors, including the quality of the raw product, the way it was processed and stored, and the length of time it's stored. So, for example, apples that you just picked are fresher and have a higher nutritional value than those on the shelves for a few days. Likewise, freshly picked herbs, if not wrapped in a moist paper towel in the fridge, will wilt in a few hours—even if placed in the refrigerator.

There's nothing worse than an overripe, mushy avocado with brownish-black spots or slimy salad greens. The solution is proper storage and using them in time. Here are the basics to get the best from your produce.

Produce Storage Basics

Fruit/Vegetable	Storage Place	Length of Time
Apples	Refrigerator	1 month
Apricots	Refrigerator	3–5 days
Avocados	Refrigerator	3–5 days
Beans	Refrigerator	3–5 days
Beets	Refrigerator	2 weeks
Berries	Refrigerator	2–3 days
Broccoli	Refrigerator	3–5 days
Cabbage	Refrigerator	1 week
Carrots	Refrigerator	2 weeks
Celery	Refrigerator	1 week

continues

Produce Storage Basics (contineud)

Fruit/Vegetable	Storage Place	Length of Time
Cherries	Refrigerator	2–3 days
Chilies	Refrigerator	1 week
Grapes	Refrigerator	3–5 days
Grapefruit	Refrigerator	2 weeks
Greens	Refrigerator	3–5 days
Lemons	Refrigerator	2 weeks
Lettuce	Refrigerator	1 week
Limes	Refrigerator	2 weeks
Mushrooms	Refrigerator	1–2 days
Onions	Pantry	1 week
Oranges	Refrigerator	2 weeks
Peaches	Refrigerator	3–5 days
Pears	Refrigerator	3–5 days
Peas	Refrigerator	3–5 days
Peppers	Refrigerator	1 week
Pineapple	Refrigerator	2–3 days
Plums	Refrigerator	3–5 days
Potatoes	Pantry	1 week
Summer squash	Refrigerator	3–5 days

Essential Takeaways

- You need a balance of both macro- and micronutrients to be healthy for life.
- The synergy of nutrients in foods is what gives them their health properties. Because whole foods maintain all their vital nutrients, they offer a host of health benefits.
- Organically grown foods and animals don't contain harmful chemicals, such as pesticides, hormones, sludge, and toxins, which can harm us and the planet.
- The Nutrition Facts Panel can help you better determine how to get the appropriate amount of nutrients in your daily diet.
- Proper storage and handling can maintain optimal nutrients and extend the shelf life of foods.

chapter 2

How Does Your Diet Stack Up?

Embracing the total diet mentality

Identifying why you eat what you do

Testing your diet recall

Putting the latest food guide system to work for you

Understanding how our environment lures us into eating more

Getting the scoop on common eating disorders

The word *diet* makes people cringe. The fact is we all live on a diet—whether it's balanced with healthy, healing foods like lean protein, whole grains, fruits, and vegetables or consists of *processed foods* full of fat, salt, and sugar. As someone who regularly advises people about all things associated with diet—weight, cholesterol, blood sugar, blood pressure, risk for chronic diseases, and libido—I say it's your *total diet* that counts!

Eating is one of the greatest pleasures in life, but when was the last time you thought about what you just ate or what you ate yesterday? We are surrounded by food, yet we don't take the time to think about what we are eating and why. Research shows us that people are more confused than ever about what *to* eat rather than what *not* to eat.

In this chapter, I delve deep into the factors that affect our eating. With food available everywhere, how do you avoid eating just because it's there? Keep reading to find out how to stay focused on the big eating picture.

<table>
<tr><td>Definition</td><td>**Diet** refers to all the food and beverages you regularly consume. **Total diet** is your overall pattern of eating over the course of a few days. No single food or meal makes or breaks a healthy diet! **Processed foods** are altered from their natural state and typically contain a lot of sugar, salt, and fat.</td></tr>
</table>

Assessing Your Total Diet

Now, let's take a look at *your* diet. Take a minute to jot down what you ate yesterday and today so far. Are there certain foods that you eat consistently? Do you always eat breakfast or do you usually skip it? Do you tend to eat a lot of food at a particular time of day? Be honest. Write down every morsel that passed your lips: food *and* drinks. (Don't forget the piece of candy from your co-worker's desk, the beer you had at your sister's birthday party, or the irresistible food samples at Costco.) It works best to write down what you eat right after you eat it, as it's easy to forget what you eat in a day, especially the small nibbles—which can add up fast!

If you found this food recall exercise challenging, you're not alone! It's tough for people to remember what they ate in a given day. That's where food logs or writing down what you eat and drink daily comes in handy. Psychologically, they might even help you cut back on how much you eat. There's something about seeing it in black and white that makes it easier to resist that mid-morning cream cheese bagel. See Appendix B for a sample food log.

In the meantime, to snap out of your eating amnesia—when you conveniently forget what you ate—take a few moments to fill out the following questionnaire. And as you answer the questions, try not to categorize foods into "good" and "bad" categories. You will find that you can fit small indulgences into your diet as long as you keep the primary focus on real, whole foods.

Total Diet Recall Questionnaire

Part I. Food	(circle yes or no)	
Finish the sentence, I eat …		
Fruits and vegetables every day	Yes	No
Sweets less than twice a week	Yes	No
Breakfast daily	Yes	No
Fish at least twice a week	Yes	No
Whole grains at least five times a week	Yes	No
Soy foods (tofu and soybeans) twice a week	Yes	No
Red meat less than twice a week	Yes	No

Part I. Food	(circle yes or no)	
Organic foods every day	Yes	No
Beans and legumes at least five times a week	Yes	No
A handful of nuts every day	Yes	No
Part II. Beverages	(circle yes or no)	

Finish the sentence, I drink …

Water throughout the day	Yes	No
Plain coffee every day (no more than 3 8-ounce cups)	Yes	No
A glass of fruit juice every day (1 glass = 4 oz.)	Yes	No
Not more than 1 to 2 glasses of alcohol daily	Yes	No
Milk shakes occasionally	Yes	No
Regular soda less than twice a week	Yes	No
Mineral water daily	Yes	No
Fruit shakes at least three times a week	Yes	No
Green tea daily	Yes	No
Diet soda less than once per day	Yes	No
Total Diet Score Card	____	____

Tally your score by counting up the number of yes's and no's. If you have more yes's, you have a balanced diet filled with real, whole foods and make room for small indulgences. If you have more no's, you should evaluate your overall diet and try to incorporate more nutrient-rich foods into your day.

Counting Calories

Do you know how many calories you need in a day to maintain your weight and health? You can calculate it on your own using a long equation or take advantage of online calculators that do the math for you, such as www.mayoclinic.com/health/calorie-calculator/NU00598.

Take a look at the table below for your daily estimated calorie needs.

Estimated energy needs in calories per day, for reference sized individuals by age, sex, and activity level.						
Age	*Male/ Sedentary*	*Male/ Moderately Active*	*Male/ Active*	*Female/ Sedentary*	*Female/ Moderately Active*	*Female/ Active*
2	1000	1000	1000	1000	1000	1000
3	1000	1400	1400	1000	1200	1400
4	1200	1400	1600	1200	1400	1400
5	1200	1400	1600	1200	1400	1600
6	1400	1600	1800	1200	1400	1600
7	1400	1600	1800	1200	1600	1800
8	1400	1600	2000	1400	1600	1800
9	1600	1800	2000	1400	1600	1800
10	1600	1800	2200	1400	1800	2000
11	1800	2000	2200	1600	1800	2000
12	1800	2200	2400	1600	2000	2200
13	2000	2200	2600	1600	2000	2200
14	2000	2400	2800	1800	2000	2400
15	2200	2600	3000	1800	2000	2400
16	2400	2800	3200	1800	2000	2400
17	2400	2800	3200	1800	2000	2400
18	2400	2800	3200	1800	2000	2400
19–20	2600	2800	3000	2000	2200	2400
21–25	2400	2800	3000	2000	2200	2400
26–30	2400	2600	3000	1800	2000	2400
31–35	2400	2600	3000	1800	2000	2200
36–40	2400	2600	2800	1800	2000	2200

Age	Male/ Sedentary	Male/ Moderately Active	Male/ Active	Female/ Sedentary	Female/ Moderately Active	Female/ Active
41– 45	2200	2600	2800	1800	2000	2200
46– 50	2200	2400	2800	1800	2000	2200
51– 55	2200	2400	2800	1600	1800	2200
56– 60	2200	2400	2600	1600	1800	2200
61– 65	2000	2400	2600	1600	1800	2000
66– 70	2000	2200	2600	1600	1800	2000
71– 75	2000	2200	2600	1600	1800	2000
76+	2000	2200	2400	1600	1800	2000

Source: Report of the DGAC on the Dietary Guidelines for Americans 2010. p. B2–18.

Your calorie needs change throughout your life. As you get older you lose lean muscle mass and gain fat mass. Because muscle mass at rest burns more calories than fat mass at rest, if you lose muscle mass, you don't need as many calories to maintain your weight. (This explains why it benefits you to build and maintain your muscle mass as you age. It's also why males typically have higher calorie needs than females.) Your activity level also plays a role in your caloric needs. The more you move, the more calories you need to provide energy to your cells, muscles, brain, and heart.

The Food Guide System: Refining the Pyramid

Now that you know what you are eating and have a target in mind for the number of calories you need, how do you determine how much of any one type of food you should eat? The Food Guide Pyramid, of course! Although, there are a variety of food pyramids, the U.S. Department of Agriculture's Food Guide Pyramid issued in 1992 is the most popular. It's a general guideline on how many servings to eat from each of the five foods groups: Grains, Vegetables, Fruits, Meat & Beans, Milk, and the *tiny* subgroup: Oils & Fats.

In 2005 the USDA created a more personalized version of the Food Guide Pyramid called the *MyPyramid Food Guidance System*. Unlike the one-size-fits-all approach of the previous system, MyPyramid is geared toward individuals. It takes your height, weight, age, and activity level into account when making recommendations for how much you should eat from every food group.

The USDA's interactive website provides more specific, personalized eating and activity recommendations. To try it out, go to MyPyramid.gov, click **Get a personalized plan,** and plug in your age, activity level, gender, and weight and height (optional). The site will issue your own eating and exercise plan.

Along with MyPyramid, came a new set of science-based nutrition recommendations, the *Dietary Guidelines for Americans*. Recently updated (as they are revised every five years), the 2010 dietary report card of America's health status revealed that people in the United States are eating too many calories, too much solid fat, added sugar, refined grains, and sodium. The latest dietary guidelines address these problems by stressing the need to balance calories in versus calories out as well as on decreasing sodium, solid fat, and added sugar in the diet while increasing other nutrients like potassium, calcium, vitamin D, fiber, and omega-3 fats. Finally, they foster an awareness of getting more nutrient-dense foods versus empty calories.

MyPyramid works hand-in-hand with the Dietary Guidelines for Americans, and it can help you …

- Make smart choices from every food group

- Find balance between food and physical activity

- Get the most nutrition out of calories

- Stay within your daily calorie needs

One of the guiding principles of the original Food Guide Pyramid and the personalized MyPyramid is total diet, promoting a good balance of essential vitamins, minerals, fiber, whole-grain carbohydrates, lean protein, and unsaturated fats into your daily diet.

Compare Your Diet to the Guidelines

Nutrient-dense foods are the cornerstone of good health. The 2010 Dietary Guidelines for Americans reveal that the following four nutrients below are lacking in our diets:

- Calcium

- Fiber

- Potassium

- Vitamin D

Although, we talk extensively about vitamins and minerals in Chapter 3, let's take a closer look at what the Department of Agriculture calls "short fall" nutrients to discover which foods contain the most of these essential nutrients.

Calcium

The mineral calcium is critical for bone development and maintenance, plus it assists with blood clotting and muscle and nerve impulses. (For more detail on calcium and bone health, see Chapter 25.) The most well-known sources of calcium are dairy products, such as low-fat varieties of milk, plain yogurt, and cheese (e.g., part-skim mozzarella, Swiss, and provolone). The mineral is also found in non-dairy sources including tofu (made with calcium sulfate), calcium-fortified soy milk, almond and rice milk, fortified ready-to-eat cereals, and dark leafy greens. A single serving of these foods contain 250 to 300 milligrams of calcium. Check the nutrition label for the calcium content of other foods.

Daily Calcium Needs	
Age	*Amount in milligrams (mg)*
Infants (0–6 months)	200
Infants (6–12 months)	260
Toddlers (1–3 years)	700
Children (4–8 years)	1,000
Tweens (9–13 years)	1,300
Teens (14–18 years)	1,300

continues

Daily Calcium Needs (continued)

Age	Amount in milligrams (mg)
Adults (19–50 years)	1,000
Adults (51+ years)	1,200
Pregnant/Lactating (14–18 years)	1,300
Pregnant/Lactating (19–50 years)	1,000

Fiber

Fiber is necessary for proper function of your intestines, and it can rid the body of excess artery-clogging cholesterol. You need a mix of both types of fiber—soluble and insoluble—for optimum health. The highest sources of soluble fiber is in oats, oat bran, and pectin in fruits; and insoluble fiber is found in beans, whole grains like bran cereals, and raw vegetables. Aim for 3 to 5 grams of fiber per serving.

A good rule of thumb for your daily fiber dose is to aim for 14 grams of fiber per every 1,000 calories you eat. So a young child may only need 14 grams a day, but as an adult you require 25 to 35 grams of fiber, depending upon your gender, calorie needs, and activity level.

Daily Fiber Needs

Age	Amount in grams
Infants (0–12 months)	No RDA*
Toddlers (1–3 years)	19
Children (4–8 years)	25
Female Tweens (9–13 years)	26
Male Tweens (9–13 years)	31
Female Teens (14–18 years)	26
Male Teens (14–18 years)	38
Female Adults (19–50 years)	25
Male Adults (19–50 years)	38
Female Adults (50+ years)	21
Male Adults (50+ years)	30

Age	Amount in grams
Pregnancy (14–50 years)	28
Lactation (14–50 years)	29

For infants, there is no established recommended daily allowance (RDA) for fiber. Normal intake of whole foods (e.g., fruits, vegetables, and whole grains) is the best source of fiber.

Potassium

Potassium is often out-shined by sodium chloride, more commonly known as table salt, in the diet; however, it makes up 5 percent of the total mineral content in your body. The Western diet has plenty of salt, thanks to its appearance in so many processed foods, but our diet all too often lacks potassium.

Potassium is nature's gift as it helps you maintain normal blood pressure levels, stay properly hydrated by balancing the water content inside your cells, stave off kidney stones, and prevents bone loss. Good food sources of potassium are potatoes (both sweet and white), beets, yogurt, halibut, and beans.

Food wise

The average adult only gets about half of the potassium required in a day. The Dietary Reference Intake (DRI) for potassium is 4.7 grams (4,700 milligrams) per day.

Daily Potassium Needs

Age	Amount in grams
Infants (0–6 months)	0.4
Infants (7–12 months)	0.7
Toddlers (1–3 years)	3
Children (4–8 years)	3.8
Tweens (9–13 years)	4.5
Teens (14–18 years)	4.7
Adults (19+ years)	4.7
Pregnancy (14–50 years)	4.7
Lactation (14–50 years)	5.1

The most common source of potassium in the American diet is milk or milk products. Young children (under 8 years) need a little more than 3 grams—that's one medium baked potato, a cup of plain yogurt, a medium banana, and ¼ of medium cantaloupe; older children and adults could get their requirement easily by eating 2 cups of cooked spinach, 1 cup of white beans, 3 ounces of cooked halibut, 2 cups low-fat milk, and 1 cup of low-fat yogurt daily.

Vitamin D

The beauty of vitamin D is that you can get it simply by walking outside during the day and letting the sunlight penetrate your skin. However, in recent years, as we protect our skin from the sun's harmful rays with sunscreen and are not outdoors as much, vitamin D levels in the body are lacking. You need it for healthy, strong bones—ongoing research shows that vitamin D may help fend off other chronic diseases. If you drink 2 to 3 cups of cow's milk, eat fatty fish like salmon, and/or foods fortified with vitamin D, such as almond, soy, and rice milks, yogurt, cheese, and mushrooms you are doing well. However, experts contend that a vitamin D supplement may be necessary to get the ideal amounts. (See Chapter 3 for your daily vitamin D needs.)

It's simple to get plenty of these "short fall" nutrients with the bounty of whole foods available to you.

What You Should Eat

The Dietary Guidelines for Americans encourage you to get the most from the five food groups every day, primarily from plant foods. Here's the lowdown: If you eat about 2,000 calories a day, you should strive to consume a variety of leafy green, orange, red, and yellow vegetables and fruits—to the tune of 2½ cups of veggies and 2 cups of fruit every day.

Even if you prefer white bread to whole grains, you should still strive to make half of your grains "whole." So that's at least three 1-ounce servings of whole grains every day.

| Munch on This | It helps to think of an ounce as one serving. So to get three servings of cooked whole grains, you could eat a slice of whole-grain bread, a half cup of whole-grain pasta, and a half cup of cooked oatmeal. |

If you eat dairy products reach for the low-fat versions of milk, yogurt, and cheese, and get at least 1 cup of milk, 1 cup of yogurt, and/or 1½ ounces of natural hard cheese every day. (You can also get calcium from other food sources; see Chapter 25 for details.)

For fat, be sure to get most of it from fatty fish, such as salmon, tuna, and halibut; nuts like almonds, walnuts, and pistachios; vegetable oils like extra-virgin olive oil and/or canola oil; and fruits such as avocadoes.

Go low-fat for protein by eating dry red beans and legumes, lean red meat (trim all visible fat) and use at least 93 percent lean ground meat, and skinless, white-meat poultry, and loin cuts of pork and beef.

What about extras? There is room for some "discretionary calories"—from fats, added sugar, and alcohol—but just a few—and only after you've met all of your nutrient needs for the day!

> **Munch on This**
>
> If you know you're going to want a piece of pie for dessert later, maybe you should pass on that high-calorie, high-fat banana nut muffin in the middle of the day.

For example, on a 2,000-calorie diet you are allowed 265 extra calories a day. That's not much: a half cup of Ben & Jerry's ice cream or a medium bagel without cream cheese or butter. These extras can also come from salad dressings, sauces, syrup, and butter. Remember, the more physically active you are, the greater amount of extra calories you have to play with in a day.

Your Extra Calorie Allowance for a Day

Age/sex	Not physically active*		Physically active**	
	Estimated total calorie need	Estimated discretionary calorie allowance	Estimated total calorie need	Estimated discretionary calorie allowance
Children 2–3	1000	165***	1000–1400	165–170
Children 4–8	1200–1400	170***	1400–1800	170–195
Girls 9–13	1600	130	1600–2200	130–290
Boys 9–13	1800	195	1800–2600	195–410
Girls 14–18	1800	195	2000–2400	265–360

continues

Your Extra Calorie Allowance for a Day (continued)

Age/sex	Not physically active*		Physically active**	
	Estimated total calorie need	Estimated discretionary calorie allowance	Estimated total calorie need	Estimated discretionary calorie allowance
Boys 14–18	2200	290	2400–3200	360–650
Females 19–30	2000	265	2000–2400	265–360
Males 19–30	2400	360	2600–3000	410–510
Females 31–50	1800	195	2000–2200	265–290
Males 31–50	2200	290	2400–3000	360–510
Females 51+	1600	130	1800–2200	195–290
Males 51+	2000	265	2200–2800	290–425

*For those who get less than 30 minutes of physical activity a day.

**For those who get 30 minutes (lower calories level) to 60 minutes (high calorie level) of moderate physical activity a day.

***Children 8 years and younger warrant more discretionary calories than older children and adults, as their nutrient needs are lower with less food needed from basic food groups.

Source: Courtesy of USDA's Mypyramid.gov. Accessed at www.mypyramid.gov/pyramid/discretionary_calories_amount_table.html.

So how does what you eat stack up to the guidelines? Let's take a look at what a typical day looks like based on the Dietary Guidelines for Americans. Remember, the guidelines are not a one-size-fits-all deal—your eating plan is unique to you. Remember, the amount of calories you need every day depends on your age, gender, size, and level of physical activity. Eating for health and healing does not rely on how you eat on one day, but a series of days, weeks, and months. Your total diet counts!

Sample One-Day Meal Plan (Based on 2,000 Calories)

Breakfast: *Breakfast burrito and a glass of milk:*

> 1 flour tortilla (7" diameter)

> 1 scrambled egg (in 1 tsp. butter)

> ⅓ cup black beans*

2 TB. salsa

1 cup orange juice

1 cup fat-free milk

Lunch: *Tuna fish sandwich, a pear, and a glass of milk*

2 slices rye bread

3 oz. tuna (packed in water, drained)

2 tsp. mayonnaise

1 TB. diced celery

¼ cup shredded romaine lettuce

2 slices tomato

1 medium pear

1 cup fat-free milk

Dinner: *Spinach lasagna*

2 oz. dry lasagna noodles

⅔ cup cooked spinach

½ cup ricotta cheese

½ cup tomato sauce tomato bits

1 oz. part-skim mozzarella cheese

1 oz. whole-wheat dinner roll

1 cup fat-free milk

Snacks:

> ¼ cup dried apricots
>
> 1 cup low-fat plain yogurt

Our Seductive Eating Environment

If Adam thought it was tough being tempted by an apple, how are you expected to fend off the allure of that same apple covered in chocolate, caramel, and peanuts? Every day our senses are bombarded with the look, smell, and flavor of delicious culinary combinations. In the face of this endless temptation, it's hard to stay disciplined, as evidenced by the high number of overweight and obese people in this country.

Think about it: if you smell freshly baked cinnamon buns at the airport or greasy burgers and fries when walking by a fast-food restaurant, aren't you more apt to seek out that food? The sight of food works, too—even if you have just eaten. There is a reason diners display their cakes, pies, and muffins in a glass case by the cashier. You can't resist! It's food seduction at its best.

The danger of living in a seductive eating environment—one where food is tempting you everywhere—is that people don't pay attention to feelings of hunger and fullness. If you eat whenever you see (or smell) food, then you are most likely overeating. Although food is meant to be enjoyed, there is a line between enjoyment and overindulgence—and far too many of us cross that line every day.

Healing Foods Pyramid

Although there are a number of food pyramids to refer to for what foods to eat and how much, the Healing Foods Pyramid developed by researchers at the University of Michigan in its Integrative Medicine group offers a culmination of what we preach in this book—a focus on mindfully eating whole, healing foods like plant foods (i.e., beans, lentils, peas, nuts, and soyfoods), moderate alcohol (if you choose to drink), proper fluids with water and tea, ample herbs and spices, a weekly dose of fish and seafood, and fewer animal products (i.e., full-fat dairy, red and processed meats) as part of an eating plan that not only fuels your body well, but can heal it, too.

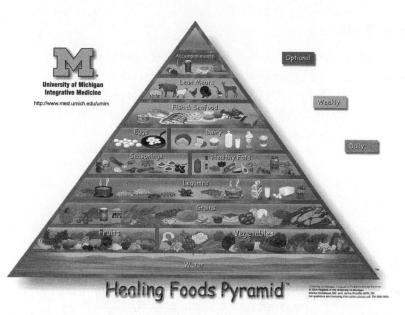

Use the Healing Foods Pyramid as a guide for choosing what foods to eat in what quantities.
(Source: University of Michigan Integrative Medicine)

For more information and to take a look at the interactive website for the Healing Foods Pyramid, visit www.med.umich.edu/umim/food-pyramid/index.htm.

Disordered Eating

With food everywhere, it's understandable that people sometimes suffer from *eating disorders*. Often the pressures of everyday life—such as stress, poor self-image or esteem, too many food restrictions (i.e., can't eat this or that), and a desire to be thin—only serve to exacerbate existing eating issues.

> **definition**
>
> **Eating disorders** are a group of serious conditions in which an individual is so preoccupied with food and weight that he or she can't focus on anything else in life.

Binge eating disorder, bulimia nervosa, anorexia nervosa, and orthorexia nervosa are all forms of disordered eating patterns that can lead to death and serious health problems down the road. The following sections examine each of these disorders and explain why they occur.

Binge Eating Disorder

At one time or another you have probably overeaten to the point of being stuffed. In other words, you binged. That doesn't mean you have an eating disorder. With binge eating disorder (BED) there are definite markers, such as eating unusually large amounts of food when alone and not being able to stop eating, followed by strong guilt and disgust afterward. In addition, people with BED often suffer from depression and anxiety, and feel out of control with food. If this happens at least twice a week over the course of 6 months, then it's classified as BED.

If you think you have BED, contact your health-care provider and/or consult with a registered dietitian and health psychologist who specialize in eating disorders.

Bulimia Nervosa

After bingeing comes efforts to reduce the effect of the excessive calories, by forced vomiting (purging) as a way of ridding the body of the excess calories, fasting, or overexercising. Like BED, bulimia nervosa (BN) can be life threatening and can seriously affect health. Symptoms of BN include eating abnormally large amounts in one sitting and typically when alone (e.g., a whole cake rather than one piece, or an entire gallon of ice cream versus a couple of scoops). Excessive vomiting manifests itself with throat and mouth sores, swollen salivary glands in the cheeks, damaged teeth and gums, dehydration, irregular heart beat, and abnormal bowel function. BN is also linked with feelings of depression, anxiety, and frustration.

It is important to note that people with BN sometimes induce vomiting even after small snacks and regular-size meals. Experts aren't sure why BN develops—it might stem from genetics, emotional problems, our culture of thinness, and/or excessive calorie restriction. Whatever the cause, it's important that people with BN get mental health and nutrition support.

Anorexia Nervosa

In our society where thin is in, people are starving themselves to fit in. Anorexia nervosa (AN) is an unhealthy obsession with food and body weight. AN is characterized by extreme weight loss, thin appearance, fatigue, dizziness or fainting, brittle nails, dry skin, intolerance to cold, low blood pressure, dehydration, absence of a regular period, and osteoporosis.

AN not only leads to malnutrition and death, it also causes social isolation, depression, reduced interest in sex, and lack of emotion. The irony of AN is that an obsession with food leads to a refusal to eat it and a denial of the need for it—by ignoring hunger (both physical and emotional hunger!). Treatment of AN can be difficult as victims do not always want help. Putting a person suffering from AN in the hands of an interdisciplinary team of medical, psychological, and nutrition professionals is vital.

Orthorexia Nervosa

You would think that eating 100 percent healthy foods 24/7 is a good thing, but this can actually be an unhealthy fixation. Imagine eating a normal-size piece of birthday cake and feeling like you had to repent by eating only "pure" foods from that point on. Dietary purity is the cornerstone of orthorexia nervosa, an unhealthy obsession with eating the right types of food. By being righteous about food, orthorexics often feel superior to others. They praise themselves when they are vigilant and condemn themselves for even the most minor indulgences. Healthy food becomes a conviction instead of a source of enjoyment and social respite.

As with other eating disorders, orthorexia causes isolation, depression, anxiety, guilt, and extremes in eating. Although, the lines are less clear with orthorexia, if healthful eating gets out of control to the point where you don't have a life, psychological and nutrition therapy are essential.

munch on this

Got a chocolate craving? Eat some dark chocolate as one of your snacks. Not only does it have less sugar and more antioxidants, but a small bar (about 0.8 oz.) has only 100 calories.

Surefire Strategies to Just Say No

There are surefire strategies to help you just say no to food seduction.

First, change your environment. If there is a candy dish on or near your desk, move it. If you drive by a Dunkin Donuts on your way to work and pull in all too often, take another route to work. Convenience is one of the main factors that lead to overeating.

food wise

In his book, *Mindless Eating: Why We Eat More Than We Think* (Bantam Books, 2006), Cornell University professor Brian Wansink points out that no one is exempt from the power of convenience—especially when it comes to food!

Secondly, know how to visualize portion sizes. It's so easy to misjudge how much is on your plate. To help you grasp appropriate portion sizes, consider these comparisons to everyday objects:

- 1 cup = baseball

- ½ cup = cupped hand

- 1 oz. = golf ball

- 2 TB. = golf ball

- 1 TB. = poker chip

- 1 slice of bread = playing card

- 3 oz. chicken or meat = deck of cards

- 3 oz. fish = checkbook

- 1 oz. lunch meat = compact disc

- 3 oz. muffin or biscuit = hockey puck

- 1½ oz. cheese = 3 dice or cubes of cheese

Lastly, people are more tempted to eat whatever is around when hunger strikes, so *do not* skip meals and *do* plan regular snacks. Many people suffering from weight problems complain about overeating when they get home from work or stopping at the vending machine or a fast-food restaurant on the way home because they haven't eaten anything since lunch. The problem is that they waited too long to eat.

The typical person should eat every three to four hours to keep their body happily humming along. If your body doesn't get a regular stream of calories or enough calories over the course of a day, it will ask for it at some point. So my advice is bring healthy snacks with you to stave off hunger and to avoid being tempted by whatever is available as an impulse appetite fix.

Think of snacks like a bridge to the next meal—not a full-blown meal—so they should only be about 150 calories. Here are some healthy snacks to keep blood sugar stable, hunger pangs away, and impulse eating at bay:

- 3 rye crisp crackers with ½ cup low-fat cottage cheese + 1 small piece of fruit

- Half of a whole-grain English muffin + 1 TB. hummus + ½ cup fresh berries

- 1½ oz. roasted salted soy nuts + 1 medium fresh orange

Healing Hints

Keep a food log every day for a week. It works! Not only will it add structure to your eating, but it will help you make better food choices. The good foods will crowd out the junky ones automatically!

Essential Takeaways

- Your total diet or overall eating pattern is the most important aspect of healthy eating.
- The Food Guide Pyramid has morphed into the MyPyramid Food Guidance System, a more personalized, interactive approach.
- The Dietary Guidelines are the foundation of our national nutrition recommendations. Check out the latest 2010 version at www.dietaryguidelines.gov.
- The USDA has identified "short fall" nutrients that we all need to get more of in our diets.
- Disordered eating can be serious and life threatening, so know the signs and symptoms and seek professional help.
- Your environment shapes how and what you eat. Be aware and take necessary precautions.
- Don't wait for hunger to strike; eat at least two balanced and healthy, 150 calorie snacks a day to stave off hunger between meals.

chapter 3

Vitamins and Minerals for Total Body Wellness

How vitamins and minerals help maintain health

Water-soluble vs. fat-soluble vitamins

Getting your daily nutrient requirements

The inside scoop on supplements

The best things in life do come in small packages, especially when it comes to vitamins and minerals. Although your body requires only small quantities of these micronutrients, they perform a host of minimiracles in your body. Micronutrients are Mother Nature's way of keeping you healthy.

Given how important these compounds are for health, it makes sense that not getting enough of them can lead to serious deficiency diseases. As well as hidden hunger, a chronic lack of vitamins and minerals can lead to mental retardation, poor health and productivity, and even death. Vitamin and mineral deficiencies account for 10 percent of the global health burden!

Nutritionists have learned a lot since 1913 when vitamin A was first discovered. Vitamins and minerals are not only powerful inside your body, but on the outside they keep your hair, nails, skin, and teeth looking great!

How much of a good thing do you need? With a variety of ways to quantify how much of a vitamin or mineral to get each day, this chapter clears up some confusion by defining the U.S. Institute of Medicine's Dietary Reference Intakes (DRIs) for each of the vitamins and minerals.

Vital Vitamins

Vitamins are *organic compounds* that your body needs in small doses. Because your body can't make most vitamins on its own, you have to get them from your diet. That's why it's important to hone in on vitamin-rich foods in your everyday eating.

definition

Organic compounds contain carbon atoms and are considered natural (not man-made) as they are made from plants or animals.

Vitamins are either water-soluble, meaning they dissolve easily in water and are eliminated from the body quickly, or fat-soluble, meaning that they are better absorbed by the body in the presence of dietary fat and they hang around in the body for longer periods of time. How a vitamin is absorbed in the body in part determines how much you may need.

Whether a vitamin is water-soluble or fat-soluble is a factor in how foods containing that vitamin should be prepared. Water-soluble vitamins lose their potency when heated or boiled, so go easy on the heating and cooking to retain more water-soluble vitamins. Fat-soluble vitamins thrive when heated and do not lose their potency. For example, the popular fat-soluble carotenoid, lycopene, found primarily in tomatoes, diffuses into the body better when heated; adding a little olive oil or canola oil helps the body absorb it better as well!

Thirteen vitamins are essential for health: the eight B-complex vitamins, and vitamins A, C, D, E, and K. Each of these vitamins perform different functions in your body.

Water-Soluble Vitamins

Water-soluble vitamins include the B-complex vitamins and vitamin C. These vitamins are eliminated by the body easily, which means you need to eat them on a daily basis. And keep in mind that these water-soluble vitamins lose some of their potency when cooked.

Just because these water-soluble nutrients don't hang around too long, you still need to pay attention not to overdo it. Getting too much (or too little) of one B-vitamin can affect the function of others.

Throughout this section, I provide Recommended Daily Allowances (RDAs) for vitamins and minerals, if there is one available. RDA is the average daily level of intake sufficient to meet the nutrient requirements of 97 to 98 percent of healthy individuals in the United States. Some vitamins and minerals have Adequate Intake (AI) levels rather than an RDA because of lack of evidence to establish a concrete recommendation, thus the AI is set to forecast the best possible nutrition outcomes. Either way, these amounts are based on the dietary reference intakes (DRIs), which are the general nutrition recommendations that vary by age and gender developed by the Institute of Medicine and used to create the USDA Dietary Guidelines for Americans.

Food wise Food is the best source of vitamins, but your body does make some on its own. Vitamin D is made by your skin from sunlight, and some vitamin K and vitamin B_7 (biotin) are produced in your intestines.

Thiamin (B_1)

Thiamin (B_1) is considered the energy vitamin because its main function is to help your cells use carbs for fuel. Thiamin deficiencies are rare if you eat a balanced diet that includes whole foods such as brown rice, whole-grain rye, oatmeal, flaxseed, sunflower seeds, kale, eggs, and lean meats.

Alcoholics typically have low levels of thiamin because their diets either lack this nutrient or they can't absorb it as well. A B_1 deficiency is a leading cause of dementia in the United States. Lack of thiamin can lead to mental confusion, muscular wasting, bloating (water retention), paralysis of the legs, and an enlarged heart—classic symptoms of beriberi, a thiamin-deficiency disease.

Recommended Daily Allowance for Thiamin

Age	Milligrams
Infants and toddlers (0–3 years)	0.5
Young children (4–8 years)	0.6
Tweens (9–13 years)	0.9

continues

Recommended Daily Allowance for Thiamin (continued)	
Age	*Milligrams*
Female teens (14–18 years)	1.0
Male teens (14–18 years)	1.2
Female adults (19+ years)	1.1
Male adults (19+ years)	1.2

Riboflavin (B_2)

This vitamin is a yellowish-orange color, which makes it the ideal ingredient in food coloring. Riboflavin can also be colorless when naturally occurring in foods such as cow's milk. This vitamin is extremely sensitive to light, thus foods high in riboflavin, such as milk, yogurt, eggs, feta cheese, and cottage cheese must be packaged in opaque containers or stored in dark places.

A low level of riboflavin is linked with low thyroid levels or hypothyroidism—since riboflavin is regulated by thyroxine, the main hormone secreted by the thyroid gland. If another water-soluble vitamin falls low, so does riboflavin.

Low levels of riboflavin—which is rare—isn't immediately obvious. It takes a few months before signs occur. Physical signs of a riboflavin deficiency are chapped and cracked lips, inflammation of the lining of the mouth and tongue, mouth ulcers, and cracks at the corners of lips. An internal sign is anemia, or low iron levels in your blood.

Recommended Daily Allowance for Riboflavin	
Age	*Milligrams*
Infants and toddlers (0–3 years)	0.5
Young children (4–8 years)	0.6
Tweens (9–13 years)	0.9
Teens (14–18 years)	1.0
Female adults (19+ years)	1.1
Male adults (19+ years)	1.3

Niacin (B₃)

Unlike the first two B-vitamins, niacin is very resistant to the elements of heat, light, and air. Yet, a small amount may be lost in cooking water. Niacin plays a role in heart health as it works to reverse hardening of the arteries (atherosclerosis) by helping to lower LDL (bad) cholesterol.

Low levels of niacin are rare in the United States, especially if you eat foods like avocados, dates, tomatoes, broccoli, sweet potatoes, asparagus, tuna, salmon, and/or eggs regularly—they all contain significant amounts of niacin.

food wise

Malnutrition, chronic alcoholism, or lack of niacin-rich foods in the diet can lead to a disease called pellagra. Extreme cases of pellagra cause diarrhea, dermatitis, and dementia (called the 3-Ds of pellagra), as well as a "necklace of lesions" around the neck, and inflammation of the mouth and tongue. Pellagra is rare in most parts of the United States today.

Recommended Daily Allowance for Niacin

Age	Milligrams
Infants and toddlers (0–3 years)	6
Young children (4–8 years)	8
Tweens (9–13 years)	12
Female teens (14–18 years)	14
Male teens (14–18 years)	16
Female adults (19+ years)	14
Male adults (19+ years)	16

Pantothenic Acid (B₅)

This vitamin is vital for all living things. It helps your body use "the big three" nutrients (carbohydrates, proteins, and fats), plus it makes coenzyme-A (CoA), a compound that energizes your cells.

Whole foods are fabulous sources of this B-vitamin. If you eat plenty of whole grains (refining of grains strips them of this and other B-vitamins), avocados, and broccoli, you will get plenty! The calling card of a deficiency in this nutrient are low energy levels, low blood sugar (hypo-glycemia) as there's an increase in sensitivity to insulin, muscle cramps, nausea, and sleep disturbances.

Recommended Daily Allowance for Pantothenic Acid

Age	Milligrams
Infants and toddlers (0–3 years)	1.7
Young children (4–8 years)	3
Tweens (9–13 years)	4
Teens (14–18 years)	5
Adults (19+ years)	5

Pyridoxine (B$_6$)

Vitamin B$_6$ balances the minerals, sodium, and potassium in your cells plus it helps form red blood cells, which give you energy. It's good for heart health, as it has been shown to decrease levels of homocysteine, an amino acid that is linked to chronic inflammation. For women, this nutrient helps balance changes in hormones. Plus, it's a great immunity booster!

It's not found in plants, but the skin of some vegetables (e.g., potatoes) may contain some from the soil. Drinking milk and eating meat are the best ways to get it in. Low levels of vitamin B$_6$ can cause seizures, anemia, nerve damage, skin problems, and mouth sores.

food wise Don't discard your vegetable or fruit skins or peels just yet. The outer protective layer on produce is where you get a hefty dose of fiber, plant-based nutrients, vitamins and minerals, and antioxidant power. So only peel if absolutely necessary!

Recommended Daily Allowance for Pyridoxine

Age	Milligrams
Infants and toddlers (0–3 years)	0.5
Young children (4–8 years)	0.6
Tweens (9–13 years)	1
Female teens (14–18 years)	1.2
Male teens (14–18 years)	1.3
Adults (19+ years)	1.3
Older females (50+ years)	1.5
Older males (50+ years)	1.7

Biotin (B$_7$)

This vitamin is important for growth of your cells. It helps keep blood sugar levels steady, and assists your body in using fats and proteins. Biotin has been known to strengthen hair, nails, and skin. Check your cosmetics and shampoo bottles for this vitamin!

Because this is one of the vitamins your intestines can make in adequate amounts, there are not many natural food sources, but egg yolks, liver, and a few veggies do contain biotin. If for some reason your body doesn't make it (due to a metabolic disorder) supplements can help. Symptoms of low levels of biotin are hair loss, pink eye (conjunctivitis), scaly skin (dermatitis) on face and/or genital area, depression, lethargy, hallucinations, and numbness or tingling in hands and feet.

Recommended Daily Allowance for Biotin

Age	Micrograms
Infants and toddlers (0–3 years)	5 or 6
Young children (4–8 years)	12
Tweens (9–13 years)	20
Teens (14–18 years)	25
Adults (19+ years)	30

Folic Acid (B$_9$)

Folic acid is essential for maintaining healthy red blood cells and fending off anemia. All women of childbearing age are advised to get plenty folic acid because it's a vital nutrient for the healthy development of the neural tube—spinal cord and brain—of a fetus.

Folic acid keeps homocysteine levels low, and low levels of this amino acid can protect your heart. Getting enough folic acid (or folate from foods) may even improve fertility in both men and women.

FOOD wise

Too much folic acid may pose a risk for certain cancers. If you are at risk for cancer because of a history of adenomas or harmless tumors, you are a man with a high prostate-specific antigen (PSA) level, or you are harboring precancerous or cancerous cells, be careful not to get an excess of folic acid from fortified foods and/or supplements.

Too much folic acid can also hide a vitamin B$_{12}$ deficiency and lead to other future health problems. So don't eat more than 1,000 micrograms per day.

Experts advise that anyone over 40 should think twice before taking in more than the DRI of 400 micrograms. (Studies show that 10 percent of the population over 40 is getting way more than the DRI from fortified foods.) The good news is you don't have to worry about getting too much folate (the naturally occurring form of folic acid in foods), because your body doesn't absorb it from food as easily.

As with most micronutrients, whole foods are your best choice for getting folic acid. So chow down on folate in leafy greens, spinach, asparagus, and turnip greens; dried and fresh beans, legumes, peas, and lentils; and fortified cereals, grains, and seeds.

Recommended Daily Allowance for Folic Acid

Age	Micrograms DFE*
Infants and toddlers (0–3 years)	150
Young children (4–8 years)	200
Tweens (9–13 years)	300
Teens (14–18 years)	400
Male teens (14–18 years)	400
Female adults (19+ years)	400
Male adults (19+ years)	400
Pregnant females	600

Dietary Folate Equivalent

Cobalamin (B_{12})

Cobalamin, or B_{12}, is an essential vitamin for the formation of blood and the function of the brain and nervous system. Like some of the other B-vitamins it gives cells energy and assists with production of DNA, the genetic code contained in most cells. B_{12} levels are linked to folic acid levels, so if your blood levels are low in B_{12}, check your folic acid level—it may be low, too. When both are low this can lead to a type of anemia called megaloblastic anemia. High levels of folic acid can hide a B_{12} deficiency, which may be dangerous over time.

Unlike some of the other water-soluble vitamins, your body can store a lot of B_{12} in the liver and kidneys, thus daily requirements are very small. Signs of deficiency may not be noticed for 5 or

6 years! In older adults, chronic low levels can cause permanent nerve damage and might seem like Alzheimer's disease.

What foods are high in B_{12}? Animal-based foods like meat, poultry, fish, shellfish, and milk products. Vegans or nonmeat eaters can get B_{12} from nutritional yeast, fortified cereals, or fortified soy products. However, vegans might need to take supplements to get enough B_{12}.

Recommended Daily Allowance for Cobalamin

Age	Micrograms
Infants and toddlers (0–3 years)	0.9
Young children (4–8 years)	1.2
Tweens (9–13 years)	1.8
Teens (14–18 years)	2.4
Adults (19+ years)	2.4

Vitamin C

Also known as ascorbic acid, vitamin C takes center stage as a defender of cell health as an antioxidant. It has come a long way from its link to the sailor's bleeding gum disease called scurvy! Because sailors didn't eat citrus fruits, collagen was not properly formed, causing poor wound healing eventually leading to death. Today vitamin C is one of the cosmetic industries go-to nutrients as an elixir for youthful skin. Because it enhances collagen formation in the skin leading to improved elasticity, it's put in serums, lotions, and creams to promote smoother skin. If those sailors only knew! It's also been shown to do wonders for reducing the severity of common cold symptoms and boosting immunity, but it's not a complete cold defender, so be sure to still wash your hands frequently!

Foods that are known for their vitamin C power are citrus fruits, such as oranges, grapefruit, lemon, limes, and kiwi. Other vitamin C heavy-hitters are guavas, red peppers, strawberries, and potatoes.

Recommended Daily Allowance for Vitamin C	
Age	*Milligrams*
Infants and toddlers (0–3 years)	15
Young children (4–8 years)	25
Tweens (9–13 years)	45
Female teens (14–18 years)	65
Male teens (14–18 years)	75
Female adults (19+ years)	75
Male adults (19+ years)	90

Fat-Soluble Vitamins

Just like their name implies, fat-soluble vitamins are stored in the body's fatty tissues and stay in the body for longer periods of time. They include vitamins A, D, E, and K. Your daily doses of these may vary, but what's important is that you get enough through the course of a week. Although getting too much is rare, be careful not to overdose on these fat-soluble nutrients as they can create health problems.

Healing Hints

Eating kale, a delicious leafy green, will give you a lot of bang for your bite as it's high in A, C, K, and calcium.

Heat from cooking does not destroy these fat-soluble vitamins.

Vitamin A

Also called retinol, vitamin A is a powerful player in the health of your eyes, particularly your retinas. Vitamin A converts into two groups of carotenoids, xanthophylls and carotenes, which act as sunscreen for your eyes by absorbing the sun's damaging blue light. Lack of vitamin A in your diet can lead to night blindness. (As a matter of fact, the RDA for vitamin A was set based on the amount of vitamin A required to reverse night-blindness in vitamin A–deficient people.) Vitamin A is also needed for healthy teeth, bones, cell membranes, and skin. It's also useful for reproduction. Retinol is the active form of vitamin A.

Food sources of vitamin A include liver, whole milk, eggs, and some fortified foods. Other forms of vitamin A are carotenoids, dark coloring found in plant foods, such as leafy greens, pumpkin, carrots, apricots, sweet potatoes, and kale. Beta-carotene is a type of carotenoid that acts as an antioxidant to fend off chronic diseases and keep you looking and feeling younger!

Recommended Daily Allowance for Vitamin A (in retinol equivalents [RE] in micrograms)	
Age	*Micrograms (RE)*
Infants and toddlers (0–3 years)	300
Young children (4–8 years)	400
Tweens (9–13 years)	600
Female teens (14–18 years)	700
Male teens (14–18 years)	900
Female adults (19+ years)	800
Male adults (19+ years)	1,000

Vitamin D

Typically, referred to without a number attached to it, vitamin D comes in five forms. The one that works in your body to regulate calcium and phosphate levels and keep your bones strong, is vitamin D_3. Vitamin D_3, or cholecalciferol, is produced by the skin from sunlight. Unless you want to gulp down a tablespoon of cod liver oil every day (that's 1,360 IU of vitamin D right there!), vitamin D is only found in a small range of foods, such as fatty fish like salmon, eggs, fortified milk and yogurt, and white button mushrooms that have been exposed to sunlight. In children, vitamin D_3 fends off a serious bone disease called rickets (in adults it's called osteomalacia).

food wise

Vitamin D may be tough to get from food alone, as experts contend that in order for adults to get the RDA of 600 IU a day, you would have to eat salmon three times a day and drink 2 gallons of milk daily!

Recommended Daily Allowance for Vitamin D*	
Age	*International Units*
Infants (0–12 months)	400**
Toddlers (1–3 years)	600**
Young children (4–8 years)	600***
Tweens (9–13 years)	600***
Female teens (14–18 years)	600
Male teens (14–18 years)	600
Female adults (19+ years)	600
Male adults (19+ years)	600
Older adults (71+ years)	800
Pregnant, lactating women	600

Upper limits for vitamin D are as follows: Adults 4,000 IU a day, children (ages 4–8) 3,000 IU, toddlers (1–3 years) 2,500 IU, infants (6–12 months) 1,500 IU, and newborns (0–6 months) 1,000 IU.

**Between birth and one year old, infants who are breast fed or get less than 17 ounces of formula per day, should take a vitamin D supplement, such as 1 ml of Trivisol or Polyvisol.*

***Older children and adolescents who drink less than 20 ounces (or 2½ cups) of cow's milk or fortified soy or nut milks should take a multivitamin supplement, too.*

Vitamin E

Also called alphatocopherol, vitamin E is also a powerful antioxidant, but it's not the wonder nutrient once thought. Studies have shown that it doesn't prevent heart disease, stroke, or prostate cancer. You won't lose much vitamin E in cooking, however freezing and deep-frying will kill most of it. Getting enough vitamin E is a good thing as it works in your intestines to enhance the activity of other vitamins, such as vitamin A.

Good food sources of vitamin E come from polyunsaturated fatty acids (PUFAs) found in foods like vegetable oils, avocados, and nuts. Deficiencies of vitamin E are rare because it's found in a wide variety of foods.

Recommended Daily Allowance for Vitamin E

Age	Milligrams
Infants and toddlers (0–3 years)	6
Young children (4–8 years)	7
Tweens (9–13 years)	11
Teens (14–18 years)	15
Female adults (19+ years)	15
Male adults (19+ years)	15

Vitamin K

This vitamin is necessary for wound healing by helping your blood clot and it also helps build healthy bones. One form of vitamin K is made in the intestines, so deficiencies are rare—except in cases of intestinal surgery, inflammatory bowel disease, and in people with cystic fibrosis. Heavy bleeding can indicate a deficiency.

Food wise   If you are on a blood thinner, such as Warfarin (or Coumadin), taking in too much vitamin K can interfere with the drug's action. For more information on vitamin K and Coumadin, see the National Institute of Health's information sheet at www.cc.nih.gov/ccc/patient_education/drug_nutrient/coumadin1.pdf.

Vitamin K is in a variety of foods, such as spinach, Swiss chard, kale, cabbage, mustard greens, avocado, and kiwi.

Recommended Daily Allowance for Vitamin K

Age	Micrograms
Infants and toddlers (0–3 years)	10–20
Young children (4–8 years)	15–100
Tweens (9–13 years)	15–100
Female teens (14–18 years)	15–100
Male teens (14–18 years)	15–100
Female adults (19+ years)	90
Male adults (19+ years)	210

Mighty Minerals

Minerals are mighty nutrients, too. Although, some are needed in larger amounts than others, it doesn't mean any one of them is more important. The minerals needed in larger amounts are called macrominerals and include calcium, phosphorus, magnesium, sulfur, sodium, chloride, and potassium. I talk about these more in the coming chapters.

The ones I focus in on here are microminerals, the minerals needed in smaller amounts by the body. Microminerals are a family of trace elements that consist of iron, cobalt, chromium, copper, iodine, manganese, selenium, and zinc. They are essential for supporting the chemical reactions in the body for proper functioning of organs, bones, and hormones.

Iron

Iron offers a powerhouse of functional value to your body. Iron deficiency anemia is the most common nutritional deficiency in the world; severe anemia kills up to 50,000 women a year during childbirth. In the United States iron levels are commonly checked at annual visits with your health-care provider.

Eating plenty of iron-rich foods is vital to the healthy functioning of your immune system. The brain also needs iron to function at its best. Studies have shown that iron deficiencies in children at a young age have long-term effects. Adequate iron levels enable children to focus, remember things, and learn better!

There are two types of iron, *heme* and *nonheme.* The body absorbs heme iron much better than nonheme iron. However, how much and how fast your body absorbs either type of iron depends on the food source. Animal foods like meat, fish, and poultry are easily absorbed heme iron sources; whereas plant-based foods contain nonheme iron, which is not as easily absorbed. Adding vitamin C–rich foods to your meals and snacks will help your body absorb nonheme iron. The ideal iron absorption scenario would be to eat an iron-fortified breakfast cereal with some diced strawberries on top, a mixed greens salad along with a handful of cherry tomatoes, or a baked potato topped with a few broccoli florets.

Recommended Daily Allowance for Iron

Age	Milligrams
Infants and toddlers (0–3 years)	7
Young children (4–8 years)	10
Tweens (9–13 years)	8
Female teens (14–18 years)	15
Male teens (14–18 years)	11
Female adults (19+ years)	18
Female adults (50+ years)	8
Pregnant females	27
Male adults (19+ years)	8

Cobalt

This mineral is a cozy component of B_{12} (hence B_{12}'s scientific name, cobalamin), and so not getting enough B_{12} leads to a deficiency in cobalt. Your body relies on cobalt to help your red blood cells grow and mature and for every cell in your body to function properly. You cannot get cobalt from foods per se, although it's present in teeny tiny amounts in the normal bacteria present in some veggies. You get cobalt by eating foods that contain sufficient amounts of B_{12}, such as meat, fish, and poultry. Just like with B_{12}, vegans or nonmeat eaters can get cobalt from nutritional yeast, fortified cereals, or fortified soy products.

The RDA for cobalt is based on B_{12} needs; for adults the RDA is 2.4 micrograms of B_{12}.

Chromium

This mineral is well-known for helping the body use insulin and keep blood sugar under control. Chromium is often paired with a chemical agent called picolinate in supplements to fend off chromium deficiency, which may be especially beneficial to people who have prediabetes or type 2 diabetes (see Chapter 21 for more on this). Chromium also appears to be beneficial for heart health as it's been found to keep cholesterol and triglyerides (a type of blood fat) within normal range and fend off plaque in the arteries.

You get chromium in your food when you eat seafood, whole grains, chicken, red meat, bran, apples, broccoli, basil, and garlic. Practice caution when using supplements to get chromium and consult with your health-care provider before using them.

Adequate Intakes for Chromium*	
Age	*Micrograms*
Infants (0–6 months)	0.2
Infants (7–12 months)	5.5
Toddlers (1–3 years)	11
Young children (4–8 years)	15
Female tweens (9–13 years)	21
Male tweens (9–13 years)	25
Female teens (14–18 years)	24
Male teens (14–18 years)	35
Female adults (19+ years)	25
Male adults (19+ years)	35
Female adults (50+ years)	20
Male adults (50+ years)	30
Pregnant women (14–18 years)	29
Pregnant women (19–50 years)	30
Lactating women (14–18 years)	44
Lactating women (19–50 years)	45

There are no RDAs for chromium, only Adequate Intake levels based on studies that showed the average consumption of foods containing chromium.

Copper

This micromineral is everywhere in your body—in your liver, brain, bones, heart, and kidneys. It's vital to the functioning of your organs and your metabolic processes. It may be part of your DNA, too! The supply of copper in your body teeters on a fine line from low to high, but your body does a daily balancing act of keeping it in equilibrium to sustain your health. Copper and another trace element, zinc, are interrelated and compete with one another for absorption in your digestive tract. If you take in more copper; zinc will fall low and vice versa. In order to get enough copper, enjoy some oysters, cocoa, lobster, nuts, sunflower seeds, and avocados.

Recommended Daily Allowance for Copper	
Age	*Micrograms*
Infants and toddlers (0–3 years)	200–220
Young children (4–8 years)	340–440
Tweens (9–13 years)	700
Teens (14–18 years)	890
Female adults (19+ years)	900
Male adults (19+ years)	900
Pregnant women	1,000
Lactating women	1,300

Iodine

Iodine is essential for the proper functioning of your thyroid gland, a large gland located just below the "Adam's Apple" in your neck, which is vital to how your body burns energy; it also controls how various hormones work. Iodine is a component of thyroid hormones, such as thyroxine (T4). How many calories you burn while at rest is truly affected by your thyroid hormones. If your thyroid hormones are low (a condition called hypothyroidism), your metabolism can drop by as much as 50 percent; on the other end of the spectrum, if your thyroid hormones are high (called hyperthyroidism) your metabolic rate can increase by 100 percent! So balancing thyroid hormones is a key to good health.

Munch on This

Lack of iodine in the diet is the number one preventable cause of mental retardation in the world. Every year 18 million babies are born mentally impaired due to iodine deficiency.

What foods contain iodine? It's found in seaweeds such as kombu, kelp, nori, and wakame; cow's milk and human breast milk; grains; eggs; and certain fruits and veggies grown in iodine-rich soil. It is also found in any table salt that has iodine added.

Recommended Daily Allowance for Iodine

Age	Micrograms
Infants (0–6 months)	110*
Infants (7–12 months)	130*
Toddlers (1–3 years)	90
Young children (4–8 years)	90
Tweens (9–13 years)	120
Female teens (14–18 years)	150
Male teens (14–18 years)	150
Female adults (19+ years)	150
Male adults (19+ years)	150
Pregnant women (14–18 years)	220**
Pregnant women (19+ years)	220**
Lactating women (14–18 years)	290
Lactating women (19+ years)	290

*These are Adequate Intake levels as there are no RDAs for infants.

**The International Council for the Control of Iodine Deficiency Disorders and other organizations recommend 250 mcg during pregnancy.

Healing Hints

Did you know table salt can be fortified with both iodine and iron? It can—and it kills two mineral deficiencies with a couple of shakes! Fortification of foods with micronutrients is a cost-effective way to fend off deficiency diseases and health problems. Check the labels for salt to see if it's iodized and/or ironized.

Manganese

This mineral is mainly concentrated in your bones. It is associated with the formation of connective and bony tissue, growth, reproduction, and carbohydrate and fat metabolism. Manganese is in direct competition with iron and cobalt for absorption in the body. Manganese deficiencies are rare. Foods that are rich in manganese are beet greens, blueberries, whole grains, nuts and legumes, fruit, and tea.

Recommended Daily Allowance for Manganese

Age	Milligrams
Infants and toddlers (0–3 years)	0.0003–0.6
Young children (4–8 years)	1.5
Female tweens (9–13 years)	1.6
Male tweens (9–13 years)	1.9
Female teens (14–18 years)	1.6
Male teens (14–18 years)	2.2
Female adults (19+ years)	1.8
Male adults (19+ years)	2.3

Selenium

This mineral is a popular antioxidant that's not only beneficial for fending off damage to cells. Selenium is found in a variety of foods, but the highest concentration is found in plant foods grown in selenium-rich soil. Meat, whole-grain bread, Brazil nuts, tuna, cod, turkey, eggs, and cottage cheese are some of the foods that contain selenium.

food wise

Selenium was once thought to fend off (along with vitamin E) prostate cancer in men. However, a large trial of 35,000 men age 50 and older found there was no difference in the incidence of prostate cancer among those men who took vitamin E and selenium and those who took a placebo.

Recommended Daily Allowance for Selenium

Age	Micrograms
Infants (0–6 months)	15*
Infants (7–12 months)	20*
Toddlers (1–3 years)	20
Young children (4–8 years)	30
Tweens (9–13 years)	40
Teens (14–18 years)	55
Adults (19+ years)	55

continues

Recommended Daily Allowance for Selenium (continued)

Age	Micrograms
Pregnant women (14+ years)	60
Lactating women (14+ years)	70

Adequate Intake (AI) for infants as there is no RDA available.

Zinc

Zinc is vital for normal growth and development. In the first studies of zinc deficiency, malnourished young boys from Egypt and Iran were found to be "nutritionally dwarfed" due to low iron and zinc levels. Researchers found that adding zinc to their diet helped, with some of the boys growing as much as 5 inches in 1 year! Studies in the United States have found shorter preschool children to have low levels of zinc in hair samples.

What should you and your children be eating to get enough zinc? Animal foods like oysters, red meat, chicken, and seafood like crab and lobster are good sources of zinc, however, kids tend to shy away from these foods. And drinking too much milk is not the best for getting enough zinc (and iron), as over-doing calcium can interfere with absorption of these two minerals. This does not mean to stop drinking milk, but you do need to balance milk (as well as yogurt and cheese) with other protein sources, such as meat, chicken, turkey, and fortified breakfast cereals.

Recommended Daily Allowance for Zinc

Age	Milligrams
Infants (0–6 months)	2
Infants (7–12 months)	3
Toddlers (1–3 years)	3
Young children (4–8 years)	5
Tweens (9–13 years)	8
Female teens (14–18 years)	9
Male teens (14–18 years)	11
Female adults (19+ years)	8
Male adults (19+ years)	11

Age	Milligrams
Pregnant women (14–18 years)	12
Pregnant women (19+ years)	11
Lactating women (14–18 years)	13
Lactating women (19+ years)	12

Supplements

Do you take a multivitamin, fish oil capsule, or vitamin D supplement daily? If you are anything like the average American, you probably do. *Dietary supplements* are big business—worth a staggering $23.7 billion annually. But with dietary supplements you don't always know what you are getting.

Under the current law, the Dietary Supplement Health and Education Act (DSHEA) established in 1994, supplement manufacturers have free reign of their products, and the FDA can only step in if a health or safety issue is reported *after* taking a supplement.

Manufacturers are not required to safety test their products or register with the FDA before taking their product to the marketplace. As with any product—food or supplement—that you put into your body, practice caution and know what's in it before consuming it.

definition

A **dietary supplement** is a product that is intended to add nutritional adequacy to the diet, contains one or more nutrition ingredients (e.g., vitamins, minerals, herbs or other botanicals, amino acids, and other substances) or their constituents; is intended to be taken by mouth as a pill, capsule, tablet, or liquid; and is labeled on the front panel as being a "dietary supplement."

Although replacing sound nutrition with supplements is never advisable, there are circumstances when using supplements makes sense. One case is when your health requires the elimination of certain foods or a food group due to an intolerance or allergy. Or you may need to supplement if you know you are deficient in one or more nutrients.

If a health claim on a bottle, box, or jar sounds too good to be true, it usually is. Before taking a supplement, educate yourself! One of the most reliable websites on dietary supplements is the National Institutes of Health Office of Dietary Supplements at http://ods.od.nih.gov.

Essential Takeaways

- Vitamins and minerals are powerful players in fending off diseases and disorders.
- There are two types of vitamins, water-soluble and fat-soluble. Both play a big role in your health.
- Water-soluble vitamins should be consumed daily as they are eliminated from your body regularly.
- Fat-soluble vitamins are stored in your body longer, so your daily doses can vary as long you get enough during the week.
- Dietary supplements are not regulated by the government before they go to market, so practice caution before using them.
- Focus on getting your vitamins and minerals from healthful foods rather than supplements. Only use supplements if they are absolutely necessary.

chapter 4

Evolve Your Eating

Improving your eating

Understanding your appetite

Making quality count

Saying goodbye to cravings for good

Eating healthfully is a process—a gradual shift in your food choices and eating behaviors over time. Naturally, the food you eat and enjoy changes as you age. However, infants and toddlers can teach us a lot about how to eat sensibly because they are born with built-in appetite wisdom. They intuitively know when they are hungry or full. They are masters of self-regulation with food.

It is very telling at mealtime when a child loses interest in food. It usually means the child is full. Fast forward 20 years. That child (now an adult) most likely will keep eating what's on the plate in front of him even if he's full. Studies show that grown-ups tend to eat what is put in front of them—even if it's too much. Most of us shut off our internal cues of hunger (stomach grumbling, light-headedness) and fullness (bloating, discomfort) because our natural appetite instincts are overridden by the allure of second helpings and tasty desserts. The danger in this is obvious: it leads to overeating and weight gain, neither of which are good for health!

Just as your body changes as you age, your body's nutrient needs change as well. During big growth spurts such as infancy, adolescence and, for women, during pregnancy and lactation, your body demands more calories and you're most likely more hungry, too. During slower growth times such as midlife and old age, you don't require as much fuel to maintain your energy, so your body's need for food decreases.

This chapter explores simple, realistic ways to evolve your eating habits with balance, mindfulness, and a focus on good-quality calories to alleviate cravings and foster healthy eating habits for life.

Success Strategies for Change

Change is a constant in life and—when it comes to eating—can happen daily. What, how much, and when you eat can change based on work, family, and social schedules. As one of the guiding principles of the MyPyramid Food Guidance System, *evolutionary eating* encourages you to take your food choices to a healthier plane.

Simple ways you can evolve your eating are toasting whole-grain bread instead of having white bread for breakfast, using red beans instead of red meat in your chili, or mashing parsnips in lieu of white potatoes as a fiber-packed side dish. All of these easy evolutions in your eating add up to better overall nutrition in your day.

Definition

Evolutionary eating involves gradual changes in food choices and eating habits that are good for overall health.

So what are some strategies to successfully rewrite your eating script to live a healthier, happier life? Take a look at the following list for some surefire ways to rethink what you eat and drink forever:

- Avoid meal skipping, especially breakfast. While all meals are a chance to get valuable nutrients, breakfast truly is the mac-daddy of your daily meal triad!

- Keep a daily food log in a small notebook or with the notes feature of your phone. You'll be surprised where excess, empty calories are coming in!

- Swap sliced, chopped, or diced raw vegetables for refined snacks like crackers, cookies, and chips.

- Banish the regular soda for mineral water or zero-calorie fruit infused water.

- Aim for the better butters such as nut butters like peanut or almond butter instead of artery-clogging dairy butter.

- Go meatless at least one day a week. Make meals with plant foods such as tofu, beans, nuts, whole grains, vegetables, and fruits.

Do you have some of your own strategies? Write them in your food journal or log.

Creating your own strategies can help you see how your eating is evolving in a healthy way. Remember, one small shift toward healthier eating every day adds up to positive changes in the long run!

Appreciate Your Appetite

Do you ever consider your appetite in the whole picture of your health and wellness? Chances are you don't. Believe it or not, awareness of your appetite is a big part of happiness and wellness.

As natural as feelings of hunger and fullness are, we experience them quite differently. Most of us are afraid to get too hungry, so we eat when we don't need to. However, we don't experience fullness until it's too late, and we end up eating more than we should. Paying attention to when you need (not *want*) to eat versus when you don't need to eat takes you to another level of eating awareness.

> **Healing Hints**
>
> If you are interested in paying closer attention to your appetite, look into appetite awareness training (AAT), a program designed to help people tune back into their internal eating cues (hunger and fullness) with written logs progressing to mental monitoring. To find out more about AAT, take a look at *The Appetite Awareness Workbook* by Linda Craighead (New Harbinger, 2006).

To get started, build an appreciation for your appetite by writing down how you feel before, during, and after eating. Unlike food logs, in which you write down every morsel you eat and drink, appetite logs work by allowing you to examine your *feelings* associated with eating and drinking. It's all about building a healthy relationship with food!

By keeping an appetite log you will develop a new "L.O.V.E." or appreciation for food by allowing yourself to …

- **L**abel feelings associated with certain foods.

- **O**bserve why and when you eat.

- **V**erify what your hunger and fullness means.

- **E**scape habitual or mindless eating.

You will see the L.O.V.E. principles begin to unfold through the process of asking yourself questions every time you eat or think about eating.

I've included an example of an appetite awareness log. Feel free to copy this one or create your own; if you do make your own, be sure to include the categories that I use on this log. Be as honest as possible. Remember, this is a tool for you, so organize it in a way that you'll find to be most helpful.

Keep this log every day whenever you eat or drink anything for one week and see if you recognize any recurring feelings at certain times or places and around any certain foods.

Appetite Appreciation Log

Day/Time	Hunger/Fullness*	Meal/Foods	Feelings**
Monday			
6 A.M.	1/not hungry	coffee	sleepy
8:30 A.M.	10/starving	2 scrambled eggs with cheese, toast with jam, banana	content
11 A.M.	1/not hungry	M & M's	bored

*Rank hunger and fullness based on a scale of 1 to 10. (1 = not very hungry; 5 = hungry, want to eat; 10 = starving, have to eat.)

**List your feelings associated with eating before, during, and/or after an eating or drinking episode. (i.e., happy, bored, satisfied, content, etc.)

Balance on Your Plate

As I mentioned in Chapter 1, healthy eating is all about balance. Balanced nutrition means eating appropriate amounts of nutritious foods every day.

Suppose you enjoy eating beans and brown rice—two very healthy and healing foods—so much so that you eat it every day. Even though beans and brown rice are very healthy, your diet might be out of balance.

Munch on This	If you eat a handful of almonds every day but you never snack on walnuts, get more balance by swapping walnuts for almonds every once in a while. You'll get a bit more of those beneficial omega-3 fats, not to mention a completely different flavor sensation!

Why is balance in your diet so important? Like the yin and yang in Chinese medicine, there is a harmony to eating hot and cold, animal and plant, and bland and spicy foods in balance. If one outweighs the other, your system may suffer. It's all about balancing types of food (and feeling satisfaction!) and getting that synergy of nutrients I talked about in Chapter 1.

Balance vs. Variety

Balance is different than variety. You can have fantastic balance in what you ate without a lot of variety, and vice versa. Variety may be the spice of life, but it can expand your waistline, if you are not conscious of how much you are eating. Recent research in the journal, *Obesity Research*, found that when people do not eat as much variety and eat the same foods daily, they maintain a healthy weight over the long term. However, people who eat more variety tend to increase their calorie intake and gain weight. While we need some variety in our diets, it can easily become too much of a good thing especially if those things are high calorie, artery-clogging ones!

For example, variety can be a real problem with buffets. Not only do you feel like you want to "get your money's worth," but there are so many flavors, textures, and temperatures on the table, that the average buffet-goer really wants to try it all. A lot of extra calories come into play when you are compelled to try three different types of chicken, four styles of potatoes, and six delectable desserts.

Healing Hints	When is variety a good thing? When it comes to fruits and veggies! Choose healthy buffets featuring a plethora of fruits and vegetables. People tend to eat more fruits and vegetables when they are offered them buffet-style. Create snack and meal buffets in your own home by offering at least two different vegetables and a fruit. Chances are your family and friends will eat them up.

Eating Mindfully

We are masters of mindless eating—those unconscious decisions about what and how much we eat. Think about that handful of M&M's you grabbed from the jar on your colleague's desk, the free cookie you picked up when you were at the bank, or your kid's half-finished plate of food you finished last night so it wouldn't go to waste. Experts suggest that we make up to 20 unconscious decisions about food every day—and we've got the waistlines to prove it. In our culture, where food is available all the time, there is no loss of opportunities to eat without thinking. After all, thinking about what you are eating takes work, focus, and most of all, awareness.

Do any of these habits sound familiar? Do you stand up and eat? Do you eat while on the phone, on the computer, or while watching TV? For the most part, we do not take time to *only* eat when we're eating. And that means we are doing a lot of other things as we're shoveling food in, without enjoying or even realizing what or how much we are eating.

Food is meant to be enjoyed and savored. It's meant to be eaten mindfully. Mindful eating is consciously choosing to eat food that is both pleasing and nourishing to your body; to use all of your senses to explore, savor, and taste.

As you begin thinking about mindfulness, it might be helpful to point out some of the characteristics of someone who eats mindfully:

- Acknowledges his or her eating experiences as different than others—as far as nutritional needs, taste preferences, culture, and peer-influences.

- Directs his or her awareness to all aspects of food and eats in the moment.

- Realizes personal food triggers that cause him or her to eat mindlessly.

- Understands how food relates to health and knows what to do and how to eat healthfully.

Do any (or all) of these characteristics sound like you? Perhaps you eat slowly, finish your meal last at the table, or because you're not very hungry, you only nibble a bite at dinner regardless of the gourmet dinner party food set before you. That's mindful eating.

Munch on This	Another aspect, albeit not a necessary one, of mindful eating is considering the source of your food. Some people believe that eating foods that are grown locally is better for you and the environment. They seek out smaller family farmers and organic farmers who avoid commercial fertilizers and pesticides. Eating locally also brings more dollars into your local economy, reduces soil depletion, and provides you with nourishing food closer to the source. Unless fruits and veggies are frozen, they lose nutrients day by day, so the shorter the distance from the farm to your table, the better. Of course, that doesn't mean eating only parsnips in winter if you live in Chicago. But if you haven't tried seasonal foods such as winter root veggies and hard squashes, it might be interesting to add these to your diet.

Eating mindfully also means eating more slowly. The fast-paced treadmill of society makes slowing down difficult. The need to eat fast, digest, and do it all over again takes precedence to chewing, savoring, and feeling your food. When you do slow down, you'll make some interesting discoveries: how to enjoy flavors and textures of different food, and how to be satisfied on less.

Can you really be satisfied with a half cup of ice cream or a handful of chocolate chips? Yes, you can! If you savor it instead of gobbling it down, it will be enough to satisfy your sweet tooth. Indulge in mindful eating by allowing yourself more time for nourishment (without the guilt of having to be somewhere else!), and to actually tune into what your body really needs.

An Exercise in Mindful Eating

Try this mindful eating exercise. Feel free to do it with any type of food you want.

Take one bite of an apple slice and then close your eyes. Do not begin chewing yet.

Try to focus just on the apple. Notice what comes to mind about the apple's taste, texture, temperature, and sensation.

Begin chewing now. Chew slowly, just noticing what it feels like. It's normal that your mind will want to wander off. If you notice you're paying more attention to your thinking than to your chewing, just let go of the thought for the moment and concentrate on chewing. Notice each tiny movement of your jaw.

In these moments you may find yourself wanting to swallow the apple. See if you can stay present and notice the subtle transition from chewing to swallowing.

As you prepare to swallow the apple, try to follow it moving toward the back of your tongue and into your throat. Swallow the apple, following it until you can no longer feel any sensation of the food remaining.

Take a deep breath and exhale.

Think about your experience, considering the following questions:

> What did you notice while chewing?
>
> Why did you swallow?
>
> Was the food no longer tasty?
>
> Did it dissolve?
>
> Were you bored?

This exercise is intended to help you slow down and become more objective about the food you are eating. It's about tasting, savoring, and appreciating the food in your mouth at that moment. All too often eating moments pass by unnoticed and we fail to fully enjoy the food that passes through our lips.

All Calories Are Not the Same

Calories count a lot. Although calories fill you up no matter what you eat, the quality (as well as the number) of calories you eat counts for overall health! As far as calories go, less can actually mean more from a health standpoint. Calorie restriction has been shown to not only help shed the dreaded belly bulge but also increase your time on this earth. Even if you are not trying to lose weight, it's important to be aware of your caloric intake. It's not just about how many calories you eat, but the *type* of calories you are taking in.

You can reach your weight-loss goals eating sugary cereals and donuts, but you're not doing your body much good! The better bet is to fuel your body well and fend off health problems with fewer calories from high-quality food. High-quality calories offer more volume from fiber plus healthier fats, antioxidants, minerals, and lean protein. You can actually pile your plate higher with lower-calorie foods that will be more satisfying in the long run. It's all about choosing those nutrient-dense calories I mentioned in Chapter 1 and avoiding empty calories.

You'll be surprised by how much food you can have if you are calorie smart!

Calorie Smarts (look what you can get for the same number of calories!)		
Meal/Place	*Foods*	*Total Calories*
Breakfast/ restaurant	French Toast Feast	1,010
vs.		
Breakfast/ at home	Whole-grain toast (2 slices)	200
	2 whole eggs, scrambled	140
	1 TB. whipped butter	70
	½ cup steel cut oats	300
	1 cup fat-free milk	90
	¼ cup walnuts, chopped	190
	1 tsp. agave nectar	20
		1,010

Reduce Your Cravings with Real Food

Food cravings are a natural part of life. Whether you crave salty, sweet, fatty, savory, crunchy, or creamy foods, when you've got food on the brain there's no denying it. You can blame a hormone called *ghrelin* for your intense food cravings. Because hormones are released during stressful times, cravings can creep up due to emotions, anxiety, frustration, and loneliness. Hunger is typically not part of the craving equation.

The catch with cravings is that they are usually high in fat and calories. When was the last time you craved steamed broccoli or spinach (without melted cheddar cheese or diced pancetta)?

definition

Ghrelin is the only hormone in humans that is known to stimulate the appetite and cravings for particular foods.

Giving into cravings on occasion is perfectly fine—and necessary—to do. If you deny your cravings all the time, it could lead to overeating or bingeing. When you do give in to cravings, watch your portions. If at all possible, only purchase a single serving size of the craved food. For example, if you want a double fudge brownie—go for it, but only have a small one. Want ice cream? Buy a single serving at the grocery store. Craving fries? Order the smallest size available. Eating these highly craved foods occasionally is not a problem. If it becomes more like two to three times a week then try to retrain your thinking about this food(s) or seek professional assistance from a health psychologist and/or registered dietitian. And use some of the mindful eating techniques from the previous exercise. Savor the flavor and eat slowly!

Here are more ways to help you control your cravings:

- Do not keep the craved food around. Instead, when cravings hit and you decide to give in to them, go to the store and buy an individual portion of that food.

- Eat healthy meals and snacks throughout the day so that you are well nourished.

- Drink a lot of fluids (e.g., water, mineral water, and tea) to stay hydrated and fend off liquid calorie cravings for sweetened coffee drinks and/or regular soda.

- Stay active. Activity can keep ghrelin levels in check and give you something else to focus on besides food.

- Write down your cravings and observe them. What foods are you craving? What time of day? How many times a week?

- Don't deny yourself by cutting out carbs, going fat-free, or bypassing protein. If you give up satisfying food combinations your cravings will get more intense and you'll end up bingeing!

Munch on This   Both men and women get cravings, but they tend to crave different taste sensations. Studies have shown that women have strong urges for sweets (chocolate ranks at the top for women), whereas men are all about the salty and savory indulgences.

Be smart about your cravings. Allow room from some indulgences, but then get back on your healthy eating horse. You'll be a happier and healthier person for it.

Essential Takeaways

- Evolving your eating is a gradual shift toward healthy food choices.
- Appreciation and awareness of your appetite plays an important role in building a healthy relationship with food.
- Balance on your plate is more important than getting a lot of variety. Too much variety can cause unconscious eating and lead to weight gain.
- Mindful eating allows you to remain in the moment, think objectively about your food choices, and savor good-for-you food.
- Calories are essential for life, but the type of calories you eat are essential to your quality of life.
- Cravings are a natural part of life. Enjoy a small indulgence occasionally.

chapter 5

Family Meals

| Eating well at different life stages |
| Teaching kids to eat healthfully |
| Tackling childhood obesity |
| Planning meals with children |
| Enjoying fabulous new foods |

Food plays a big role in setting the tone of your home. The family table should be a place for enjoyment, laughter, and nourishment. Adults can use mealtimes to teach children how to share meals, eat with manners, and appreciate different types of food.

This chapter highlights the importance of family meals, planning together, and experiencing the pleasure—and nourishment— behind a vast array of foods.

Eating Well Through Life

Optimal nutrition at every age is vital for health. From infancy through young adulthood, children need nutrient-rich foods for normal growth and development of the brain, eyes, teeth, bones, muscles, organs, and hormonal systems. Adults need nutritious food to maintain their good health, and pregnant and breastfeeding women have extra nutritional needs.

The middle years bring about hormonal changes for men and women. With menopause women experience many changes including shifts in weight and body composition. As men age their hormone levels change, too, though much less dramatically than in women.

Both genders lose lean muscle mass resulting in increased body fat. Because of these hormonal changes, men and women need to pay close attention to their nutritional needs, especially as it relates to maintaining bone, heart, and brain health. Foods to focus on for optimal middle-age health include whole fruits and vegetables; low-fat dairy, such as milk, cheese, and yogurt; whole-grain breads; cereals; and plenty of tea, especially green tea—it can be good for your heart, blood sugar levels, and may fend off certain cancers.

Munch on This	Studies show that, in general, men prefer high-protein foods, such as meats like veal, ham, and duck, as well as shellfish like shrimp and oysters. As far as vegetables, men prefer Brussels sprouts and asparagus. Women tend to eat more vegetables and fruits, such as carrots, tomatoes, apples, strawberries, blueberries, and raspberries. Plus, women tend to prefer eggs, yogurt, almonds, and walnuts—and crave chocolate.

Teaching Kids Healthy Eating Habits

Children formulate opinions about food early on. Scientific studies show that a child's taste preferences are established as early as conception, with solid food preferences developing before a child comes into the world!

Infants naturally prefer high-calorie, sweet-tasting foods like bananas, apples, potatoes, and peas. They provide the fuel that growing bodies need!

As infants grow into toddlers, they begin to assert independence with food preferences. This is when they begin to push peas around the plate, spit out chicken, and turn their noses up at the sight (and smell) of new foods. However, take heart, if your child is growing well, that is the best indicator of good health and nutrition. Parents still need to set good eating examples by offering vegetables, whole grains, lean proteins, and fruits at family meals and for snacks.

Munch on This	Studies have detected the presence of garlic, cumin, and curry in the amniotic fluid of pregnant women, which means the infant's first experiences with flavors are from swallowing amniotic fluid. This prenatal tasting can provide a "flavor bridge" that familiarizes infants with flavors and food preferences in the mother's womb!

When it comes to new foods, children often have a fear of trying new things, called neophobia in medical parlance. It can be tough to get children to eat up and enjoy unfamiliar foods. The best thing to do is not give up—keep introducing that food over and over again. It can take up to 25 times before a child accepts a new food! Keep it light and be patient with your child's appetite. Don't get crazy if your child is not eating a new dish.

Remember, between the ages of 2 and 5 years toddlers are growing rapidly, so appetites are high. However, their stomachs are not very large, so go with smaller meals and healthy, low-calorie snacks during these years.

Combating Childhood Obesity

The rates of childhood obesity are sky-high. The latest stats show that 10 percent of children throughout the world are overweight or obese. With high-calorie and high-fat foods and drinks readily available to children, they are gaining weight at record proportions. Obesity in children is dangerous for their health. Obese children face a greater risk for serious chronic diseases, such as type 2 diabetes, high blood pressure, heart disease, sleep problems, cancer, eating disorders, early menstruation/puberty, and asthma.

After age 2, body mass index (BMI), the ratio of height to weight is used to assess if a person is within a normal, overweight, or obese weight range.

To find out your child's BMI, refer to the Centers for Disease Control and Prevention growth charts at www.cdc.gov/growthcharts. If a child's weight is over the ninety-fifth percentile on the growth chart, then the child is considered obese.

If the growth charts indicate obesity in your child, take a look at some of the other contributing factors to childhood obesity:

- Lack of physical activity. Children should get at least 60 minutes of activity every day, even if it means limiting the amount of time spent in front of the TV, computer, and video games!

- Genetics. If parents are obese, children most likely will be as well.

- Family does not eat meals together.

- Fed formula instead of breast-milk as a baby. Breast-fed babies are less likely to be obese adults.

- Low self-esteem and/or depression.

- Medical illnesses (e.g., low thyroid function or hypothyroidism, polycystic ovarian syndrome).

Teaching Children Healthy Eating Habits

As a play on the Chinese proverb, if you give a child a healthy food, she will eat for a day, but teach her *how* to make healthy meals, and she will eat well for a lifetime. Children need support when it comes to eating healthfully. Whether you start off during the toddler years or older, one of the best things you can do is allow kids to experiment in the kitchen. Grab a small table or boost them up to the counter to observe and participate in making family meals. The art of cooking should not be reserved for adults only. Allow children to use all of their senses to see, touch, smell, and taste all types of foods.

Allowing small hands to help out in the kitchen is about more than just cooking. It's about developing other skill sets in a fun, nonthreatening fashion. Cooking should be fun for kids, so keep it simple, and don't let "rules" get in the way of enjoying cooking time with your kids. I am not implying to let your young one(s) have full reign and create a huge mess, but be prepared for a little disruption and recipes not to come out exactly as planned.

Foster learning and creativity by permitting other skills to naturally develop. For example, cooking can enhance mathematical skills by measuring ingredients with cups and spoons. It can also enhance attention spans by requiring them to follow along with recipes, expand their knowledge base of different foods and cuisines, and increase cultural competence for different flavors and scents. Finally and most important, teaching kids their way around the kitchen helps to instill a lifelong interest in healthy food.

food wise	Tasks in the kitchen that you take for granted are teaching opportunities for kids. Show kids the way liquids freeze, raw eggs become hard-boiled, or cheese melts on bread. These are new and interesting transitions in form, function, and flavor for kids!

Creating a Healthy Family Table

Family meal time is the perfect opportunity for family members to connect with one another and for parents to serve as a role-model for manners and healthful eating habits. It's true that the family that eats together sticks together. There is more family unity when meals are shared regularly. However, with the fast pace of life, varying schedules, and both parents working outside the home, family meals are often the first thing to go. To try to maintain family meals in the face of all these obstacles, it helps to create quick meals that are satisfying and healthy.

Designate a "cooking day" in your house, when you cook multiple meals to freeze for later in the week. By batch cooking you not only save time, but money.

As soon as family members are old enough, have them take turns setting the table. They not only learn the proper way to organize dishware and utensils, but they learn responsibility. Make mealtime cleanup a family job as well.

Eating Etiquette for Kids

Although the days of fine china and silver at dinner time are long gone (except maybe at holidays), table etiquette remains important. As kids grow up, take the time to teach them mealtime manners. For very young kids, the rules should be as simple as "no toys at the table" (that goes for Mom and Dad, too—no texting at the table) and "everyone must stay seated while eating."

As kids grow up, they should be taught to put their napkin on their lap, ask for food to be passed (instead of reaching across the table), and use forks, knives, and spoons (no eating with fingers) at the table. Although, you want to encourage family interaction while eating, encourage children to chew with their mouths closed. (Yes, this means that have to wait between bites to talk!) This not only fosters good manners, but encourages your family to eat more slowly. Another trick is to put utensils down between bites. Follow these tips, and you will all spend more time tasting and enjoying the food. After all, that's why you are at the table!

Healing Hints Reinforce good table manners for young children by keeping a dry erase board in the kitchen and marking down the good behavior. At the end of each week, review the board and reward good manners with nonfood items.

Menu Planning with Children

Kids like to be involved in planning their lives, whether it's where to play for the day or what to eat. When you are planning your menu for the week, ask your kids for their input. Doing so empowers them to make their own choices. Of course, if you leave it entirely up to them they'll probably suggest sugary cereals and ice cream for dinner. Instead, give them choices. Ask if they would rather have baked sweet potato rounds instead of a baked potato, or find out if they would prefer broccoli or cauliflower. A bonus of getting kids involved in the family meal planning is that they are more likely to eat what you serve.

Keep an ongoing grocery list throughout the week. Include all five foods groups: Grains, Vegetables, Fruits, Milk, Meat and Beans (and incorporate some healthy fats and oils, too). For a handy shopping list, download one from the Nutrient Rich Foods Coalition website at www.nutrientrichfoods.org. Click Living Nutrient-Rich and then click Nutrient-Rich Shopping List.

Food wise

It's true—eating before you go grocery shopping does help you save calories and cash on extra purchases. Also, wear a jacket or sweater, grocery stores are typically kept on the cooler side for good reason: people tend to feel more hungry when they are chilly. And try to ignore those tantalizing food samples at the deli!

A Place for New and Familiar Foods

There is something to be said for sticking with what works when it comes to family meals. If you're used to making turkey chili on Wednesdays and bean burritos on Fridays, then stick with it. Food conjures up memories, and familiar foods bring comfort to life. However, in order to foster acceptance for a wide range of novel foods, it is beneficial to introduce new foods into your family's eating dynamic.

So how can you broaden your family's palate for new and interesting culinary delights? Pick a new food, ingredient, or dish to incorporate into your weekly meals. For example, if you've never had quinoa, a versatile Mediterranean grain that can be used in place of couscous, rice, pasta, or bread, try adding it to your meals. Or replace the chicken in your chicken salad with baked tofu chunks for a delicious vegetarian twist (and you can use the same ingredients as the chicken version).

Add a dollop of plain Greek yogurt instead of full-fat sour cream to chili, soups, or fajitas. In lieu of lasagna noodles layer thinly-sliced zucchini with farmer's cheese and tomato sauce for a lower-calorie version of this delicious Italian staple. Instead of your average sports drink, grab coconut water—one cup has as much potassium as a banana. New foods add zest, zip, and a nice nutritional surprise to your meal planning. Expand your flavor and taste horizons. Bon appetit!

Essential Takeaways

- Men and women naturally have different food preferences.
- Babies develop food preferences from the mother's amniotic fluid before they are born.
- New foods have to be introduced to children many times before they are accepted.
- It's never too early to teach your children table manners.
- Family meal planning begins with a smart shopping list.
- Change up your weekly meal plans and incorporate novel, nutritious foods into your cooking.

Part 2

Healthy Foods in Focus

These chapters take a close look at the foods that contribute to your good health. From colorful fruits and veggies to whole grains, fabulous fats, and powerful proteins, you learn what gives certain foods their healing and healthful properties. We also explore the big eight food allergens that can make seemingly innocuous foods downright dangerous to some people, get smart about how to treat an allergic reaction, and identify where hidden allergens can lurk.

You also find interesting ways to spice up your health by swapping salt with sodium-free, flavor-packed herbs and spices. With recipes and tips on how to use these foods in your kitchen, you'll see that healthy, healing eating is all about using disease-fighting ingredients.

chapter 6

Vegetables Up Close

Discovering the myriad health benefits of vegetables

Looking at four popular veggie families: alliums, roots and tubers, cruciferous veggies, and squash

Cooking with vegetables

It's no surprise that vegetables are good-for-you foods. Yet studies show that less than half of the people in the United States eat enough veggies. It's too bad, because they are missing out on iron-rich leafy greens and beta-carotene loaded orange veggies like pumpkin, squash, and sweet potatoes. Vegetables contain a whole host of vital nutrients and plant compounds that act as nature's medicine cabinet. Besides, your plate would be rather bland without emerald leafy greens, purple eggplant, and golden squash! And those colors are more than beautiful—they're responsible for the healthy nature of vegetables.

Both organic and conventionally grown vegetables are high in antioxidants, which can defend against free radicals that can damage your cells and lead to chronic diseases, such as cancer, type 2 diabetes, and heart disease. (To avoid eating excess chemicals, choose organic produce when you can—see the "Dirty Dozen" list in Chapter 1.) Plus, vegetables have been shown to offer natural protection against some forms of bacteria, fungus, and viruses.

In this chapter, I describe several groups of vegetables and explain why they are an important part of a healthy and healing lifestyle.

Allium Family

There is no mistaking the members of this bulbous species. Each one of them has its own unique pungent aroma and characteristics. The allium family includes onions, chives, shallots, scallions, leeks, and garlic.

The allium clan, which is part of the lily family, adds strong flavors to dishes.

Chives

The smallest kids in the allium family, chives have been an important culinary herb in Europe, Asia, and Africa since the Middle Ages, and were embraced in the Americas after they were settled by the Europeans. Not used for their bulbous bottoms (as many of the other alliums), the soft, slender, tubular leaves of chives impart a more subtle onion flavor than their allium cousins. You may have seen chive's light purple flowers (they are edible, too) in dry floral bouquets.

| munch on This | Garlic chives are a type of chive that tastes more like mild garlic than like typical chives (hence its name). Its white flowers may also be used as a spice. Garlic chives are commonly used in Asian stir-fries, dumplings, and soups. |

For Your Health

The bright green leaves contain flavonoids, a type of antioxidant that studies have shown can fend off a whole host of chronic diseases, such as cancer of the stomach, esophagus, and prostate. Plus, chives also contain vitamins A and C, calcium, and iron. Although it's not common to eat large quantities of chives, people can experience stomach irritation if they eat too many.

Selection and Storage

Chive bulbs grow close together, and their skinny leaves grow like soldiers standing at attention. They typically make their appearance in early spring and can grow from 6 to 15 inches long. Chives are best used fresh, but they can be refrigerated for up to a week and be frozen for up to 1 year. Unlike other herbs, chive leaves do not work well dried as they lose their onion flavor.

In Your Kitchen

Chives can be mixed into cream cheese, cottage cheese, tomato and cucumber salads, and dips. You can toss chives into hot foods, such as soups, chili, stews, omelets, scrambled eggs, and mashed potatoes as a garnish. Chives lose their flavor when overheated, so they are usually added after the dish has been removed from the heat.

Garlic

Garlic is used primarily for its flavorful bulb, which is made up of edible sections called cloves. Garlic has been used as a medicinal herb for centuries. Internationally, China is the largest producer of garlic, with 23 billion pounds of garlic grown annually; in the United States most of the garlic comes from Gilroy, California, which calls itself, "the garlic capital of the world." Garlic is a staple in Mediterranean cuisines of Greece, southern Italy, and Croatia.

For Your Health

Garlic's sharp, pungent flavor tells you the plant-based nutrients have been released (as the chopping, chewing, and crushing of garlic releases its beneficial properties). Native Americans used garlic as a cough and cold remedy. In both world wars, garlic was used as an antibacterial and antiseptic agent to prevent gangrene. It's high vitamin C content puts it in contention with lemons for preventing scurvy, and it is believed to help with the absorption of vitamin B_6 (thiamin), which can help prevent the deficiency disease, beriberi.

Although there have been a lot of small studies showing garlic as a miracle food for fending off high cholesterol levels, high blood pressure, and certain cancers, more research is needed in the garlic-health arena.

Food wise — Some people are allergic to the sulfur compounds in garlic and other members of the allium clan, which may manifest with diarrhea, irritable bowel, nausea, trouble breathing, and mouth and throat sores.

Selection and Storage

Fresh garlic bulbs should be kept warm (about 64°F) and dry to avoid sprouting. The bulbs can be hung or braided together into strands for storage. You can buy preminced garlic packed in water or oil, but the latter has more calories and can go bad more rapidly, so if you buy it, be sure its tightly sealed, refrigerate it upon opening, and use it quickly.

Munch on This	The large bulbs called "elephant garlic" are not really garlic. They are wild leeks, which look and taste more like a mild form of garlic. They taste great raw in salads, dips, and as a topping for sliced crusty bread.

In Your Kitchen

Garlic can be roasted, baked, chopped, crushed, and diced into a variety of foods. Bake a head of garlic and spread it on bread dipped in a touch of olive oil for a delicious appetizer, or sauté minced garlic as a starter for tomato sauce, soups, stocks, and chili. Toss garlic into omelets, scrambled eggs, frittatas, casseroles, meatloaf, and meatballs. Top homemade pizza with garlic, mushrooms, spinach, and mozzarella cheese.

Leeks

Leeks are hearty allium veggies with the flavor of a mild onion. Unlike its other bulb-forming cousins, leeks have sheaths of leaves that form a cylinderlike shape. The white and light green parts are edible, but the dark green leaves should be discarded. (Chefs use it as part of an herbal bouquet garni, a bundle of herbs used to make stock.)

The leek is the national emblem of Wales—welsh soldiers wore the leek on their helmets for identification while in battle. Ironically, many of the ancient British battles took place in leek fields.

For Your Health

Leeks are jammed with healthy flavonoids; one in particular is called kaempferol, a plant-based antioxidant that has been shown to protect the blood vessel walls from damage and help produce more nitric oxide, a gas that helps dilate and relax the blood vessels to the heart. Leeks contain a significant amount of folate, the B-vitamin that helps with heart health by keeping homocysteine (a heart-damaging compound) levels in check. Leeks are also high in an antioxidant polyphenol called gallic acid, which is great for keeping the cells healthy. It's important to note that leeks contain the same sulfur-containing compounds that other alliums like onions and garlic do, thus it kicks up leeks' wellness quotient a notch.

Selection and Storage

Leeks can last through the winter months, but their peak season is early fall and early spring. Select leeks that are green, firm, and straight; not wilted or yellow. Avoid very large leeks, as they can be more fibrous and not as flavorful. Don't cut or wash them before storing them in the refrigerator; they will last for one to two weeks. When you are ready to use them, rinse them thoroughly to wash off all soil that may have gotten lodged in between the leaves. Once they are cooked, leeks go bad quickly. To freeze them, blanch them (place them in boiling water briefly and then take them out and immediately "shock" them in an ice water bath or under cold running water to stop the cooking process) and put them in the freezer; they'll last up to three months.

In Your Kitchen

Cooking with leeks is a cinch. All you need to do is discard the bottom bulb and the tough top green leaves then slice them thinly into rings or lengthwise. Leeks taste great sautéed in olive oil with other vegetables. Cook them in water to make a hearty soup or vichyssoise, a cold leek soup. You can add leeks to eggs, salads, chicken salad, pasta, and rice dishes. Toss with red potatoes or sweet potatoes and bake for a tasty side dish.

Onions

Onions are the mainstay of the allium clan. Globe onions, the mature round varieties, have been revered since ancient times. Onions were a form of currency in the Middle Ages—people gave them to their landlords as rent, and they were also highly prized gifts. Today, we prize them for their health benefits and wonderful culinary flavor.

For Your Health

Onions' sulfur compounds are jam-packed with vital, plant-based flavonoids or antioxidants, which are believed to fend off everything from inflammation to viruses, cancer, infections, and bee stings. Onions offer a fair amount of vitamin C, too. An agricultural report from Cornell University showed that Western Yellow onions have the most flavonoids—almost 11 times as many as Western White onions, which have the fewest flavonoids. Basically, the more pungent the onion, the higher the health benefits!

<table>
<tr><td>**Healing Hints**</td><td>If you want to get the healing power from onions, but want to avoid irritation to your eyes from chopping, dicing, or slicing the fresh stuff, use onion powder, a spice that's made from the most pungent onion bulbs (and it has the smell to prove it!). You can choose yellow, white, red, and toasted onion powders. A couple of other no-more-tears remedies are cutting the onion under water or leaving the root side on until the end of the cutting process, which helps keep the sulfur compounds at bay!</td></tr>
</table>

Selection and Storage

Store onions at room temperature in a dark, well-ventilated place. Onions used for cooking (e.g., white, yellow, and red) can last up to three to four weeks, while sweet onions last from one to two weeks and can be stored in the refrigerator. Be aware that other vegetables stored near onions will decay faster due to onions sapping the moisture from them. Cooking onions will take on the odor of pears and apples, if they are stored in close quarters. Wrap cut onions tightly in plastic and keep them tucked away from other vegetables and fruits; use them within a day or two for best flavor and quality.

In Your Kitchen

Onions offer boundless culinary possibilities. Slice up white onions for fajitas, dice yellow onions for tomato pasta sauce, or grill red onions to top burgers, chicken breast, or fish. Onions are the classic vegetable used in stocks; toss them into soup, sauces, and chili. Sweet onions, the most popular of which are Vidalias, are especially good sautéed.

Scallions

Also, called spring onions, scallions are milder-tasting not-quite-mature shoots of the bulb onion. The green part is hollow and the root is small. They are especially popular in Asian cuisine.

For Your Health

Similar to the other alliums, scallions are high in flavonoids, specifically one called quercetin, which can help fend off inflammation. Also, the sulfur compounds have shown promise in cancer prevention. The catch is that you have to be sure to include scallions or other alliums into your everyday eating to get the best health benefits.

Selection and Storage

When purchasing scallions look for fresh, bright green, dry, and firm tops. They should not be moist, blemished, or dried out. The bulbs should be white and firm, too. Scallions are available year-round in temperate (mild) climates. Use them as soon as possible, especially after they have been cut, because they are sensitive to oxygen and lose flavor fast. You can store them whole in a plastic bag for up to two weeks in the fridge.

In Your Kitchen

Add these delicate aromatics to Asian noodle dishes, such as Pad Thai, and soups and dipping sauces. Dice them into salads, tuna or chicken salad; add them to hummus and leafy green wraps; or sprinkle them into scrambled eggs, omelets, and quiches.

Shallots

The delicate light purple cousin of the onion has been used in classical cooking for centuries. Shallots grow in clusters of bulbs with loosely fitting copper or pinkish skin. Shallots are believed to have originated in the Palestinian city of Ascalon. Today, shallots are widely used in Thai, Cambodian, Malaysian, and Indonesian cuisine. They have a milder, sweeter flavor than other alliums, yet they can hold their own in terms of pungency.

For Your Health

Shallots are believed to contain a whole host of plant-based nutrients—even more than other members of the allium family. They offer more flavonoids like quercetin, which helps prevent heart disease, diabetes, and cancer; they contain more vitamin C and protein than other members of the allium clan.

Selection and Storage

Shallots can be stored for as long as six months in a cool, dry, dark place with plenty of ventilation. Their peak season is April through August. Choose firm shallots without blemishes or soft spots, and they should be heavy (not light) for their size. The larger the shallot, the stronger the taste.

In Your Kitchen

Shallots offer just the right amount of pungent flavor to gravies, sauces, and stir-fries. Cooking them diffuses their strong flavor a bit. Shallots are often cooked with wine for a delicious taste combination. Sauté shallots with olive oil and mushrooms as a topping for meat, fish, or poultry. Or make a reduction sauce with shallots and balsamic vinegar and pour over baked extra-firm tofu.

Roots and Tubers

These hearty, substantial vegetables grow underground and have a very long shelf life. Root veggies are the underground parts of plants, and can have a sweet flavor, such as carrots, parsnips, and beets, or a sharp, bold bite, such as radishes. Tubers are the starchy stems of plants and run the gamut from starchy, new, and sweet.

Beets

Brightly colored, smooth, tender, and packed with glorious sweetness, beets have gone from a peasant food staple to gourmet fare. Once Germans discovered how to extract sucrose (a form of sugar) from the large sugar beets in the nineteenth century, Europeans completely jumped on board and began using sugar beets as an alternative sweetener to tropical sugar cane. Beets come in many colors from ruby red, pink, golden, white, and striped. One particularly striking beet variety is the pink–and–white striped, Italian-grown heirloom Chioggia beet.

For Your Health

As their vibrant colors suggest, beets are packed with unique pigment antioxidants called *beta-cyanins.* This antioxidant compound has shown promise in cancer prevention and may fend off the development of fungi. Beet's earthy smell and taste comes from natural compounds called *geosmin*. Some of the earthier tasting beet varieties like Chioggia have greater amounts of geosmin. Beets are a low-calorie food, with about 45 calories and almost 3 grams of fiber for a half-cup serving, making them perfect for weight control. Beets are heart-healthy with a fair amount of folate, which helps keep harmful homocysteine levels down, and potassium for controlling blood pressure.

Selection and Storage

Beets are available throughout the year, but culinary experts call the best beet times late summer and early fall. When scouting out beets, look at their leaves, as they indicate freshness: they should be green and fresh, and not wilted. The actual root should be smooth and firm, not discolored or bruised. Be sure to remove the leaves from the beet root before storing them in the refrigerator—put beets in a plastic bag and they will last up to 5 days. The beet greens are also delicious and healthy, so don't throw them out!

In Your Kitchen

Beet root can be pickled, roasted (which intensifies the flavor), and chopped into salads and soups. For maximum flavor, cook beets whole (if boiling leave a bit of the stem on to avoid losing the healthful red pigment in the water) and then proceed to chop, slice, and/or mash them for all sorts of good eats. The beets greens can be sautéed in toasted sesame oil for a wonderful Asian flair or olive oil with garlic for a Mediterranean-inspired dish.

Carrots

Although commonly orange-colored, carrots come in purple, yellow, red, white, and maroon varieties, too. Both the root and leaves of the carrot are edible. Carrots have distant herbal relatives, such as fennel, dill, parsley, and cumin.

Munch on This
The maroon-colored carrot called the BetaSweet was developed at a Texas-based university. It's extremely high in cancer-fighters as well as beta-carotene, an antioxidant that is good for your eyes and fending off other chronic diseases.

For Your Health

Carrots are a good low-calorie source of fiber, with 26 calories and 3 grams of fiber for a half-cup serving. Carrots contain an abundance of beta-carotene, a fat-soluble precursor to vitamin A. (White-colored carrots lack beta-carotene, but make up for it with an abundance of vitamin E.) Like all fat-soluble nutrients, in order to reap the benefits of beta-carotene, cut up carrots and cook them with a bit of olive or canola oil to increase the absorption of beta-carotene—it can increase absorption by almost 40 percent!

Research indicates that only 3 percent of the beta-carotene from a raw carrot is released during digestion, so heat them up for maximum nutrition benefit. Keep in mind that eating too many carrots may cause your skin to turn orange.

Selection and Storage

Carrots are at their peak flavor from early winter through spring but can be purchased year-round. Look for smooth skin and brightly colored exterior with no green near the stem. Leaving about an inch of the stem on while storing will help keep carrots moist. Store them in the refrigerator in a plastic bag; some varieties can last up to four weeks. Carrots absorb odors from other foods, such as apples and pears, so keep them in a separate container.

In Your Kitchen

You can chop, slice, and dice carrots into salads. Steam baby carrots for a fun toddler snack. Roast them in the oven with a drizzle of olive oil, a dash of salt, cumin, and paprika for a delicious side dish. Purée carrots into juice and smoothies. Add slivers of carrots into baked goods like carrot cake and muffins.

Munch on This	Rutabagas are bigger and have white, yellow, or brown skins and yellow flesh. Turnips have a distinct creamy white skin with a flash of purple at the top. Roasting either of them or both brings out their sweet flavor without adding any additional calories. The two root veggies are closely related and can be substituted for one another in recipes.

Parsnips

This long, thick, straight taproot looks like an ivory carrot. Parsnips have a distinct, sweet, earthy flavor that people tend to either love or despise.

For Your Health

Like the carrot, parsnips are a fantastic, nutrient-dense food with only 55 calories and 600 milligrams of potassium in a half-cup serving. They are also a good source of fiber (3 grams per half cup), which can fill you up faster and longer. Parsnips also contain a fair amount of folate and are an excellent source of vitamin C. So they can help boost immunity as well as help to ensure healthy babies and manage your waistline.

Selection and Storage

Parsnips are a winter veggie that thrives in the cold months. Though like carrots, they are generally available year-round. Purchase parsnips that are firm, unblemished, and have a pale pallor. The green tops should look green and fresh. The larger the parsnip, the more tough the flesh and core will be. Cut off the green tops and store covered in the refrigerator; they can last up to one month.

In Your Kitchen

Before cooking parsnips, especially large ones, remove the inner, woody core. Wash thoroughly with a scrub brush, as they can have a lot of dirt residue left on them. Peel the skin if it's badly beat up from harvesting or appears to be tough. Parsnips can be eaten raw or cooked. Boil, steam, or roast parsnips; they taste great with other root veggies, such as potatoes, carrots, beets, and turnips. Purée cooked parsnips for a mash that tastes great with a pat of butter, a dash of salt, and a handful of diced chives.

Potatoes

Potatoes are the oldest vegetables of the roots and tubers clan, and today constitute the fourth largest crop in the world. The potato's ancient roots can be traced back to Peru from as early as 2000 B.C.E. These tubers contribute a lot of energy-rich fuel to the vegetable party.

Starchy potatoes such as Russet, Butterfinger, or Kennebec are great for baking, roasting, and making into French fries. Waxy varieties such as red, white, or yellow potatoes have thinner skins and are round, small in size, and have less starch than the larger, thicker-skinned varieties. Sweet potatoes have either yellowish-brown, orangey-red, or purplish skin with dark orange or yellow flesh. As their name implies, they are the sweetest of them all.

For Your Health

Potatoes often get a bad rap from a calorie standpoint, and many weight-loss programs banish them because of their high starch content. In reality, potatoes are jammed packed with a lot of good nutrition. A medium potato, such as an Idaho, has only 110 calories and 620 milligrams of potassium—more potassium than a banana—and is a good source of vitamin C, which is great for wound healing and maintaining healthy, youthful skin. There's even 2 grams of dietary fiber in a potato (if eaten with the skin on), which is good news for digestive health and weight management. And potatoes also contain 2 grams of protein in a medium-size potato. In other words, potatoes offer more balance to a meal than you think.

Sweet potatoes are blessed with a nutritional bonus: their orange-red pigment offers high amounts of beta-carotene, a powerful antioxidant. Research has shown that sweet potatoes have four times the beta-carotene as the USDA's Recommended Daily Allowance (RDA), especially when eaten with the skin. They also offer a fat-free vitamin E source, as $\frac{2}{3}$ of a cup of sweet potatoes has 100 percent of the RDA. They contain a moderate amount of calories: 1 cup has 180 calories. Sweet potatoes are also a good fiber source for a slower release of sugar in the bloodstream and greater satiety (feeling full).

Selection and Storage

Look for unblemished, smooth-skinned, mold-free potatoes. Starchy potatoes are best during the late summer; new potatoes are best in spring and early summer; and sweet potatoes are at their peak in autumn and winter. Store potatoes in a cool, dark, dry, and well-ventilated space, such as the pantry. Starchy and sweet potatoes will last for one to two weeks, but waxy, new potatoes should be used as soon as possible—within two to three days. None of the varieties keep well in refrigeration.

In Your Kitchen

Scrub potatoes under cold water to remove dirt and pesticide residue (if not organic). Be aware that it's easy to scrape off the skin from the thin-skinned varieties, so take extra care with them. Cut off any blemishes or "eyes" before cooking.

Potatoes offer many culinary possibilities: you can bake, roast, boil, mash, and sauté them. Sweet and starchy potatoes are delicious chopped thin or thick lengthwise and baked as French fries. Boil new potatoes for a cold potato salad or slice them thin for a potato casserole or pie.

Roast new potatoes with herbs and spices, a drizzle of olive oil, and a dash of salt for a fabulous side dish. Dice potatoes into scrambled eggs or sauté with other diced vegetables for a tasty hash.

Radishes

This crisp, clean-tasting, rounded root veggie is closely related to mustard greens and turnips. The color and shape of a radish can dictate its name: the slender white ones are called icicle radishes; Easter egg radishes are rounded and range from purple, pink, lavender, and white; and watermelon ones have pale green skin and pinkish-red insides. Black Spanish radishes have black, rough skin with strong, pungently flavored white inner flesh.

For Your Health

The radish is almost a zero calorie food, containing just a single calorie. A cup of sliced radishes is a mere 20 calories, making them a great any time of day snack food. They pack a nutritious punch, too: radishes are high in vitamin C (the leaves are believed to contain 6 times the vitamin C as the root!), which can help fend off certain cancers and boost immunity; folic acid for healthy babies and heart health; and a good dose of potassium for blood pressure control. One cup has 2 grams of fiber and contains a lot of water, which helps make you feel full faster and hydrate your body well.

Selection and Storage

Peak seasons for radishes are spring and early summer. Radishes should be firm, unblemished, and have smooth skin. The greens, if still attached, should be unwilted. Trim away the greens before storing and put the vegetables in a plastic bag in the refrigerator; they will last from one to two weeks, depending on the size. (Larger ones tend to last a bit longer.) Popping the rounded roots into ice water can refresh them and revive their crispness.

In Your Kitchen

Radishes are unique among other root vegetables as they offer a crispy crunch to cold food preparations but don't respond very well to heat. Slice them thin for mixed green or cucumber salads, layer them with other vegetables and hummus in sandwiches, or eat them whole with a dash of salt or feta cheese and crusty bread dipped in olive oil.

Cruciferous Family

The elite squad called *cruciferous vegetables* includes cabbages, broccoli, cauliflower, and Brussels sprouts. They are members of the Brassica group of vegetables and offer a powerhouse of nutritional value in the body.

Broccoli

Broccoli is a must-have veggie for good health. It's a versatile vegetable with a lot of culinary uses. China is the largest producer of broccoli in the world; the United States (California) ranks third in broccoli production.

> **Munch on This**
>
> There are three types of broccoli: the common green headed variety with thick stalks; sprouting broccoli, which has many heads with thin stalks; and purple cauliflower, with purple-hued flower buds in the shape of a cauliflower head.

For Your Health

Broccoli does your body good; it contains the highest amounts of carotenoids, particularly lutein and beta-carotene, of the crucifers. It's low in calories, with a mere 35 calories in a half-cup serving, plus it's low in fat and sodium. It's a good source of fiber, with 3 grams per half-cup serving, and it's jammed with vitamins C, A, and K. It aids in defense against damaging free radicals and it helps with normal blood clotting functions.

Broccoli has distinct chemical compounds that fend off diseases like cancer, particularly prostate cancer, and heart disease. One such compound is called diindolylmethane, which has been found to boost immunity, fend off viruses, bad bacteria, and cancers. It also contains another chemical compound called sulfurophane, another potent player in cancer defense.

Selection and Storage

Broccoli thrives in cooler weather and is in season from fall to early spring. But like many veggies sourced from other parts of the country and world, it's available year-round. Look for tight heads with green or purplish—not yellow—tops. Choose firm stalks that are uniformly colored with fresh green leaves. Refrigerate broccoli in plastic bags for up to five days.

In Your Kitchen

Wash broccoli in cold running water and cut the florets from the stalk into bite-size pieces. (Be sure not to discard the stems; you can peel a bit of the outer layer away and prepare the rest of the stem with the florets—it's tasty and offers the same bounty of nutritional benefits!) You can also cut them lengthwise to look like baby trees, if you are roasting them. Broccoli is a culinary dream with a plethora of possibilities including steaming, roasting, and stir-frying. You can also purée broccoli into soups, stews, or vegetable juice. Broccoli is tasty with dips, topped with cheese, dressing, or marinades. Crush peanuts over a bowl of steamed broccoli with angel hair pasta and drizzle with sesame oil for a delicious dish.

Cabbage

Cabbage leaves have a distinct wrinkly almost veinlike exterior with an elephant ear shape. The leaves are often covered with a natural waxy, powdery coating called *bloom*. Mature cabbage usually has tightly wrapped leaves around a circular body. Young cabbage leaves are typically loose and don't form a compact head. There are red and green cabbages, such as savoy and napa varieties.

Healing Hints

Brussels sprouts are mini cabbages named after the capital of Belgium, where they were originally grown. These small sprouts are a delicious way to fend off cancer with plant-based compounds like sulforaphane and indole-3-carbinol.

For Your Health

Cabbage is a highly nutritious food with significant amounts of vitamin C (there's over 60 percent of the RDA in a half-cup serving), the B-vitamin riboflavin, and a significant amount of glutamine, the amino acid that gives food it's savory quality. It's also an inflammation fighter. A half-cup serving has a mere 25 calories.

Munch
on This
Raw cabbage leaves can be placed on a breast-feeding woman's engorged breast to relieve discomfort and pain. Just remove the leaves from the core, wash them, and pat dry; place them in the refrigerator to cool, and pound them a bit with a mallet or your fist to soften before placing on the breasts. Also, raw cabbage leaves can be puréed into a paste to help relieve inflammation on any inflamed area of the body.

Selection and Storage

Green cabbage is best in fall and early winter; red cabbage thrives in the dead of winter. Look for tightly furled heads that are firm and heavy for their size; smooth leaves and vibrant color signal freshness.

In Your Kitchen

Cabbage can be eaten raw or cooked, but either way run the individual leaves under cold water and scrub lightly with a brush before eating or cooking. Coarsely chop cabbage for coleslaw and/or salads. Roll green cabbage leaves with a filling of ground meat or turkey and brown rice or barley; cook with a tomato-based sauce until tender. Use braised red cabbage as a side to pork chops, poultry, or fish.

Cauliflower

This popular crucifer with creamy white florets is closely related to broccoli. There are purple (which is different from purple broccoli), green, and orange varieties of cauliflower, too.

For Your Health

Cauliflower's health benefits are similar to broccoli. It is low in calories with a mere 25 calories per half-cup serving; a good source of fiber, vitamin C, and folate. It also contains sulforaphane, and indole-3-carbinol compounds, which fend off cancerous cell growth.

Food
wise
Be aware that boiling cauliflower diminishes its beneficial compounds significantly. After 30 minutes of boiling, 75 percent of its beneficial compounds are lost. Five minutes of boiling causes a 20 to 30 percent loss. The longer a veggie is left in boiling water the more nutrients are pulled out and left behind swimming in the water. Other cooking methods—steaming, microwaving, roasting, and stir-frying—will not cause a loss in any beneficial compounds.

Selection and Storage

Cauliflower is available in markets all year, but its peak season is late summer to early fall. Look for firm, tightly rounded heads without blemishes or brown spots. Keep cauliflower in the refrigerator, either in a plastic bag or container; it will last for up to five days.

In Your Kitchen

Cauliflower is a versatile culinary vegetable. Cut the florets from the thick stalk with a small paring knife and separate the florets into small, bite-size pieces. Cauliflower can be steamed, boiled, roasted, and eaten raw. Mash steamed cauliflower as a side dish—it's a tasty stand-in for potatoes. Purée it and make creamy soup (minus the cream), or roast the florets with garlic, olive oil, and rosemary. The florets are tasty raw with dips and on crudité platters.

Squashes

This family of gourd veggies grow on vines and vary widely in size, shape, and color. The squashes we eat and grow today, such as zucchini, acorn squash, butternut squash, and pumpkin, have roots dating back up to 10,000 years ago. Squash comes in two types: summer and winter squash. Winter squash, such as acorn and butternut, mature longer and have thicker skins; summer squash, such as zucchini and yellow squash, have thinner skins and a more delicate flavor.

Acorn Squash

This winter squash is shaped like an acorn with a thick-ribbed, dark green shell and pale orange, soft flesh. In the center of the acorn squash is a round vessel of seeds. When you cut it into two halves, it's a cinch to scoop the seeds out from both sides. The seeds are edible.

For Your Health

As its orange flesh indicates, acorn squash is packed with carotenes, specifically beta-cryptoxanthin, which is a powerful antioxidant in reducing risk for cancer, specifically lung cancer—even among smokers! Acorn squash also are high in vitamin A, which research has shown to be particularly beneficial to smokers and people exposed to second hand smoke because a common element in cigarette smoke can rob the body of vitamin A. Acorn squash is a good source of fiber, potassium, and omega-3 fats, which are all good for heart health.

Selection and Storage

Like all winter squashes, acorn squash is at its best during the wintertime. Choose squash that is firm, heavy for its size, and has a dull outer shell; it shouldn't be glossy, soft, or moldy. If you store acorn squash properly it can last as long as 6 months. Store in a dark place with moderate temperature (about 50°F–60°F). Refrigerate individually wrapped in pieces for up to four days.

In Your Kitchen

Acorn squash is simple to cook. Just cut the squash in half and remove the seeds from the inner cavity. Drizzle olive oil or a pat of butter onto the flesh, sprinkle cinnamon or brown sugar over it, and bake until soft and piping hot. Scoop out the flesh as a side dish, stuff it into ravioli or pasta shells, or purée into a creamy squash soup. The hollowed out shell halves make a unique serving vessel, too!

Butternut Squash

Butternut squash has a characteristic round bulb at one end with smooth, pale beige skin. Its flesh has sweet, nutty flavors and a deep-orange hue.

For Your Health

Butternut squash is packed with vitamin A and its precursor beta-carotene (specifically beta-cryptoxanthin). It's a good source of fiber with 3 grams per half-cup serving. Plus it's high in potassium and vitamin C, which are good for healthy blood pressure and boosting immunity. As with all squash, it's a low-calorie food, with about 50 calories in a half-cup serving, and contains a fair amount of folate, which is great for healthy babies and fending off high homocysteine levels, a marker of inflammation and potential heart disease.

Food wise Contact with butternut squash may cause an allergic skin reaction called *contact dermatitis,* in which skin on the hands cracks, tightens, and may tingle and/or feel numb. Wear rubber gloves when handling squash (as this can happen with acorn squash, too); if a reaction has begun, apply cortisone cream to the area and it should be better within a day. If you have this kind of reaction, it's still okay to eat the squash, just be careful when touching it.

Selection and Storage

Butternut squash is best in the winter months. Choose squash that is firm, heavy for its size, and has a dull outer shell; it should not be glossy, soft, or moldy. Store in a dark, moderate temperature (about 50°F–60°F). Under the right conditions, butternut squash can last as long as six months. Refrigerate individually wrapped in pieces for up to four days.

In Your Kitchen

Butternut squash is easy to cook, but cutting it up can be challenging. Cut it in half lengthwise with a sharp chef's knife. If you need to cut it into smaller pieces, do so carefully. Once it's cut, scoop out the seeds from the small cavity and drizzle the flesh with olive oil, a dash of salt and rosemary, and bake it. Once it's baked, scoop out the sweet flesh and enjoy plain or with a dollop of butter. Use it to fill pasta shells or ravioli; as a side for meat, poultry, or fish; add it into soups; or cube it into stews or stuffing. For a special sweet treat, drizzle a bit of maple syrup on it.

Zucchini and Yellow Squash

Botanically speaking, the zucchini is actually a fruit, but it's treated like a vegetable in the culinary world. They have thin green skin and a soft and silky, ivory-colored flesh. Zucchini can be eaten raw or cooked in many different ways. Zucchini became widely used in the United States in the 1920s; it's grown mainly in California today.

Yellow squash may have bumpy skin and some varieties have a crooked necked. They have creamy white, soft flesh with a hint of seeds distributed in the center. Another type of yellow squash is patty pan squash, which is round with a scalloped (almost doily-like) edge.

For Your Health

Like most summer squashes, zucchini and yellow squashes are low-calorie with about 35 calories per cup. Summer squash contains a fair amount of magnesium, which research has shown can reduce the risk of heart attack and stroke. They also have a fair amount of potassium, which helps regulate blood pressure. These warm weather culinary beauties may also boost immunity and fend off hardening of the arteries, as they have a fair amount of vitamin C and beta-carotene in their sleek bodies. These two nutrients have been shown to defend against certain cancers, too.

Selection and Storage

As the name implies, summer squash is best in the summertime. Choose squash that are heavy for their size with unblemished, shiny skin. Medium-size varieties have the best flavor. Unlike winter squash, summer squashes do not keep long. In general, they can keep for up to three days covered in a plastic bag in the refrigerator.

In Your Kitchen

Summer squash works well in all culinary applications. Slice them thin and sauté with a little olive oil, or cut them into chunks and roast them with herbs and spices in the oven. Cut them lengthwise and grill them. (They make a great plate presentation complete with grill marks.) Ribbon them over pasta or rice dishes, or use them raw in salads and party platters with dip.

Veggie Health Benefits at a Glance

Many vegetables offer fantastic health benefits. The following table lists some key veggies that you should add to your kitchen's "medicine cabinet."

More for Your Health! Leafy Greens, Fungi, and Flower Buds		
Vegetable Name	Type	Health Benefit
Arugula	Leafy green	High in vitamins A & C, potassium, and fiber

Vegetable Name	Type	Health Benefit
Chard	Leafy green	High in vitamins K, A, C, magnesium, potassium, fiber, and iron
Kale	Leafy green	Chock full of fiber, flavonoids (antioxidants), and vitamins K, A, C
Spinach	Leafy green	High in vitamins K, A, C, folate, iron, potassium, and fiber
Mushrooms	Fungi	Contains selenium, riboflavin, niacin, potassium, and phosphorus; vitamin D (if exposed to ultraviolet light); and soluble fiber (some varieties)
Artichokes	Flower bud	High in potassium, vitamin C, folate, magnesium, and fiber

Healing Hints

Kale is considered a cruciferous vegetable with a myriad of marvelous health benefits from fending off certain cancers to lowering cholesterol. It's a must-have healing food.

Shiitake mushrooms contain a beta-glucan fiber called lentinan, which has shown benefit in boosting immunity, fighting infection, and preventing the growth of cancerous tumors.

Essential Takeaways

- Vegetables are nutrient-dense foods that are high in fiber, vitamins, and minerals.
- Vegetables come in many shapes, colors, and sizes—enjoy at least 2 to 3 cups a day.
- Whether vegetables are starchy, leafy, or aromatic, they all have health benefits that can fend off chronic diseases, such as cancer, heart disease, obesity, and type 2 diabetes.
- From a nutritional standpoint, organic and conventional (nonorganic) vegetables do not differ much; however, organic produce are grown without chemicals.

chapter 7

The Sweet Nature of Fruit

Looking at four fruit types

Grasping the healthy nature of fruit

Satisfying your sweet tooth with fruit

Using fruit in the kitchen

Fruit is a delicious part of a healthy diet. The flavorful flesh surrounding the seeds of plants, fruit is a culinary and nutritious staple. Whole fruits come in seemingly endless varieties and types; the best part is they are naturally free of cholesterol and saturated fat and low in sodium.

Fruit can keep your cells healthy, fend off chronic diseases, and provide a nutrient-rich source of calories. Whole fruits are an ideal way to restore good nutrition while at the same time control weight.

In this chapter, I take you through four families of fruit and explore ways to fit fruit into your life in new and delicious ways.

Berry Family

Every member of this popular sorority of fruits has a healthy reputation as a powerful disease defender. The skins and seeds of berries are the keepers of the health-enhancing goods, such as polyphenols (antioxidant compounds) that help keep your cells healthy. Due to their high antioxidant levels, berries are one of the highest among plant foods in oxygen radical absorbance capacity (ORAC). The ORAC scale is used in laboratories to determine the antioxidant capacity of certain foods. The United States Department of Agriculture (USDA) uses the ORAC scale to rank foods for potential health benefits.

Food wise
Although fruit juice contains vitamins and minerals, you're far better off eating whole fruit. It provides you with the whole package of fiber and plant-based nutrients—plus chewing is always more satisfying!

Avocado

Many people are surprised to learn that the avocado, also called an alligator pear, is a large berry with a large seed. Avocados grow on trees and can be pear-shaped, egg-shaped, or spherical. Avocados originated in Pueblo, Mexico, and the earliest records reveal that they date back to 10,000 B.C.E. Early Mexicans thought of the avocado as the "fertility fruit" (avocado means *testicle* in the Aztec language). Today California produces 90 percent of the U.S. avocado crop.

For Your Health

Avocados contain a ton of heart-healthy fat (a.k.a. monounsaturated fatty acids, or MUFAs). They contain more potassium than bananas and are rich in B-vitamins as well as vitamins E and K. The fiber in avocados is amazing, too—it contains 75 percent insoluble fiber and 25 percent soluble fiber, so it's great at ridding the body of excess cholesterol; some studies also show that it raises HDL (good) cholesterol. MUFAs have been shown to keep blood sugar in check, too. There are only 50 calories in a serving (one fifth of a medium-size avocado).

Selection and Storage

Avocados ripen a few days after picking. If you store them with bananas or apples they will ripen more quickly thanks to ethylene gas naturally produced by these fruits. Grocers sometimes preripen avocados by exposing them to ethylene gas; this does not pose a health risk, but allowing a fruit or vegetable to ripen in the sun on its own time table is the best way to get the most nutrients out of it.

Leave avocados at room temperature to ripen or refrigerate them to slow down ripening. After you cut an avocado open, leave the pit in the part you are not eating—this will help it from turning brown—and store it, covered, in the refrigerator.

<table>
<tr><td>Food wise</td><td>Don't cook avocados, at least not for very long. Prolonged exposure to heat will render the fruit bitter and inedible.</td></tr>
</table>

In Your Kitchen

Buy avocados ripe if you want to make a dip, such as guacamole. Look for firmer ones if you want to use them sliced into salads, sandwiches, wraps, or scrambled eggs. Avocados work well in sushi rolls and as a dessert mashed up with a hint of sugar. In Indonesia it's a popular ingredient in smoothies with a drizzle of chocolate sauce.

Banana

Bananas are a common starchy staple in many tropical cultures. They are believed to have originated in Papau, New Guinea. Technically, bananas are not berries, but are referred to as "leathery berries." Bananas are usually seedless or have tiny seeds. They have similar growing properties as avocados in that they mature on the tree, but ripen off of it. Depending upon how ripe they are, bananas can vary from starchy to sweet.

For Your Health

Bananas get a bad rap as a starchy food to avoid, but they pack a lot of good nutrition. Known for their potassium, bananas are an athlete's go-to fruit for replenishing this important electrolyte. They also have a fair amount of vitamins B_6 and C. One cup of mashed banana is packed with 6 grams of fiber. A small banana only has 90 calories, so it won't hurt your waistline either.

Selection and Storage

Store bananas at room temperature on their own or with other fruits to ripen more quickly. Like avocados, bananas can be artificially preripened with man-made ethylene gas at grocery stores. The green ones at the stores were most likely not treated with this gas.

In Your Kitchen

They can be baked, grilled, and pan seared for numerous dessert-type dishes. Instead of baking bananas into high-calorie muffins and quick breads, split a whole banana, add a dollop of low-fat yogurt, a drizzle of honey, and sprinkle of cinnamon for a fun and healthy Banana Split.

Blackberries

Blackberries are not true berries but actually considered caneberries—each berry is made up of drupelets, or individual parts. Because it takes two years to complete a life cycle, blackberries have biennial stems, also called "canes." There are over 375 different species of blackberry. Blackberries are mainly grown commercially in Oregon.

For Your Health

Blackberries' deep purple flesh contains a lot of beneficial anthocyanins, which give them their high antioxidant power. And one cup has a mere 62 calories. Blackberries are also high in fiber, vitamins C and K, folic acid, and manganese. Blackberries offer extra protection against cancer and heart disease due to their high amount of ellagic acid, a powerful antioxidant. Their large seeds are packed with nutrients, including high amounts of essential fatty acids, such as omega-3 and omega-6, as well as protein, carotenoids, and fiber.

Selection and Storage

Buy fresh, whole blackberries in any grocery store or at farmers' markets in the warm, summer months. They are available frozen and as jam, jelly, and syrup. Look for fresh blackberries that are dry and firm and not leaking or soft. Blackberries can be pricey; look for seasonal deals at farmers' markets or buy them frozen in large bags to save money.

In Your Kitchen

Blackberries are a delicious way to add variety and nourishment to your culinary world. Throw fresh blackberries into low-fat plain yogurt, hot or cold cereal, salads, pasta salad, or a fruit smoothie.

Blueberries

Small, round, and packed with juicy flavor, blueberries don't start off indigo-blue, but end up that way. Young blueberries are pale-green and they mature to reddish-purple before ripening to a vibrant blue. Maine is one of the world's largest producers of low-bush, or wild, blueberries.

For Your Health

Blueberries are jammed with antioxidant powerful *anthocyanins.* They also contain a good amount of vitamin C, fiber, and manganese. Studies show that blueberries may lower brain damage in stroke patients, prevent urinary tract infections, and lower total cholesterol levels. Other promising studies show that blueberries may enhance memory and control blood sugar levels in older adults. All that in only 80 calories in a cup!

Definition

Anthocyanins are water-soluble pigments that appear blue, red, or purple in fruits and vegetables that have been found to prevent chronic diseases.

Selection and Storage

The prime season for harvesting blueberries in North America is mid-May through September. Store fresh blueberries in your refrigerator or freeze them. Wait to rinse them until right before eating them, as they turn bad quickly if they get too moist. Instead of buying high sugar jams and jellies, make your own blueberry fruit-spread by boiling blueberries with lime juice, water, lime rind, powdered pectin, and a bit of sugar.

In Your Kitchen

Bake blueberries into muffins, pancakes, and breads. Toss fresh berries into salads, ice cream, yogurt, pizza, cereal, and oatmeal. Spread blueberry jam on toast, waffles, English muffins, and crackers. Use blueberry syrup in smoothies, over ice-cream sundaes, and as a topping for rice pudding or tapioca pudding.

Grapes

Yeast occurs naturally on the skins of grapes, which makes this an ideal fruit for wine making. Ancient Egyptians used grapes for both food and wine. The first mention of grapes in the Bible was a reference to Noah (of the Ark) growing them on his farm.

For Your Health

Although wine has received a lot of attention for its health benefits (which is discussed in Chapter 15), the antioxidant-packed skin of grapes is another rich source of disease prevention. With only 62 calories per cup, grapes are the perfect food for waistline management, too.

Research has shown that the plant-chemicals in grape skins can keep blood vessels open wide by producing nitric oxide, a hormone that has been shown to cause blood vessels to dilate (or open). This is great for healthy blood flow to and from the heart! Plus grape skins have resveratrol, the powerful antioxidant that studies have shown to fend off cancer, heart disease, progressive nerve disease, and viral infections. Some studies also strongly support resveratrol's role in staving off Alzheimer's disease. As we've seen with other richly colored fruits, grapes contain anthocyanins, which are beneficial for chronic disease prevention.

Selection and Storage

Buy grapes organic if you can, as conventional grapes are on the Environmental Working Group's "Dirty Dozen" list of fruits and vegetables (more on this in Chapter 1). Grapes are sold on their vines in bunches. Twenty-seven percent of the world's grapes are sold as fresh fruit, while 2 percent are sold as dried fruit such as raisins, currants, and sultanas. The rest—a whopping 71 percent—is used for wine making. Seedless grapes are typically sold for eating, but we recommend going for the seeded variety, as the seeds contain a lot of plant-based nutrients.

MUNCH ON THIS

Raisins, currants, and sultanas are all dried grapes. A raisin is made from the Thompson seedless grape variety. A currant is a specific grape variety called Zanthe Black Corinth. Sultanas, the sweeter and less acidic dried grape, were originally made from a special Turkish grape, but now they come from common raisin grapes and are treated (with sulphur dioxide and heat) to take on a golden, plumper, and moister appearance and taste.

In Your Kitchen

Grapes are the perfect finger food. They're delicious whole and fresh, or you can chop them up into mixed greens, chicken salad, pasta, quinoa, brown rice, and over yogurt. Grapes taste great frozen, too—just wash grapes, put them on waxed paper, and freeze them for at least an hour for a quick burst of refreshment.

Guava

Guavas come from tropical trees that were originally grown in South America, Mexico, and Central America. There are more than 150 varieties of guava. The Apple guava is the most common type of guava and the one most widely used today. In general, when guava matures its skin turns from green to yellow to maroon. The skin can be soft or tough depending on the variety.

For Your Health

Guava are superior for your health. They have more vitamin C than any other fruit—four times more than oranges! Eating one guava provides an adult male 100 percent of the RDA for vitamin C. Plus, guavas are high in vitamin A (especially carotenoids), folic acid, potassium, and soluble fiber, particularly pectin. Pectin is effective in ridding the body of excess cholesterol—that's good for heart health! The red-orange varieties are especially high in antioxidants, carotenoids, and retinol (the active form of vitamin A). One small guava has only 60 calories, which makes it perfect for waistline watchers.

Selection and Storage

Guava can be found fresh but they are also commonly found in the frozen food section. They are also sold as juice and in candy, jelly, jam, preserves, and marmalade. The peak season for guava is November through March. When buying guava look for clean skin that is free of blemishes, bruises, or blotches. Smell it. If the fruit has a floral, fragrant aroma, that's good. Steer clear if it's soft, mushy, and has a funky odor. A large guava yields a half cup of fruit. Store guava at room temperature until ripe (soft to the touch); at that point you can eat them, refrigerate them for up to two days in a plastic bag, or freeze them.

In Your Kitchen

Guava is deliciously succulent and has many culinary uses worldwide. It's eaten with soy sauce and vinegar in Hawaii. It's eaten raw and dipped into cayenne pepper in the Middle East. In Asia it's dipped in prune powder or salt. The red guava can be used in sauces as a substitute for tomatoes, which is helpful for people sensitive to acidic foods. Put guava over hot oatmeal, fold it into a whole-grain crepe, include it in a fruit salad, or serve it with a mild or sharp low-fat cheese after dinner.

Papaya

This tropical, pear-shaped fruit is grown in a treelike plant. Papaya is susceptible to the ringspot virus, thus it is commonly genetically modified (GM) to be resistant to viruses. That's why 80 percent of the papayas in Hawaii are GM fruits. There are two types of papaya: Mexican and Hawaiian (both are found in grocery stores). Papaya fruit grows rapidly, but is highly susceptible to frost.

For Your Health

Papayas are the perfect weight watcher food with only 55 calories and 2.5 grams of fiber in one cup. This tropical fruit is used medicinally as a supplement to help with digestion. It's active enzyme, papain, is used topically for cuts, burns, rashes, and stings. It's also used in meat tenderizer, as the papain enzyme softens protein fibers well. Studies indicate that papaya and its juice are an immune booster and the fruit's high level of the carotenoid, lycopene, may ward off cancer cell growth in the liver. It contains high levels of beta-carotene, the carotenoid derived from vitamin A.

Food wise

Eating too much payapa can turn the soles of your feet and palms of your hands yellow.

Selection and Storage

Papayas ripen well after a few days at room temperature. When they are fully yellow and soft to the touch they are ready to be eaten. They can be stored in the fridge for up to three weeks.

In Your Kitchen

Use papaya in tropical frothy drinks, diced up in salads, in quinoa and pasta salads. Papayas can be cooked to make chutney or other desserts. Green papayas should not be eaten raw as it can cause allergic reactions for people susceptible to its natural latex content.

Persimmon

Persimmons are grown on beautifully flowering trees. Although not considered a common berry, it is a true berry—a fleshy fruit made from a single ovary. There are two types of persimmons: the astringent Hachiya variety, which causes a dry, puckering taste in the mouth; and the more mild tasting, nonastringent Fuyu. The taste of the Hachiya persimmon is likened to a super ripe apricot with a slippery, smooth texture. It's best eaten ripe. On the other hand, the Fuyu persimmon is hard on the inside and tastes like a crunchy apple. Its looks like a squat tomato with its orange-red skin and flat bottom. These are getting more popular in the United States, although Hachiya constitute 90 percent of the market.

For Your Health

The two persimmon varieties hold a host of health benefits, but different ones. The Hachiya persimmon has a mere 32 calories, whereas the Fuyu persimmon has 118 calories. The Fuyu is high in fiber with 6 grams in each one; plus significant amounts of vitamin A, beta-carotene, and vitamin C. Much of these values are not known for the Hachiya, yet its vibrant orange color indicates it's potentially high vitamin and antioxidant content. In general, persimmons contain high levels of betulinic acid, which has been shown to have anti-inflammatory effects and is good for keeping your organs and cells functioning well.

FOOD wise

Eating unripened persimmons may cause masses in the stomach that have to be surgically removed.

Selection and Storage

Persimmons can typically be found in November and December. Store persimmons at room temperature until they ripen. Some Asian cultures store unripe persimmons outside during winter—freezing them is supposed to make them ripen more quickly. The Hachiya variety is ripe when it's mushy, very orange, and has a jellylike texture. Fuyus maintain firmness and are very orange when ripe; they are eaten whole like an apple.

In Your Kitchen

Persimmons can be eaten fresh, dried, or raw—but make sure they are ripe! The flesh of Hachiyas can be scooped out like a pudding making it perfect for desserts and smoothies. Hachiya persimmons can also be baked, sliced over salads, or stirred into hot or cold cereal.

Pomegranate

The pomegranate is a berry with almost 600 seeds in it; each seed is surrounded by a watery shell called an aril. The arils are white, deep red, or purple and are the edible part of the fruit. Pomegranates are grown in California and Arizona specifically for its popular juice. More than 500 varieties of pomegranates are grown worldwide.

For Your Health

This fruit has received quite a bit of attention lately for its health benefits. In ancient Ayurvedic medicine, all parts of the pomegranate from the fruit and the bark of the tree were believed to help with mild diarrhea and potentially fatal dysentery from intestinal parasites or bacteria. The seeds and juice are considered a tonic for the heart. It's packed with vitamin C, potassium, and powerful antioxidants, including tannins and polyphenols. The pomegranate also contains a good amount of fiber and "good" fats in the arils.

Selection and Storage

You can buy pomegranates in your produce section from September through January. Pomegranate concentrate is available year-round. The fruit is ready to eat when purchased, but it can be stored at room temperature out of direct sunlight for a few days. The whole fruit or just the seeds can be stored in the refrigerator in plastic bags, and the seeds can be frozen.

In Your Kitchen

Here's one way to get the arils out: cut off the top and then cut the pomegranate into sections. Place the sections in a bowl of water and roll the arils out with your fingers. Strain out the water and enjoy the arils. The arils are delicious in salads, smoothies, desserts, cakes, marinades, and glazes. Toss the arils into pancakes, waffles, oatmeal, and low-fat ice cream or yogurt. Use the juice in smoothies, yogurt drinks, or drink it straight up over ice.

Raspberry

Raspberries are also called caneberries because they are grown on plants called canes.

For Your Health

Raspberries are a powerhouse of good nutrition with only 64 calories and 8 grams of fiber in one cup. This ruby red fruit is high in antioxidants, which studies have shown can promote a healthy heart. The berries' signature red color is packed with anthocyanins—the water-soluble plant pigments that have shown to be beneficial for your blood vessels and heart health. Raspberry leaves can be steeped fresh or dried for herbal teas. They have been used through the ages to quicken childbirth and to soothe sore throats and upset stomach. Raspberry extract is used in the artificial sweetener xylitol.

Selection and Storage

Grown from June through October, raspberries are available in grocery stores and farmers' markets. The fruit is very delicate. Remove spoiled, moldy, or rotten berries before storing them in the refrigerator so they don't contaminate others. Keep them in their original container or place them on a paper towel in a single layer on a plate covered with plastic wrap. They can be frozen for up to a year. To freeze them, place them in a single layer on a cookie sheet or plate, adding a little lemon juice can preserve the red color longer. Once the berries are completely frozen, they can be stored in a container or freezer bag.

In Your Kitchen

Raspberries' vibrant color adds life to your diet. The healthy pigments in raspberries have been shown to be sensitive to processing, so eat the whole fruit, fresh or frozen, to get the most nutrition. Eat them plain or toss them into low-fat yogurt or ice cream, high-fiber cereal, salads, and homemade sorbet. Instead of baking them into high-calorie pancakes or muffins, purée them into soups and fruit compotes to drizzle over fish, chicken breast, or lean beef.

Strawberries

Strawberries are named for the original mulch—straw—used near the plants. The United States is the largest strawberry producer, growing more than 4 million tons each year.

For Your Health

A cup of strawberries has only about 45 calories, 3 grams of fiber, and provides 93 percent of your recommended vitamin C. Studies have shown that strawberries have over 40 active anti-oxidant compounds, including anthocyanins, making strawberries a key fruit for preventing chronic diseases. It may also enhance memory.

FOOD wise

An allergen that ripens strawberries can cause oral allergy syndrome, a reaction that affects the mouth, lips, tongue, and throat. White-fruited strawberries are allergen-free.

Selection and Storage

Buy strawberries that are plump and have a rich red color and vibrant green caps. Store them loosely covered in the fridge, and don't wash until you about to eat them.

In Your Kitchen

Strawberries are a versatile fruit. Dice them up for a burst of vitamin C in cereal, yogurt, low-fat ice cream, salads, and soups.

Tomato

This fruit, sometimes thought of as a vegetable, was brought to the United States by the Spanish in 1492. It's one of the most common garden fruits in the United States. There are believed to be more than 700 varieties of tomatoes! Some of the most sought-after tomato varieties are called heirlooms, which are passed down through the generations typically by small family farms; they are grown with open-pollination (not controlled pollination) and are not genetically modified.

> **Munch on This**
>
> Big Rainbow, Baby Special, Black Krim, Brandywine, and Cherokee Purple are just some of the heirloom varieties of tomatoes out there. These tomatoes have unusual colors, shapes, and sizes, but they are delicious and just as nutritious as any other tomato!

For Your Health

Tomatoes are lauded for their high lycopene levels. Lycopene is a carotenoid with powerful healing properties. Research has shown that cooked tomato products can fend off prostate cancer in men. Cooking tomatoes with some olive oil or canola oil will enhance the absorption of lycopene. Some studies show that up to 10 servings a week of tomato products is protective. Tomatoes are high in vitamins A and C as well as anthocyanins. A cup of cherry tomatoes has a mere 27 calories, so feel free to pop these in your mouth as a healthy snack.

Selection and Storage

Tomatoes are available in most grocery stores and farmers' market worldwide. When selecting this fruit, be sure they are plump with no blemishes or soft spots. Store them at room temperature away from direct sunlight for a week after ripe. Refrigerating them tends to break down the flesh, making them mushy.

In Your Kitchen

Whether tossed raw in a salad or bitten into with a shake of salt, they are a quick and easy burst of flavor. Heat them up in sauces, gravies, and pasta dishes. Tomatoes are perfect puréed, chunked, diced, and stewed.

Citrus Family

Fruits in the citrus family are flowering plants of the rue family called Rutaceae. Citrus fruits are grown in trees that originated in southeast Asia. Brazil, China, and the United States are among the top citrus-producing countries in the world today. Citrus fruits are juicy, flavorful, and packed with antioxidants, such as vitamin C. The four that we describe in the following sections are part of the "superspecies" of citrus, meaning that all other citrus varieties originate from these four fruits.

Grapefruit

Another one of the "superspecies" of citrus fruits, grapefruits were elevated to fame for their starring role in The Grapefruit Diet from the 1930's, which advocated eating half a grapefruit before every meal and limited dieters to 800 calories per day. Needless to say, this excessively restrictive diet was deemed dangerous. Grapefruits have a bitter flavor that is an acquired taste. Common varieties of grapefruit are Ruby Red, Pink, Thompson, Marsh, and Duncan. They come in red, white, and pink. The red is the sweetest, followed by pink and then white.

For Your Health

Like all citrus, grapefruits are an invaluable source of vitamin C, a powerful antioxidant. With a mere 74 calories in 1 cup of the sectioned fruit, you can be sure your weight will not go up eating it! Be careful with grapefruits as they can interact with medications, such as blood pressure drugs, chemotherapy drugs, and organ transplant medications. Grapefruit contains plenty of soluble fiber and pectin, which help lower cholesterol levels; pink and red varieties contain the antioxidant, lycopene.

Selection and Storage

Grapefruit season runs from October through June. Grapefruits should be heavy for their size and firm, but slightly soft to the touch; their surface should be shiny and smooth. The riper they are, the more antioxidants they have. Store them at room temperature for up to a week.

In Your Kitchen

Grapefruit tastes especially good when cut and sprinkled with sugar and cinnamon. Peel and quarter a grapefruit and toss the fruit into salads, or try adding a little to poultry stuffing.

Lemon

Lemons are 5 to 6 percent citric acid, giving them their acidic (sour-tasting) flavor. They are used as a culinary additive across the globe.

For Your Health

A medium lemon contains 88 percent of your RDA for vitamin C, a powerful antioxidant. Researchers at The Ohio State University found that lemons may not affect the immune system as once thought, but there is a link between lemons and enhanced mood.

Selection and Storage

Choose lemons that are heavy for their size with firm, thin, and blemish-free peels. Lemons left at room temperature for too long will mold. Refrigerate them if you're not going to use them within a day or two. They can be refrigerated for up to two weeks.

In Your Kitchen

Lemons' pungently sour flavor is often the perfect accompaniment to other flavors. Accent dressings, sauces, and marinades with lemon zest or juice. Add the zest to pancake, muffin, and quick bread batter. Toss the juice over grilled calamari, fish, or shrimp. Steep tea with a sliver of lemon for a soothing hot beverage. Jazz up plain water—with or without bubbles—with a couple of lemon slices.

Lime

Limes come in sour and sweet varieties, but those found in most grocery stores in the United States are sour. These small green fruits contain more sugar and citric acid than lemons but are used for similar flavoring purposes. Lime zest has a floral aroma. India is the biggest producer of limes.

For Your Health

With a mere 20 calories, these green goodies offer outstanding health benefits in small doses. Limes contain a glycoside called limonin, which is a powerful antioxidant that fends off disease, particularly some cancers. Due to their plant chemicals, limes are used as an antibiotic for bites and stings—drink lime juice to fend off internal toxins and prevent infection. Limes are also used to fend off cholera, a bacterial disease typically found in underdeveloped countries. Although they have less vitamin C than lemons, limes are believed to have enough vitamin C to fend off damaging free radicals and help support the immune system. They can also reduce inflammation and help prevent hardening of the arteries.

Selection and Storage

Choose very ripe limes (as they ripen they become higher in antioxidants!) that are round and free of mold. Avoid fruits with brown spots, which usually indicate decay. Keep them at room temperature for up to a week or put them in the fridge in a loose plastic bag for up to two weeks.

In Your Kitchen

Lime is perfect in Mexican-inspired dishes. Squeeze the juice into grilled chicken, onions, and peppers to add a little zest to your fajitas; capture the essence of guacamole by adding plenty of lime juice; and add the tangy juice to mixed drinks such as Mojitos for a fun cocktail. Cut up limes as a garnish and self-seasoning accompaniment for seafood rice dishes like paella and ceviche (a diced raw seafood medley). Lime juice can also be added to plain or carbonated water and fruit smoothies for an extra flavor burst.

Orange

The orange is a hybrid of the pomelo and mandarin, which is grown on a small flowering tree. The seed of an orange is called a pip; the white threadlike material inside the peel is called the pith. Some familiar orange varieties are Blood, Navel, Persian, and Valencia.

For Your Health

One raw orange contains 75 percent of the daily recommended amount of vitamin C. Studies have shown that vitamin C can help shorten the symptoms of a cold, but may not ward it off all together. One medium orange has only 46 calories. They contain a lot of pectin, the soluble-fiber that helps lower cholesterol. Oranges contain herperidin, a powerful plant-based nutrient shown to have the potential to lower blood pressure and cholesterol. The nutrient is found in the peel and inner white pulp so you need to eat the whole fruit (zest the peel, of course) to get these beneficial plant nutrients.

Selection and Storage

Oranges have a shelf life of one week at room temperature and one month when refrigerated. Store them loose or in a bag with air holes. Be careful about storing them with meat, eggs, and dairy products as they produce odors that these other foods may inherit.

In Your Kitchen

Oranges are fabulous peeled and eaten raw. Add them sliced or diced into green salads, chicken salad, stuffing, and casseroles. Squeeze them into sauces, soups, dressings, and syrups.

Stone Family

Stone fruits are also called drupes. These fruit have an outer fleshy part surrounding a hard pit or stone. Other flowering plants that produce drupe or stone fruits are coffee plants and palms. (The fruit of these plants are coffee beans, coconuts, and dates.)

Apricot

This golden orange stone fruit looks a lot like a small peach. The apricot is native to China and was believed to be first cultivated in India around 3000 B.C.E. Persians have cultivated apricots for ages and are particularly fond of them dried. Apricots can withstand cold and warm climates and so are grown all over the world.

For Your Health

Apricots contain beneficial cyanogenic glycosides, chemical compounds that may help lower blood pressure and open up the arteries to allow greater blood flow. They also contain high amounts of beta-carotene (a precursor to vitamin A), which has been shown to be effective at fending off heart disease and eye diseases, such as cataracts and age-related macular degeneration. They are high in fiber and eating as few as three apricots can relieve constipation (but they can cause diarrhea if you eat too many). They are low-calorie, too: one apricot has a mere 16 calories and 3.6 grams of fiber!

Selection and Storage

Apricots are in season from May to August. Buy them golden orange, not pale yellow. Choose fully ripened ones for better taste and higher antioxidants. Be aware dried apricots are often treated with sulfur dioxide to preserve them. This can cause allergic reactions in some people, primarily those who suffer from asthma. If you are at risk or have had a reaction in the past, choose unsulfured dried apricots; they tend to be brownish in color, but they will be safe to eat.

Healing Hints

Dried organic apricots do not contain sulfites, as these preservatives are not allowed under organic regulations.

In Your Kitchen

Middle Eastern dishes like curried rice and couscous taste great with small bits of dried apricots. Toss dried apricots into trail mix, oatmeal, and salads. Fresh apricots offer a few bites of sweetness to your day. Cut an apricot (discard the tiny pit) and put it on the grill for a tasty fruit accompaniment to meat, chicken, or fish dishes. Sauté diced apricots in a pan with honey and cinnamon for a delicate sauce for yogurt, ice cream, or crepes.

Cherry

Cherries are grown on beautifully flowering trees primarily in Washington, Oregon, California, and Michigan. Cherries come in sweet and sour varieties. Some common sweet cherries varieties are Bing, Rainier, and Queen Anne. Cherries are popular all over the world. Turkey is the world's leading producer of cherries.

For Your Health

The color of this vibrant red small fruit is filled with powerful antioxidants called anthocyanins. These pigment chemicals have been shown to reduce pain and inflammation. A cup of sweet cherries has a mere 74 calories with no saturated fat, cholesterol, or sodium. Some animal studies have shown that cherry powder fends off weight gain and lower levels of inflammation related to heart disease and diabetes.

Selection and Storage

Cherry season is in the early summer months. Look for firm, shiny, and nonbruised fruit. Store loosely packed unwashed cherries in a plastic bag or in a single layer on a tray in the fridge. Wash them right before eating. Freeze washed cherries on a cookie sheet then transfer them to a plastic bag. They will keep for up to one year.

In Your Kitchen

Cherries are tasty fresh or frozen. However, fresh cherries require extra culinary work since they have tiny pits that can be removed with a paring knife or a small device called a cherry pitter. Use cherries to top low-fat ice cream, plain yogurt, and cottage cheese. Toss pitted sliced cherries into mixed green salads, over oatmeal, and over roasted chicken breast or grilled fish.

Mango

This yellow or orange fruit originated in India and is still considered a staple food there. Mangos thrive in tropical, frost-free zones. There are more than 1,000 varieties of this so-called "apple of the tropics." Mangos have a single flat pit or stone. The pit can be hairy and rough; and it sticks to the mango flesh, making it a bit of work to remove.

For Your Health

Mango fiber is a valuable prebiotic, meaning that it's food for immune-boosting bacteria in your intestines. Mangos have many other healthy properties as well: they are high in vitamins C and A and carotenoids. One medium mango has 130 calories and 4 grams of fiber. Mangos contain a powerful antioxidant, gallic acid, which helps keep cells healthy. Mangos also contain heart-healthy omega-3 and omega-6 fatty acids.

Selection and Storage

Ripe mangos give off a pleasant, floral fragrance. When choosing, don't go by color as mango colors can vary. Instead, buy them when they are a bit soft to the touch and store them at room temperature until ripe. Their delicious fragrance will scent your kitchen. To ripen mangos more quickly, place them in a brown paper bag on your counter. Store ripe fruits in the refrigerator for up to five days.

In Your Kitchen

Mangos impart unique tropical flavors to food and drinks. To access the fruit, cut the cheek, score it, and peel back the skin. The cubes will fall away. They are very smooth and can be a bit slippery, especially when very ripe. Enjoy mangos in salads, pasta, quinoa, and rice dishes. Mangos are tasty mixed into plain yogurt and cottage cheese. It's a perfect fruit in cold drinks like smoothies and slushy-type drinks.

Peach and Nectarine

Peaches are fuzzy yellow or white fruit that originated in China, where they are revered as a symbol of longevity. Nectarines are peaches with smooth skin; they are usually slightly smaller and sweeter than peaches as well. They are called clingstones or freestones depending on how easy it is to get their pit out.

For Your Health

A medium peach or nectarine is about 30 calories, making them great for your waistline. They contain cyanogenic glycosides that are excellent disease fighters. A specific one called amygdalin is purported to be a cancer-defender.

food wise

Peach pits are very toxic, so be careful not to eat one or let your pet gobble up one either (as animals can have reactions, too). Some people suffer from oral allergy syndrome after eating fresh peaches, but if the fruit is peeled or canned it usually doesn't have allergic effects.

Selection and Storage

July and August are peak season for these stone fruits. Choose peaches or nectarines that are firm and contain no blemishes or dark spots. Store them in a paper bag until ripe; once ripe they should be fine at room temperature for one to two days. They are both highly perishable so buy them in small quantities.

In Your Kitchen

There's nothing more satisfying than biting into a juicy peach or nectarine! They are great grilling fruits, too. Serve them warm from the grill with meat, chicken, and fish. Dice them up into salads and as a sauce for pancakes and low-fat plain yogurt, cottage cheese, or part-skim ricotta cheese. Stuff grape leaves with thin slices of peaches, brown rice, and feta cheese for an interesting appetizer.

Food wise	Olives are a stone fruit. You can eat them whole as an appetizer with cheese or make a meal out them with crusty bread. Olives can be sliced into pasta sauce, baked into breads, or tossed into chili, stews, and salads. The oil from the olive is a good fat for a healthy heart by promoting optimal cholesterol levels. A serving of 10 small black olives is only 36 calories. Watch the sodium, particularly in the green ones, as 10 small ones contain about 450 milligrams of sodium!

Plum

These small grayish-blue fruits come in a wide variety of shapes and sizes. Many have a tart-sweet flavor. The dried version is called a prune or dried plum. They are popular worldwide.

For Your Health

Plums have a laxative effect due to their relatively high dietary fiber and compounds called sorbitol and isatin. That's why dried plums, also known as prunes, are a great constipation aid. Plums are often used to help regulate the functioning of the digestive system. Like other stone fruits, they contain beneficial antioxidants called cyanogenic glycosides. They are high in vitamin A and potassium, and have a mere 30 calories in a medium-size plum.

Selection and Storage

Plums are available from May to late October. Choose wrinkle-free, even-colored, smooth skinned fruit. Their greyish sheen is normal and perfectly fine to eat. Leave plums at room temperature to ripen. Wash them right before using. Store ripe plums in the refrigerator or freeze them for later use.

In Your Kitchen

Plums are delicious raw or sliced into fruit salads and mixed green salads. Slice plums thinly and serve with low-fat cheese and go European-style for dessert. If you feel like a sweet treat, bake a plum in the oven and serve it warm with a dollop of low-fat Greek yogurt.

Pome Family

The Pome family produces fruit from flowering plants in the Rose family. The most common pome is the apple.

Apple

This crunchy, red, green, or yellow fruit is the most widely grown tree fruit in the world. China is the leading producer of apples; the United States is second. The apple tree is one of the oldest trees known to be cultivated, with records dating back to Asia Minor in 300 B.C.E.

For Your Health

An apple a day really can keep the doctor away. Research has shown that apples provide a whole host of health benefits. The fiber content from apples can help reduce high cholesterol and regulate bowel movements. Apples are particularly high in an antioxidant called quercetin that's been found to fend off inflammation and cell damage. A small apple has only 50 calories.

Selection and Storage

The freshest apples are available September through November, but you can usually buy them all year long. Be sure to look for firm bruise-free skin. Scrub apples before eating under cold water to take off the waxy coating and any pesticide residue. Store apples in a cool, dark place; they can also be refrigerated or frozen whole or sliced (to avoid browning dip apple slices in lemon juice beforehand or blanche them for 90 seconds before refrigerating or freezing).

In Your Kitchen

Apples make a great sauce with a dash of cinnamon as a snack or as part of a meal with baked pork chops and sauerkraut. Slice apples and bake them. Sauté apples, sugar, and cinnamon for a delicious sauce to eat with oatmeal, cold cereal, and/or low-fat plain yogurt.

<table>
<tr><td>munch
on This</td><td>A quince looks like a small, red-hued pear but it has a tart taste. It's a unique fruit in the kitchen. Slice and bake quinces or dice them into salads, soup, and stews. Poach quinces and eat them with a dash of cinnamon. Sauté them in gravy for lean meat, chicken, turkey, and pork chops. Bake whole quinces in the oven until soft and serve with warm chocolate sauce or maple syrup.</td></tr>
</table>

Pear

Pears originated in the foothills of western China, and that region is still the largest producer of pears today.

For Your Health

With 100 calories and a whopping 6 grams of fiber in a medium pear, they are a perfect snack. Pears contain a fair amount of vitamin C (10 percent of RDA) and are loaded with beneficial antioxidants and pigments. The darker red the skin, the more antioxidants.

Selection and Storage

Pears can be stored at room temperature until ripe. Apply gentle pressure to the neck with your thumb; if it yields to pressure the pear is ripe and ready to eat. Ripe pears should be refrigerated, uncovered, in a single layer for two to three days.

munch
on This

To stop sliced pears from browning, put them in a solution of lemon juice and water. This works for apple slices, too.

In Your Kitchen

Pears are tasty eaten whole and fresh, but when ripe they add a succulent juiciness to salads and grain dishes. Pear sauce (puréed pears) tastes great with meat, chicken, and fish. They are perfect on pancakes, waffles, and crepes. Pears are fun in tarts, pies, cobblers, or baked whole served with a drizzle of caramel or chocolate on top. Pears are also great with celery in soup, omelets, and as a bruschetta with creamy goat cheese on toast points.

Essential Takeaways

- Whole fruit is a fantastic source of fiber, vitamins, minerals, and plant-based nutrients for overall wellness.
- Whole fruits are nutrient-dense, which means they offer a lot of nutrients for a small number of calories.
- All families of fruit offer a myriad of delicious and healthy culinary opportunities.

chapter 8

Power up with Protein

Distinguishing between plant and animal proteins

Harnessing the power of protein

Planning for protein in the kitchen

Satisfying protein-packed recipes

Like the support beams of a building, protein makes up the structure of every cell in your body. It's an important energy source and is vital for overall wellness. Your body needs protein on a daily basis. Ideally it should be high-quality protein containing all the essential amino acids. If you don't get all the protein you need, your body robs it from your muscles and organs in an effort to maintain energy balance, which ultimately can lead to malnutrition and serious illness.

Protein is available in both plant and animal foods. So whatever your cultural, ethical, environmental, or nutritional ideologies are, there is a protein source out there for you. In this chapter, I explore the wide array of proteins available for your culinary and nutritional needs.

Plant Proteins

The protein in plants comes from a diverse group of vegetables, grains, beans, legumes, and nuts. Although you may not always think of plants in your protein mix, they contribute a significant amount of high-quality protein without much saturated fat but with a lot of good-for-you fiber. Studies show that lower cholesterol and blood pressure is linked to eating plant proteins such as whole grains, beans, and nuts.

Beans

Beans belong to the *Leguminosae* (Legume) plant family. The oldest recorded bean plant dates to the second millennium B.C.E. Beans were a main source of protein in the world back then *and* they still are now.

There are over 4,000 varieties of beans grown in the United States alone! Beans include soybeans, peas, lentils, chickpeas, azuki, mung, black-eyed peas, lima, pinto, kidney, black beans, and many more. Fresh beans are either edible pod beans, such as green (string) beans, or shell beans, such as lima.

For Your Health

Beans are superstars as far as soluble fiber, the type of fiber that has been shown to lower total and LDL (bad) cholesterol levels. On average, 1 cup of cooked beans has between 9 and 13 grams of fiber—that's almost half the fiber an adult women needs for the day! The fiber in beans makes them a natural waist-trimming food because fiber fills you up on fewer calories.

Munch on This

Dietary fiber has 1.5 to 2.5 calories per gram. Carbs and protein have 4 calories per gram. Fat has 9 calories per gram.

Beans are also a great source of folate, the plant food version of folic acid, the B-vitamin that protects fetuses from spinal cord birth defects and prevents anemia (low-iron levels) in children and adults. Beans contain a significant amount of iron, too.

Be careful with raw beans—particularly red and kidney beans—as they can contain a harmful toxin. Place raw beans in boiling water for *at least* 10 minutes to destroy the toxin. The longer you keep the beans in boiling water, the better. Some countries, such as Africa, ferment beans to destroy potential toxins.

munch on This What about the bean's reputation for flatulence? Beans naturally contain oligosaccharides (sugar molecules) that our bodies lack the enzymes to break down. Instead, bacteria in our digestive system have to break them down, which causes gas. There are products, such as Beano, that you can either add to food or take separately to reduce flatulence. You can also add herbs and spices such as anise, cumin, and coriander as they are carminatives that help prevent the formation of gas.

Selection and Storage

Dried beans and peas will last up to a year. Keep them in their unopened bag; if opened, place them in an airtight container in a cool, dry, dark space. You can also buy bean and pea flour, which are particularly useful for people with gluten intolerances.

In Your Kitchen

You have to plan and prep a bit when using dried beans. You should first sort through dried beans and discard any debris, pebbles, wrinkled or discolored beans. Rinse the beans in cold water and soak them overnight. Soaking will not only soften the beans but also help destroy some of the gas forming carbohydrates. If you're in a hurry you can rinse the beans, bring them to a boil, then turn off the stove and let the beans sit in the hot water for at least an hour.

For a quick bean dish, use canned beans, but rinse off the salty solution and drain them before adding them to your dish. To make a delicious meatless meal toss beans into garlic and onions sautéed in olive oil with mushrooms and diced tomatoes.

Nuts

Nuts are the hard-shelled fruit of plants. They are not only a fantastic protein source, but they contain a lot of "good" fat, which is good for heart health. According to anthropologists, nuts have been a part of the human diet since the Stone Age. It's been suggested that prehistoric humans developed special tools for the sole purpose of cracking open nuts.

True nuts include the beech nut, chestnut, hazelnut, and filberts. Many foods that we consider nuts, including almonds, pecans, and walnuts, are the edible seeds of fruits with pits called drupes. These fruits are typically grown on trees and so the seeds are often called tree nuts. The cashew, macadamia, pine nut, and pistachio are also seeds.

For Your Health

Nuts, in particular almonds and walnuts, have received a lot of attention because of their positive effects on heart health, blood sugar control, and weight management (if portion controlled). Nuts have quite a good health story to tell.

Walnuts contain a lot of omega-3 fats, which can help lower LDL "bad" cholesterol levels. Plus, their thin, waxy skin just under the shell holds a whole host of healthy compounds, including flavonoids, tannins, and phenolic acids. Almonds are packed with monounsaturated fatty acids (MUFAs), which may help raise the HDL "good" cholesterol.

Many nuts, including almonds and pistachios, have been found to have high levels of disease-fighting antioxidants. One study found that an ounce of almonds has as many polyphenols—a type of antioxidant—as a half cup of cooked broccoli. In addition, raw nuts are generally low on the glycemic index (GI), meaning they don't raise blood sugar after eating them alone or combined in other foods. Thus, they are great for people who have prediabetes or have been diagnosed with diabetes. Because nuts tend to be high in calories, it's important to eat them in moderation.

Nuts & Protein		
Nuts	Portion (1-ounce)*	Protein (grams)
Almonds	23	6
Brazil nuts	6	4
Cashews	18	4
Hazelnuts	21	3
Macadamia	10–12	2
Pecans	19 halves	3
Pine nuts	167	4
Pistachios	49	6
Walnuts	14 halves	4

*An ounce portion of nuts is between 160 and 200 calories, so it's very important to measure portion sizes.

Source: The International Tree Nut Council (www.nuthealth.org)

Selection and Storage

Nuts can be purchased boxed, bagged, and canned. They are also sold combined in trail mixes, granolas, and cereals. Store raw, roasted, or toasted nuts in a cool, dry place in an airtight container; due to their high unsaturated fat content nuts can spoil quickly, so put nuts without shells in the refrigerator for up to six months or freezer for up to one year. Nuts in the shell can be stored in a cool, dark place or refrigerator for up to six months. You can buy nuts crushed into butter form (though called butter they do not contain dairy), such as almond butter, cashew butter, and peanut butter. Nut butters are a great substitute for regular butter as they contain a lot less saturated fat and no cholesterol, plus they give you a dose of "good" fats! But watch your portion as a tablespoon of nut butter can have up to 100 calories.

In Your Kitchen

Use your imagination when cooking with nuts. Almond flour is commonly used in cookies and bread, and it's gluten-free, which is a good alternative for people with celiac disease and gluten intolerance. To get an ounce a day, toss toasted nuts into mixed green salads or top low-fat yogurt or low-fat ricotta cheese with a touch of honey and nuts. Encrust lean beef, chicken, or fish with crushed or slivered nuts before baking.

Healing Hints	In the ancient Indian system of healthcare called Ayurveda, almonds are considered beneficial to the central nervous system. Plus, they are believed to improve intellectual levels and longevity.

Seeds

Except for root vegetables, all plants start out as a seed. As a matter of fact, seeds are believed to be the most important nutrition component of the six plant parts. (The others are roots, stems, leaves, flowers, and fruits.) The term *seed* actually encompasses beans or legumes, cereal grains, and nuts. Seed foods you are probably most familiar with include sunflower, flax, chia, hemp, sesame, and pumpkin seeds.

For Your Health

Although most seeds are eaten as snacks (because they are high in calories), they offer a lot of good-quality protein. A half cup of sunflower seeds contains about 22 grams of protein, which is like eating a 3-ounce portion of chicken breast! Seeds are also a great source of "good" unsaturated fats.

<table>
<tr><td>Munch on This</td><td>Flaxseed is one of the most popular seeds for heart health. Two tablespoons (the recommended daily dose) of flaxseed have 4 grams of dietary fiber, which a recent study in the *American Journal of Clinical Nutrition* found may contribute to flaxseed's cholesterol-lowering properties. The special fiber in the flaxseed called lignans is believed to help defend against breast cancer as well. Flaxseed made the list of the top 100 foods rich in polyphenols, which have been shown to ward off several chronic diseases.</td></tr>
</table>

Selection and Storage

Seeds are sold prepackaged and in bulk as well as in butter or paste form, such as pumpkin seed butter, sesame paste (tahini), and sunflower seed butter. All forms are great protein sources, but watch your portion sizes, as a tablespoon of seed butter is around 100 calories. Store seeds in a cool, dark, and dry place. Natural seed butters should be refrigerated.

In Your Kitchen

You can toss any type of seed into salads, soups, chili, or low-fat yogurt. For an Asian flair, add sesame seeds to chicken salads and noodle and rice dishes. Sprinkle ground flaxseed onto cereal, smoothies, and tomato sauce. The fats in whole flaxseed are better absorbed in your body if you grind the flaxseed first. Grind a tablespoon or two as you need it with a coffee grinder. You can add a dash of flaxseed oil to cold foods, such as salads and steamed, but cooled veggies (heating flaxseed oil makes it go bad quickly).

Soyfoods

Soy protein-rich foods are made from the soybean, a native legume to East Asia. In China and Japan, the soybean plant is referred to as "greater bean." It didn't become popular in the U.S. food supply until after 1920. Although typically green in the United States, soybeans can also be black, brown, blue, and yellow.

<table>
<tr><td>Food Wise</td><td>Soybeans—along with corn, canola, sugar beets, and cotton—are a big biotech food crop in the United States. Recent estimates indicate that 93 percent of U.S. soybean crops are genetically modified (GM), meaning the plants' genes are altered to tolerate herbicides and resist insects. GM foods are controversial from an ecological, health, and economic standpoint. You can also seek out non-GM soybean products. Look for labels that say so.</td></tr>
</table>

For Your Health

Soybeans are complete proteins, meaning they contain all of the essential amino acids (the ones your body can't make on its own). They also pack a lot of protein—40 percent—in each little bean. These qualities mean that soyfoods can replace some, or even all—of the animal protein in your diet. Soy is also a high-fiber and low-calorie food, with 9 grams of fiber and 120 calories per half-cup serving.

Selection and Storage

Soy protein is found in a variety of foods and can be found at any major grocery store. Tofu, the white block of soybean curd, is usually stocked in the refrigerated produce section. It comes in silken (soft), firm, and extra-firm varieties. You can also find whole shelled or unshelled soybeans, called edamame, in the refrigerated and frozen sections. Be sure there's nothing added to them so you can add your own salt or seasonings at home. Soy also comes in milk form and is often in the cow's milk or in the natural foods section of the store. It comes in plain and flavored varieties (but watch sugar levels in flavored soymilk). Soy also comes in cheese form and is flavored in familiar choices like cheddar and American.

Food wise	Before cooking with firm or extra-firm tofu, pat the entire block dry with a clean paper towel to get the excess water out of it. Because tofu requires moisture, completely immerse the unused portion in cold water, cover, and store it in the refrigerator. Change the water every other day; if it starts turning cloudy or the tofu takes on a yellow hue, it's time to change the water or discard the tofu. With proper care, tofu can last up to 10 days in the refrigerator.

In Your Kitchen

Soyfoods can be used in a myriad of culinary endeavors. Incorporate silken tofu into smoothies, pudding-type desserts, sauces, and dips. Toss soybeans with diced fresh tomatoes, scallions, and diced cucumbers with a tablespoon of olive oil and balsamic vinegar for a delicious fresh salad. Add a dash of salt to steamed whole soybeans (edamame) for a delicious appetizer. Marinate extra-firm tofu, cut it into chunks, and bake it for a protein-packed addition to pasta, rice, or quinoa. Add steamed soymilk to a latte or cappuccino. Crunch on roasted soynuts for a high-protein snack attack!

Animal Protein

The animal kingdom is full of high-quality protein. Meat, fish, milk, and eggs offer a complete source of essential amino acids and easily (for most people) digestible protein. But not all animal proteins are equal. High-fat red meats, the dark meat (and skin) of poultry, and processed meats such as bacon, hot dogs, and lunch meats are high in artery-clogging saturated fats.

Meat can fit into a healthy and healing lifestyle as long as you maintain a balance of animal and plant proteins. Try eating fewer saturated fat and cholesterol-laden animal proteins in favor of more plant proteins, which have heart-healthy fats and a generous helping of fiber, which can trim your waist without leaving you feeling hungry!

Dairy Foods

Dairy foods, such as low-fat and fat-free milk, yogurt, and cheese, are an ideal source of protein. Although most Americans eat too much protein, evidence shows that it's not coming from milk or milk products. That doesn't bode well for calcium needs: large, long-term nutrition studies have shown that people over age 12 are not eating or drinking enough calcium-rich food sources. Experts believe this may be linked with increased heart disease, type 2 diabetes, and poor bone health.

For Your Health

Drinking enough milk and milk products is not only about calcium—as you can get it from other foods, such as dark leafy greens, tofu (made with calcium sulfate), and fortified orange juice. It's about getting all of the other nutrients in milk and milk products, such as potassium, magnesium, vitamins A and D, and—of course—protein. Fat-free milk has 8 grams of protein per cup and only 90 calories for a cup serving.

> **Munch on This**
>
> The RDA for low-fat dairy products for children ages 2 to 8 is 2 cups; for people 9 and over, 3 cups. Keep in mind one serving is 1 cup of milk, 1 cup of yogurt, and/or 1.5 ounces of cheese.

Selection and Storage

When buying milk, yogurt, and cheese look for low-fat or fat-free products to avoid the high levels of saturated fat and cholesterol found in full-fat "regular" versions.

Munch on This

Going back to the basics by grass-feeding dairy cows (rather than feeding them corn) has been found to be better for the planet, the cows, and the consumer. Organic, grass-fed cows release less methane into the air, they are not given hormones and/or antibiotics, and their milk is nutritionally superior with higher levels of polyunsaturated fats, particularly, conjugated linoleic acid (CLA). CLA has been found to reduce risk for heart attacks, obesity, and cancer.

Grass-fed cows produce meat and dairy products that have 300 to 500 percent more CLA than grain-fed cows.

In Your Kitchen

Stir skim milk into your morning oatmeal with a handful of walnuts, a drizzle of honey, and a few raisins. Dollop low-fat plain yogurt over chili, enchiladas, and crab cakes—it's the perfect substitute for high-fat sour cream. Drizzle honey and sprinkle cinnamon on top of fat-free plain Greek yogurt. Choose low-fat cheese (part-skim mozzarella, provolone, or Swiss) as a topper for homemade vegetable pizza along with fresh tomatoes, bell peppers, red onion, and mushrooms.

Eggs

Eggs have been a part of the human food supply since around 1500 b.c.e. Since eggs are a complete protein source, the U.S. Food Guidance System includes eggs in the Meat food group.

For Your Health

Eggs are a neat little package of all of the essential amino acids, plus they provide vitamins A, D, E, B-vitamins, choline—a water-soluble essential nutrient for proper brain development—iron, calcium, phosphorus, and potassium.

The egg white contains most of the protein (the yolk contains slightly less than half of the protein); the yellow or yolk contains the fat-soluble vitamins (A, D, E) and cholesterol. There's about 300 milligrams of cholesterol in a large egg yolk; for people with high cholesterol or heart disease, that's more than the recommended intake of cholesterol for a day. However, studies have shown that eggs don't necessarily raise cholesterol levels. The yolks also contain lutein and zeaxanthin, two fat-soluble carotenoids that are great for eye health. From a weight management standpoint, eggs are low in calories with about 70 calories for one medium-size egg. Eggs from hens that are fed a diet of kelp (seaweed) meal are high in omega-3 fats.

Selection and Storage

Eggs are an inexpensive food staple. Consider looking for "free-range" or "cage-free" eggs as this means that the laying hens were allowed to roam outdoors freely and most likely treated humanely. Handle eggs with care as proper storage is vital to ensuring the safety of eggs. Raw eggs in the shell can keep in the refrigerator for three to five weeks; if the whites and yolks are separated, then they can last two to four days in the refrigerator. Do not freeze whole eggs in the shell. Be sure to check the carton for the expiration date.

In Your Kitchen

From frittatas to omelets to soufflés, eggs are a culinary miracle. They are versatile and adaptable in all types of dishes. You can whip up two scrambled eggs, a hard-boiled egg, or egg salad in minutes. Eggs pair well with all sorts of veggies, too. Dollop Dijon mustard and/or salsa on scrambled eggs or make an egg sandwich with whole-grain bread, a slice of tomato, and a sliced hard-boiled egg.

> **Munch on This**
>
> For the perfect hard-boiled egg, cover eggs completely in cold water in a pot. Bring water to a rolling boil and immediately turn down to a simmer for 10 minutes. When the time is up, turn off heat, immediately spill the hot water out and replace with cold water from your faucet. You have to cool the eggs immediately to complete the process.

Red, White, and Dark Meat

Red meat is a complete source of protein. Any meat that is red when raw falls into this category, including bison burgers, steak, lamb chops, ostrich, duck, and goose meat. The flesh of mammals with red meat has more iron and oxygen-binding proteins called myoglobin, which causes its red color. Processed meat found in ground beef, hot dogs, and lunch meats is considered red meat, too.

White meat comes from chicken, turkey, rabbits, veal calves, sheep, and pigs. White meat is any meat that is white or light when raw; it turns even whiter when cooked. In chicken and turkey the white meat comes from the breast area, which doesn't require much muscle movement.

A turkey or chicken's dark meat comes from the leg and thigh area of the bird. Because this is where the greatest muscle activity takes place, these areas need more oxygen and so more myoglobin.

For Your Health

Red meat is a good source of iron, protein, zinc, phosphorus, B-vitamins, and creatinine, a nitrogen-based organic acid that supplies energy to muscles. Red meat is also high in the saturated "bad" fats and cholesterol. Studies show that high-fat red meat (and processed meats from ground beef, lunch meat, and hot dogs) raises blood pressure levels. Heart disease experts contend that eating leaner cuts of meat, such as loin cuts of red meat and trimming visible fat from meat, are better choices for overall health. White meat, particularly breast meat, contains less saturated fat and cholesterol than red and dark meat.

Munch on This

Fish is not considered a red or white meat or dairy, but it is a great source of protein. See Chapter 10 for more on the health benefits of incorporating fish into your diet.

Amount of Protein in Meat

Type of Meat (4 oz.)	Protein (grams)
Fish	20–25
Chicken breast	28
Lamb	30
Steak (beef top round)	36
Steak (beef T-bone)	25

Selection and Storage

Always refrigerate or freeze meat when storing it. Temperatures are important for food safety. Keep all meats out of the danger zone (40°F–140°F). Store meats on the bottom shelf of the refrigerator or freezer to avoid cross-contamination with other foods. Choose grass-fed, eco-friendly meats when you can. You'll probably get higher-quality fresh meat and fish at specialty meat and seafood markets; you'll also likely find a better selection and seasonal varieties as well. So it might be worth the extra trip to such a market.

In Your Kitchen

Go for lean meats in your culinary endeavors. Choose loin cuts of meat, such as tenderloin, pork loin, or chops. Get sirloin steak, which is low in saturated fat, instead of prime rib. Bake, broil, or roast meats to allow the fat to drip off and away!

Food wise

Cook chicken and turkey breast to 180°F and ground chicken or turkey to at least 165°F. Ground beef should be cooked to at least 160°F.

Purchase skinless chicken and turkey breast whenever possible. Ground beef, chicken, and turkey are processed meats, so beware of additives, preservatives, and hormones in the meat.

Healthy, Healing Meat Recipes

The following protein-packed meat, chicken, and egg recipes are easy to make and will get you started preparing healthy, healing meals in your kitchen.

Steak with Warm Tomato Salsa

Blanketed by the earthy tomato and onion salsa, this lean cut of meat offers a delicious meal with a leafy green salad and whole-grain rice.

Yield:	Serving size:	Prep time:	Cook time:
2 servings	1 steak	5 minutes	15 minutes

Each serving has:			
323 calories	22 g total fat	9 g saturated fat	0 g trans fat
28 mg cholesterol	111 mg sodium	6 g carbohydrates	1 g fiber
4 g sugars	24 g protein	17 percent iron	

2 lean sirloin steaks, about ¾-in. thick	2 TB. balsamic vinegar
4 large plum tomatoes, peeled and diced	2 tsp. water
2 spring onions or scallions, chopped	Salt and pepper

1. Trim excess fat from meat and then season both sides with salt and pepper. Heat a nonstick frying pan over medium heat and cook steaks for about 3 minutes on each side for medium rare.

2. Transfer steaks to plates and keep warm.

3. Add vegetables, balsamic vinegar, water, salt, and pepper to cooking juices in the pan and stir briefly until warm, scraping up any meat residue. Spoon salsa over steaks to serve.

munch on This

Serve with steamed broccoli with a touch of olive oil and minced garlic.

Soy & Citrus Chicken

This light citrus chicken has a hint of an Asian flair and is delicious with steamed veggies and brown rice.

Yield:	Serving size:	Prep time:	Cook time:
4 servings	1 chicken breast	10 minutes	30 minutes

Each serving has:			
316 calories	6 g total fat	2 g saturated fat	0 g trans fat
146 mg cholesterol	395 mg sodium	7 g carbohydrates	2 g fiber
4 g sugars	55 g protein	18 percent iron	

4 skinless chicken breast fillets	2 TB. soy sauce, low sodium
1 large orange	16 medium asparagus spears

1. Preheat the oven to 350°F. Place each chicken breast in a single layer in a shallow, oven-proof dish.

2. Halve orange, squeeze juice from one half, and mix juice with soy sauce. Pour sauce mixture over the chicken.

3. Cut remaining orange into wedges and place on chicken. Cover and put in the refrigerator to marinate for a couple of hours, turning a couple of times.

4. Bake chicken, uncovered, for 20 minutes. Turn chicken over and bake for another 15 minutes, or until cooked through. Place a thermometer in a chicken breast; when the temperature reaches 180°F, it's done.

5. As soon as the chicken goes into the oven, place asparagus with tough ends cut off in an oven-safe dish. Roast in the oven with the chicken. Stir it after 10 minutes and put back in the oven for another 15 minutes. Once tender, arrange the asparagus on plates, then top with chicken and orange wedges. Spoon cooking juices over the chicken. Serve immediately.

Spicy Egg and Bean Scramble

This jazzy egg dish has notes of fiery jalapeno peppers with the cooling balance of basil and tomatoes. Enjoy for brunch or a simple dinner date.

Yield:	Serving size:	Prep time:	Cook time:
1 scramble	1 cup	5 minutes	25 minutes

Each serving has:			
486 calories	21 g total fat	5 g saturated fat	0 g trans fat
218 mg cholesterol	424 mg sodium	44 g carbohydrates	10 g fiber
11 g sugars	33 g protein	30 percent iron	

½ cup (1-in.) sliced asparagus

2 tsp. fat-free milk

⅛ tsp. salt

Dash freshly ground black pepper

2 large egg whites

1 large whole egg

1 tsp. jalapeno pepper, diced

1 TB. extra-virgin olive oil

¼ cup canned black beans, rinsed and drained

1 TB. chopped red onion

2 tsp. chopped fresh basil

2 tsp. grated parmesan cheese

2 grape or cherry tomatoes, quartered

1. Preheat oven to 400°F. Drizzle ½ tablespoon of olive oil on asparagus and roast in the oven for 10 minutes; toss, and cook for 10 more minutes.

2. Combine milk, salt, ground pepper, egg whites, egg, and jalapeno pepper, stirring with a whisk.

3. Add the remainder of olive oil to an 8-in. nonstick skillet and heat over medium-high heat. Add beans and onion; sauté 30 seconds. Add egg mixture; reduce heat to medium, and cook for 1 minute. Sprinkle asparagus and basil evenly over egg mixture and scramble. Sprinkle with cheese and tomatoes and serve immediately.

Essential Takeaways

- Protein is an essential nutrient for growth, development, and health.

- Some plants are great sources of protein without the saturated fat, cholesterol, and calories found in many animal sources of protein. So boost your plant proteins while downgrading your animal protein for optimal health.

- Complete proteins contain all of the essential amino acids. Food sources for complete proteins include eggs, milk and milk products, meat, chicken, fish, soybeans, and some whole grains.

- Your protein needs are based on your age, weight, and activity level. To get yours, go to www.mypyramid.gov.

chapter 9

The Goodness of Grains

Discovering the whole-grain family

Uncovering the healing properties of grains

Identifying whole grains in foods

Enjoying whole grains in your kitchen

Whole grains are the original health food. The entire grain seed, called the kernel, holds a tidy package of goodness in its bran, germ, and the endosperm—where all of the fiber, vitamins, minerals, antioxidants, and healthy fats are stored.

Whole Grains

The relationship of whole grains in preventing diseases such as heart disease, type 2 diabetes, and obesity is proof positive that eating whole grains is a huge healthy step in the right direction. This chapter looks at the history, healthfulness, care, and culinary uses of these powerful whole grains from A to Z. You'll be amazed at the wide variety of grains available for your culinary pleasure and health.

Amaranth

This whole grain dates back dozens of centuries to the Aztec civilization in South America. It's still grown there today, where it's popped like corn and peddled in the streets as a healthy snack. Amaranth was once regarded as a "seed sent by God." It's a "pseudo-grain" as it's really a seed, but tastes and acts like a grain when cooked. Amaranth's tiny brown kernels have a nutty, highly palatable flavor.

For Your Health

Amaranth is loaded with protein—it's one of the only grains (besides quinoa, which we discuss later in this chapter) that's a complete protein package. It has 30 percent more protein than other cereal grains. Not only does 1 cup of amaranth contain over 28 grams of protein (that's more than three ounces of chicken), but it contains all of the essential amino acids—the necessary parts of protein, which you have to get from food, making it a perfect protein alternative for vegans and vegetarians. Amaranth also conveniently fits into a gluten-free lifestyle, which makes it a go-to grain for people with gluten intolerance or a diagnosis of celiac disease.

As with all grains (and seeds), be sure to measure out what you put on your plate. The calories can add up—½ cup of dry, uncooked amaranth is a whopping 358 calories!

Selection and Storage

Amaranth can be found in natural food stores and grocery stores as well as online. Because it does contain oils that may become rancid or bad if exposed to sunlight, air, and moisture, it should be stored in an airtight container in a cool, dark, and dry area or in the refrigerator.

In Your Kitchen

Amaranth seeds can be used as a grain and added to soups and stews, tossed with steamed or roasted vegetables for additional flavor, texture, and nutrition. The seeds can also be sprouted and used in salads, or ground and used in combination with other flours for baking.

food wise

Just because a product claims to be "made with whole grains," doesn't mean that it's 100 percent whole grain. In order for a product to be considered whole grain, the U.S. Food and Drug Administration standards say that it has to contain at least 51 percent whole grains by total weight. Check the label, look for the word "whole" before the first grain listed, or look for the black and gold "100% Whole Grain" stamp.

Barley

Barley is the fourth most grown crop in the world. It is used from Scotland to Africa in food and beverages. It can grow in most climates, but it prefers cool temperatures.

munch
on This
Barley beer is believed to be the first drink developed by Neolithic humans, and it's still popular today! As a matter of fact, barley is considered to be the best grain for malting.

For Your Health

Due to its tough hull, it's hard to keep the whole barley grain intact but hull-less varieties are now available. You're probably most familiar with pearled barley, which is not considered a whole grain. It has high fiber and iron but less than the whole-grain variety.

Studies have shown that whole-grain barley can control high blood sugar levels up to 10 hours after eating a meal. The grain also fends off hemorrhoids and constipation. In addition, barley has an ample amount of soluble fiber called beta-glucan, which has been shown to lower cholesterol levels as much, if not more than, oat fiber.

With a high-fiber content of over 15 grams per $\frac{1}{2}$ cup, barley is considered a low glycemic index (GI) food. (You can read more on GI foods and diabetes in Chapter 21.) Barley also fills you up faster on fewer calories, which is great for weight management. Half a cup is a mere 97 calories!

food
wise
Many people enjoy roasted barley grains as a coffee substitute without the caffeine. The barley grains are left whole, boiled, and steeped like tea. You can also just add hot water to instant barley beverages, such as Pero brand.

Selection and Storage

As with most grains, store barley in an airtight container and keep it in a cool, dry, dark place—either the refrigerator or a pantry closet away from the stove or oven. You can buy barley in bulk, but it's not a good idea to overbuy as you don't want to store the grain longer than 9 months to 1 year (for maximum freshness and nutrient content).

In Your Kitchen

Mushroom barley soup is a perennial culinary favorite, but barley—either in kernel or flake form—is fabulous in many recipes. Mix it into hot oatmeal for a great flavor and texture variety. Boil the barley and use it in place of rice in paella-type dishes or as accompaniment to vegetables and lean meat, chicken, or fish in a meal. It can also be used in place of rice and rolled into cabbage leaves or stuffed into green, red, or yellow peppers.

Buckwheat

Buckwheat is used in everything from Japanese soba noodles to French crepes to Eastern Europe's beloved kasha. Even though it's technically the fruit of a plant, it has been adopted into the grain family as a "pseudograin" to whole grains because of similarities in appearance, nutrients, and nutty taste flavor. You would never guess that its real botanical relation is rhubarb!

Buckwheat is grown all over the world, and it was one of the first crops introduced to North America. Buckwheat grows in poor soil, on rocky hillsides, and without chemical pesticides.

For Your Health

For people who have celiac disease or gluten intolerance, buckwheat is ideal.

Food wise	Some studies show that buckwheat may be an allergen for some people. There have been reports of buckwheat causing mild allergic reactions and sometimes serious anaphylaxis, which requires immediate medical attention.

Buckwheat is close to being a complete protein and contains lysine—which is an amino acid often missing in grains—making it great for vegans and vegetarians. A protein in buckwheat has been found to cling to cholesterol and help bring it down in people with high cholesterol levels. With ½ cup serving at 77 calories and almost 3 grams of fiber, it's great for your waistline, too.

Selection and Storage

Buckwheat groats (hulled grains), grits, or flour can be found in most grocery stores, typically in the natural foods section. It may be more expensive because it takes special equipment to mill it (due to its triangular shape). Groats come whole or in coarse, medium, and fine grinds. Roasted groats are called kasha. Cracked groats that are very finely ground are called grits—you can buy these as "cream of buckwheat" cereal. When buying buckwheat flour choose darker varieties because they contain the hull and many of the vital nutrients and fiber along with it.

As with other grains, buckwheat can go bad quickly—so store it in a cool, dark, dry place such as the refrigerator or freezer.

In Your Kitchen

Whole groats have a nutty flavor that works well mixed with vegetables as a side dish to fish or baked tofu. The medium and finer ground grits can be used in cereals or as a topping for yogurt or low-fat ice cream.

Bulgur

Bulgur is a mixture of parboiled, dried, and cracked wheat kernels that are sorted by size and served up as a base for all sorts of dishes. Bulgur has been a culinary staple in the Middle East for centuries. Also, called "Middle Eastern pasta," bulgur is a common whole grain in many Mediterranean, Middle Eastern, Turkish, and Indian dishes. It has a light, nutty flavor, which is sometimes mistaken for rice in dishes. Bulgur is similar to couscous, another wheat-derived food.

Munch on This

Bulgur is often confused with cracked wheat, but they are different. As the name implies, cracked wheat is just that—the crushed wheat grain—but it isn't parboiled like bulgur.

In the United States bulgur is most widely recognized in tabbouleh salad.

For Your Health

Like most whole grains, bulgur is a fiber-packed, vitamin- and mineral-rich food source. It has more fiber than quinoa, oats, millet, buckwheat, or corn. One cup of dry bulgur has 25 grams of fiber—that's a day's worth of fiber for an adult woman right there. Be aware that you probably won't eat that much at one time (that would be about 2 cups cooked) because not only will it create gas, bloating, and discomfort, but it would be almost 500 calories by itself! So reach for a measuring cup and dollop a $\frac{1}{2}$ cup on your plate for half the calories and still a ton of fiber and plenty of blood-pressure friendly potassium.

Healing Hints

Remember, when eating a high-fiber grain like bulgur, be sure to drink fluids (water is the best bet) to adequately move the fiber through your body.

Selection and Storage

Although more mainstream grocers are carrying bulgur, you might have to go to a natural food store to find it. It comes in three different grinds: coarse, medium, and fine. Use the coarse variety for pilaf or stuffing for poultry or vegetables (e.g., peppers or zucchini), the medium grind in cereals, and the fine grind for dishes such as tabbouleh salad. Store bulgur in the refrigerator in an airtight glass container and use as needed.

In Your Kitchen

Bulgur is a very versatile grain, and because it's so easy to make, it's ideal for people who haven't cooked with whole grains in the past. Since bulgur is already parboiled, it literally takes minutes to make: to make $\frac{1}{2}$ cup, just simmer it in a cup of water for about 15 minutes. Turn the heat off, cover the pot, and let it sit for a couple of minutes. It will triple in volume, so it's a great grain to share.

Corn (Maize)

Corn crops are hearty and can grow in most climates—it's the most commonly grown crop in North and South America today. Corn is available dried as popcorn or corn meal or fresh as "sweet corn."

For Your Health

Although corn has gotten a bad rap in the health department, its reputation is being re-evaluated lately. Several studies have shown that corn has higher levels of antioxidants than any other grain or vegetable. There are only 86 calories in a half-cup serving, so corn is not fattening unless you eat too much of it (as with any starchy food).

Healing Hints

Corn is processed into high-fructose corn syrup (HFCS) and used as a sweetener (just *not* a low-calorie one). HFCS is in many processed foods, such as breads, cereals, breakfast bars, lunch meats, soups, and condiments. Displacing whole foods in your diet with processed, high-calorie ones is not a good idea for your health in the long run!

Selection and Storage

When you are scouting out whole-grain corn, if it says "degerminated" on the label, skip it as its not whole grain. Fresh corn can be bought at any grocery store, farm stand, or market. When buying fresh corn, pull the husk back and look at the kernels, if they are tight and rows are even—that's good. The husk should be wrapped tightly, be grass green, and have a slightly moist husk and silks—not dried out. Corn can be stored in the refrigerator with or without the husks for five to seven days.

When it's frozen or canned, check labels for no added salt, sugar, or flavorings.

In Your Kitchen

Use cornmeal to make a hearty polenta with a dash of jalapeno—this is a flavorful comforting side dish. Fresh corn can be husked and put on the grill, boiled in water, and baked in the oven. Thaw frozen corn and add to a chunky guacamole of diced avocado, tomatoes, red onion, and black beans. Drizzle with plenty of lime juice and serve up with baked tortilla chips. Pop dry kernels for a whole-grain snack—just keep the butter to a minimum!

Farro (or Emmer)

Emmer is an ancient strain of wheat that was a popular cereal grain over 7,000 years ago in the Orient. It was slowly abandoned when durum wheat, which was easier to hull, came into the picture. Although Ethiopia is one of the only countries to use emmer as one of their main grains, the ancient grain is staging a comeback in Italy with their version of emmer called farro. Farro is the wheat grain in semolina flour, which is in traditional Italian soups, pasta, and other dishes. It's become an Italian gourmet go-to grain.

For Your Health

Emmer, although a close cousin of durum wheat, is believed to be safe for people with wheat allergies as it supposedly doesn't carry the genes that initiate an allergic reaction. However, practice caution if you have genuine gluten intolerance. Emmer (farro) is perfect for regulating blood sugar. It's not totally a complete protein, but eating emmer with beans or legumes rounds it out to nutritional completion. It's also fairly high in magnesium, which can help with blood pressure, too.

Selection and Storage

Semolina flour made from farro or emmer wheat is found in most grocery stores. Store wheat flour or grains in a cool, dark and dry place in an airtight container. The refrigerator is the perfect place and can fend off little bugs and insects from invading it.

FOOD wise Wheat flour should not be stored near apples, onions, or potatoes as they will cause the flour to have an odor or "off" flavor.

Wheat is classified by color and texture. Common types are hard red spring, hard red winter, soft white spring, and soft white winter. Although red and white wheat are the most common colored kernels in the United States, they also come in amber, red, purple, or creamy white.

In Your Kitchen

You can use farro wheat flour to make homemade bread, pasta, or ravioli as well as hot (farina) cereal such as Cream of Wheat. To make Cream of Wheat, boil water (or milk for a creamier texture) and stir in the farina until thickened; it can take as little as 1 minute to make. Serve it with dried fruit, nuts, and a dash of brown sugar for a delicious treat.

Oats

This grain is popular for its soluble fiber content, which helps keep cholesterol levels in check. The many forms of oats—from the hearty steel cut to old-fashioned rolled oats to the finer regular and instant varieties—are all whole grain, but there are significant differences in cooking time and texture among the different forms. They all contain significant amounts of beta-glucan—the soluble fiber which makes oats heart healthy. Look for plain, unflavored oats whenever possible as it's always a healthier bet to add a touch of sweetness or flavor on your own.

For Your Health

The soluble fiber in oats can do wonders for ridding the body of excess cholesterol. Oats also have a lot of potassium, which studies have shown to help keep blood pressure in a healthy range. Plus, they are perfect for weight management by providing satiety or fullness with fewer calories. Oats contain an antioxidant called avenanthramides, which has been shown to keep blood vessels healthy. Watch your portions of oats, as $\frac{1}{4}$ cup dry steel cut oats contains 150 calories. Measure out your portions, keeping in mind that the serving will at least double once it's cooked. You can always doctor it up with fresh berries, walnuts, and diced banana to add volume without a lot of extra calories.

FOOD wise	Oats are naturally gluten-free, but they can be contaminated with wheat during growing and processing. Check food labels for uncontaminated oats.

Selection and Storage

Oats are widely available. Typically, they are in cereals, oatmeal, or baked into cookies, crackers, and bread. If you buy oats in bulk, store them in a cool, dry, airtight container. Always look for "whole" oats on the product label; oats typically never have their bran or germ removed in processing, which means you'll get whole-grain oats almost all the time!

Healing Hints	No matter which way you buy oats: steel cut, old-fashioned, regular, quick, or instant, you are still getting plenty of the heart-healthy soluble fiber. However, watch the added sugar—keep it under two-digits (less than 10 grams) per serving!

In Your Kitchen

Try adding volume and texture to lean turkey meatloaf by adding $\frac{1}{4}$ cup of whole oats with some diced onion, garlic, and minced basil to the meat mixture for a flavorful dish. Toss raw oats into salad greens for a crunchy fiber boost. For a vegetable course, scoop out two zucchini halves and stuff them with a mixture of whole oats, chopped tomatoes, marinated artichokes, garlic, and onions. Top with a dash of part-skim mozzarella and bake.

Quinoa

This is another one of those "pseudograins" (like buckwheat), that's not really a true grain but looks, tastes, and adapts to dishes like a grain. It's related to beets, Swiss chard, and spinach and originated in South America. The Incas thought quinoa was sacred and called it the "mother of all grains."

For Your Health

Quinoa is a complete protein, so you don't have to go anywhere else to get your protein needs fulfilled. It has 12 to 18 percent protein by weight, which is high. It's high in fiber, with over 7 grams in a half-cup serving; there are about 110 calories in $\frac{1}{2}$ cup cooked, so be sure to get your measuring cup out. It can be an ideal grain for helping with weight management and blood sugar control. Quinoa also contains a fair amount of phosphorus, magnesium, and iron. It's gluten-free quality makes it a good go-to grain for people with celiac disease and gluten intolerance.

Selection and Storage

It used to be that you could only find quinoa in natural food stores, but now it's available in many grocery stores. You might have to look in the natural foods section, though. Store it in a cool, dry, dark place.

In Your Kitchen

Quinoa takes only minutes to make. Just add water, bring it to a boil, let it simmer until the water is dissolved (about 15 minutes), and remove from the heat and flake it with a fork. Be sure to rinse it before cooking, as quinoa may have the bitter residue of saponins, a plant-defense that wards off insects. Enjoy it as a side dish by adding a touch of cumin, olive oil, and chick peas for a Mediterranean twist.

Rice

Rice is a food staple all over the world. White rice has been refined (the bran and germ removed). Whole-grain rice can be brown, black, red, and purple. Rice is the most popular grain after corn in the world, with more than 100 varieties of rice produced in the United States alone.

> **FOOD wise**
>
> Wild rice is not really rice. It's actually the seed of a marine grass. Due to its high cost and strong flavor, it's usually blended with other grains and types of rice. Wild rice has double the protein and fiber of brown rice!

For Your Health

Rice is the most important grain for nutrition around the world, making one fifth of the calories consumed worldwide. Brown and wild rice offer more nutritional value than white rice. Although brown rice is not as high in fiber as other grains, it still offers a great gluten-free alternative for people who are gluten intolerant or have celiac disease. It's very easy on the digestive system and works well as an infant's first food. Be sure to measure out rice, as the calories can add up fast. (A cup of cooked brown rice contains 220 calories!)

Selection and Storage

Rice can be found in all grocery stores. When you go down the rice aisle check out all of the varieties available. Try a new one! You can buy it in bulk, plastic bags, containers, and boxes. Store it in a cool, dry place.

Food wise

Be careful, cooked rice can contain Bacillus cereus spores, a dangerous bacteria, which can produce a toxin when left out of the refrigerator. When storing cooked rice for use the next day, quick cooling is advised to prevent foodborne illness.

In Your Kitchen

Rice is simple to cook. Just boil it in water and simmer until all the water is dissolved. Usually, the ratio is 1 cup of rice to 2 cups of liquid. Low-sodium broth works well to give rice added flavor. You can also throw rice into soups and stews or use it as a stuffing in grape or cabbage leaves. You can also add sugar and milk to cooked rice for a delicious rice pudding. Use rice flour in batters and breading for meat, chicken, and fish. Rice milk is a good alternative to cow's milk.

Rye

This cereal grain is a close cousin of barley and wheat. It's a hearty grain that grows in areas that are too wet and too cold for other grains. Rye is used all over the world in food products.

For Your Health

Rye contains a ton of fiber (especially soluble fiber) in its endosperm, which is the inner most part of the kernel. This is unusual, as the fiber is typically located in the bran layer. Rye's high fiber content makes it a lower GI food that may help with better blood sugar control and feeling full faster, which can help with weight management. As with most grains, the calories in rye add up fast: there are 566 calories in a cup of dry, uncooked rye. Rye contains gluten.

Selection and Storage

Rye is a popular grain in crisp breads, such as Ry-Vita and Wasa. Pumpernickel breads contain rye, and many stores sell rye flour.

In Your Kitchen

Hearty rye crackers are a great accompaniment to cheese, avocado, and hummus. Use rye flour in place of some all-purpose flour in baking. For a healthy twist on all old favorite, the rueben sandwich, make a sandwich with two pieces of hearty rye bread, two slices of lean turkey breast, a slice of low-fat Swiss cheese, a tablespoon of sauerkraut, and light spicy Thousand Island dressing (two teaspoons of low-fat mayo, a dollop of ketchup, and a dash of horseradish); grill the sandwich until cheese is melted, and enjoy!

Spelt

This close cousin of common wheat was originally grown in Iran back around 6000 B.C.E. Spelt is an eco-friendly crop that requires few fertilizers to grow.

For Your Health

Spelt is higher in protein than common wheat. It has a tougher husk, which is believed to hold in a lot of its nutrients. It's loaded with dietary fiber, which makes it good for your waistline (it has 3 grams per slice of bread). Spelt contains gluten (as it's related to wheat), which puts it on the list of grains to avoid for people with celiac disease or gluten intolerance. It's a great source of niacin (B_3), which can help reduce LDL (bad) cholesterol levels. The calories are moderate; a slice of spelt bread contains 131 calories and $\frac{1}{2}$ cup cooked spelt has 144 calories.

Selection and Storage

You can find spelt flour in natural food stores, although some mainstream markets carry it, too. You can buy the whole spelt grain and grind it into flour. Buy spelt flour, bread, and pasta. Store it in airtight containers, preferably in the refrigerator, although cool, dry pantries work well, too.

In Your Kitchen

Spelt has a nutty taste that's sweeter than wheat. Cook up spelt pasta to make a baked pasta dish by adding marinara sauce, basil, oregano, diced zucchini, onions, and mushrooms. Top with a dash of part-skim mozzarella and bake.

Wheat

Wheat originated near Babylon in a region known as the Fertile Crescent around 9000 B.C.E. Wheat was one of the first grains to be used widely thanks to its ability to self-pollinate easily. Wheat is the number one source of plant protein in our food supply. It's the third most produced cereal grain in the world after corn and rice.

For Your Health

Whole wheat holds a triad of health benefits from the grain's bran, germ, and endosperm. Wheat contains more protein than corn or rice. When the whole grain is refined or milled into white flour, it is stripped of some of its protein and fiber; plus, many essential B-vitamins—like riboflavin, thiamin, niacin, and folate—and minerals—like iron—are lost. It is high in gluten—so it's not appropriate for people with celiac disease and gluten intolerance. Hard wheat has even more protein and gluten; it is commonly used in bread making. Soft wheat contains less protein and is used in cake flour. One cup of whole-wheat hot cereal has 150 calories and almost 4 grams of fiber. Whole-wheat bread ranges in calories from 50 to over 200 calories per slice, so check your labels and try to choose bread that's around 100 calories a slice.

Selection and Storage

You can find whole-grain wheat products in any grocery store. You can buy it in bulk, flour form, or processed in snacks, pastas, and baked goods. Store it in a cool, dark, dry place.

In Your Kitchen

Use whole-wheat flour to dredge chicken breast in and then lightly bread the chicken with whole-wheat breadcrumbs. Bake the chicken and serve it with a side of freshly steamed veggies. Spread crushed whole-wheat cereal flakes over a casserole of cut-up carrots, celery, onions, and garlic in a lite cheese sauce.

Essential Takeaways

- Whole grains are a powerful tool for fending off chronic diseases, such as heart disease, diabetes, and obesity.

- Although some grains are "pseudo-grains" they have health benefits similar to whole grains and a plethora of culinary uses.

- Aim for three 1-ounce servings of whole grains a day. That's one slice of whole-grain bread, $\frac{1}{2}$ cup cooked whole-wheat pasta, and 1 cup 100 percent whole-grain ready-to-eat cereal.

- Grains containing gluten, such as wheat, rye, barley, spelt, khorasan (Kamut), farro (emmer), bulgur, and sometimes oats should be avoided by people with celiac disease and gluten intolerance.

chapter 10

Fabulous Fats

Understanding why you need fat for health

Identifying "good" fats and "bad" fats

Knowing the difference between MUFAs and PUFAs

Determining how much "good" fat you need every day

This chapter gives you the green light to indulge in some fat. When eaten in moderation fat is a fabulous nutrient with amazing healing properties. It's one of what I call The Big Three nutrients.

Why do you need fat? Every cell in your body gets its structure from membranes made of fats called lipids. Lipids are fats, oils, waxes, and related compounds found in foods and the human body that facilitate the absorption of fat-soluble vitamins (A, D, E, K, and carotenoids). If your body's fat levels are kept within a normal range, fat also cushions your internal organs and stores fatty acids, which provide energy to every cell in your body. Fat also serves as a secondary fuel source for your brain, blood cells, and kidneys when there is not enough glucose (sugar) available. And there's no question that fat makes food taste good.

You probably already know that the type of fat you eat makes a difference. The "bad" fats, which threaten health, are saturated fats. These include the solid fats, such as butter, bacon, cheese, and marbling in meat; and trans fats—those partially hydrogenated vegetable oils found in store-bought baked goods.

Unsaturated fats are the "good" fats, and they are typically liquid fats, such as vegetable and fish oils, as well as the fat found in plant-based foods such as avocados, nuts, seeds, and small amounts in dark leafy greens. In this chapter, we focus on "good" fat and how to get more of it to improve the quality of your diet and life. Most packaged foods have a combination of unsaturated (good) fat and saturated (bad) fats.

Unsaturated "Good" Fats

Unsaturated fats distinguish themselves chemically from their saturated fat sibling by carrying one or more double bonds of hydrogen, which is what makes them less saturated, or less apt to clog arteries and cause damage in your body.

Unsaturated fats offer a whole host of health benefits. They help guard you against heart disease and fend off inflammation, certain cancers, and depression.

Good fats come in two forms, monounsaturated and polyunsaturated. Your body needs both.

Food wise

Because the nature of fat makes it high in calories (9 calories per gram) compared to carbohydrates and protein (4 calories per gram), it's important to watch your total fat intake.

Monounsaturated Fats

If you think of the Mediterranean diet when we say monounsaturated fats (MUFAs), you're right! The traditional Mediterranean diet is based on the scientific theory that the foods of countries like Crete, Greece, and southern Italy are especially healthy. People there tend to eat lots of fresh vegetables, fruits, olive oil, olives, fish, nuts, yogurt, and cheese. Such diets contain a wide variety of foods that are high in MUFAs, such as olives, avocados, almonds, olive oil, and canola oil.

So what is it about MUFAs that make them so desirable? MUFAs decrease the detrimental low-density lipoprotein (LDL) "bad" cholesterol and possibly raise the better-for-you high-density (HDL) cholesterol. On the other hand, saturated fats (such as most deep fried and highly processed foods) can raise cholesterol levels and your risk for heart disease.

MUFAs have gained more of a foothold in the American diet. According to a large national nutrition survey of over 8,500 people in 2005 to 2006, MUFAs were found to make up the highest part of the respondents' total fat calories. That's great news!

Healing
Hints
The Mediterranean diet includes olive oil. The healthiest olive oil is referred to as "first-cold pressed, extra-virgin olive oil." It's the least processed and made from virgin (young) olives, which are known to have superior taste. The "first press" means that the olive was only crushed one time with a press. Plus, during processing the oil is not heated over 80°F, preserving its high-MUFA profile.

Here are some ways to get more MUFAs into your daily eating plans:

- Spread ⅓ (2 TB.) of a ripe avocado on a whole-grain tortilla with a few slices of tomato and cucumber and mixed greens.

- Drizzle olive oil (1–2 TB.) over salads and soups and/or use for dipping.

- Grab a handful of raw almonds (one serving is 23 almonds) for a quick pick-me-up snack, or purée almonds for a vegan ricotta cheese filling for lasagna or pasta shells.

- Toss chopped olives onto a pizza, in marinara sauce for whole-grain pasta, or serve them whole.

Food
wise
Be careful to watch your fat portions as the calories can add up fast!

Polyunsaturated Fats

Foods high in polyunsaturated fats, or PUFAs, also contribute to the Mediterranean style of eating. This group of fat contains more than one (a.k.a. *poly*) double bond, which makes it unsaturated *and* a liquid oil versus a solid fat. Liquid fats have been shown to be better for overall health. Two main PUFAs are considered essential fatty acids (EFA), meaning that you need to eat these because your body cannot make them on its own. They are omega-3 (alpha-linolenic acid) and omega-6 (linoleic acid) fatty acids.

Omega-3 fats are found in the fatty flesh and oil of cold-water fish, such as salmon, tuna, halibut, mackerel, herring, and sardines; krill or shrimplike marine life; algae (e.g., algal oil); and dark leafy greens, such as spinach, kale, and collard greens. You can also find ample amounts of omega-3s in flax, chia, and hemp seeds.

Omega-3s in fish and shellfish are different from the omega-3s in plant sources. Seafood contains two omega-3 fats called eicosapentaenoic acid (EPA) and docosahexaeoic acid (DHA). Plant foods contain another type called alpha-linolenic acid (ALA). Although they are all omega-3 fats, DHA and EPA have been found to be more potent than ALA in the body, thus offering more precise health benefits, especially when it comes to your heart, eyes, brain, and mood!

food wise	The best way to get omega-3 fats is in the DHA form found in fish. Aim to get at least two 6-ounce servings of oily fish every week. Don't rely on foods fortified with the plant form of omega-3 fat, called ALA, found in bread, mayonnaise, pizza, yogurt, orange juice, pasta, milk, and eggs. Although a small amount of ALA converts to DHA, the health benefits are greater from the pure marine-life sources.

Your Daily Omega-3 Dose

Fish and seafood are among the best sources of omega-3s, but they also pose a real danger of exposure to contaminants such as mercury, which has been linked to brain and heart problems, especially in developing babies. So what should you do? According to the 2010 Dietary Guidelines for Americans up to 12 ounces (2 average meals) per week of low-mercury, cooked fish is safe and healthy to eat, even for pregnant and nursing women, young children, and women of child-bearing age.

Everyone should steer clear of the large predatory fish including shark, swordfish, king mackerel, and tilefish because of their high mercury levels. The larger the fish and the longer they live in contaminated waters, the more mercury and other pollutants build up in their bodies. Check with your state seafood advisories for information about the safety of eating locally caught and harvested seafood.

Take a look at the list below for seafood that contain low levels of contaminants as well as the daily minimum of omega-3s (at least 250 milligrams per day):

- Albacore Tuna (troll or pole caught)

- Arctic char

- Barramundi (farmed, from United States)

- Dungeness crab (wild-caught, from California, Oregon, or Washington)

- Freshwater Coho Salmon (farmed in tank system, United States)

- Longfin squid (wild-caught, from the U.S. Atlantic)

- Mussels (farmed)

- Oysters (farmed)

- Pacific Sardines (wild-caught)

- Rainbow Trout (farmed)

- Salmon (wild-caught, from Alaska)

munch on This For safe seafood choices anywhere in the United States, log on to www.montereybayaquarium.org for downloadable regional pocket guides and mobile phone applications.

Omega-3 Supplements

If you are thinking of getting your daily dose of fish oil from a soft-gel capsule or liquid oil, be careful. As with all supplements, the FDA does not test omega-3 supplements. A recent report from Consumerlabs.com, an independent organization that tests health and nutrition products for quality and effectiveness, looked at 24 omega-3 supplements and found that only 17 passed testing for purity and freshness and the right amount of omega-3 listed on packaging. Seven of the supplements failed due to incorrect amounts of omega-3s, three brands were spoiled upon opening, and one of the brands didn't have an effective coating on the pills and so released the oil too early.

Be careful of misleading label lingo on supplements. A few terms don't mean much but seem to carry a lot of weight on omega-3 supplement labels. "Pharmaceutical grade" is not a useful term as there is no FDA standard for pharmaceutical grade fish oil products. Another meaningless term is "Tested in FDA approved laboratories" as the FDA does not approve laboratories.

Also, keep in mind that taking omega-3 supplements cannot make up for a diet that is high in saturated fat, cholesterol, and processed food.

Food wise Consuming high levels of omega-3s can result in internal bleeding. The FDA has set safety limits for omega-3 fats from fish and supplements. You should aim for eating no more than 3 grams (3,000 milligrams) of fish per day and no more than 2 grams (2,000 milligrams) of supplemental omega-3 per day.

As much as omega-3s are a good thing, you still need to be careful and consult a registered dietitian and your physician, before taking fish oil supplements, especially if any of the following conditions apply:

- You take blood thinners, such as Coumadin (warfarin), as omega-3s may cause internal bleeding.

- You are immunity-compromised, as high doses (over 3 grams per day) can suppress your immune system.

- You are allergic to fish or krill. Labels may not always reflect if the product contains any potential allergens.

- You are taking blood pressure medications. Fish oil supplements might lower blood pressure even more, resulting in dangerously low pressure.

The Scoop on Omega-6 Fats

Also an EFA, omega-6 fats are essential as they work well with omega-3 fats in the body. With its anti-inflammatory properties, moderate doses of omega-6 protect us from a whole host of diseases and disorders, and might fend off type 2 diabetes and lower blood pressure. But for optimum health you need to balance omega-3s and omega-6s. Omega-6 is found in foods that contain oils, like nuts and seeds, and vegetable oils, such as safflower, sunflower, soybean, and corn oil.

The problem is many people in the United States consume more omega-6 fats than they need. If you eat a lot of fast and processed foods, most of which is cooked and fried with oils rich in omega-6 fats—like palm, soybean, rapeseed (canola), and sunflower oil—you're getting a lot of processed omega-6 oil, and the calories can add up fast! Ideally, you should eat more omega-3 fats than omega-6 fats for optimum health.

The American Heart Association recommends that most people consume 5 to 10 percent of their daily calories from omega-6 fats. Depending upon your age, gender, and level of physical activity, aim for getting between 12 and 22 grams of omega-6 fat daily. Instead of reaching for processed, fast, and fried foods, opt for natural sources of omega-6 fats like canola oil, nuts, and seeds.

Fat Figures Made Simple

The nutrition guidelines recommend swapping the saturated and trans fats in your diet with the healthier unsaturated fats like MUFAs and PUFAs. And there are some easy ways (and websites) to help you determine your total fat needs—which for adults should not exceed 20 to 35 percent of total calories. To calculate how many fat grams you need per day, figure out how many calories you need at your current weight first.

Total Fat Needs Every Day	
Age (years)	*Total Fat Percentage*
Children (2–3)	30%–35% of total calories
Children and adolescents (4–18)	25%–35% of total calories
Adults (19+)	20%–35% of total calories

So let's say you are moderately active (you're active, but don't work out formally), it's as easy as 1, 2, 3:

Write your current body weight in one of the scenarios:

Male: _____ pounds × 15 calories = total calories per day

Female: _____ pounds × 10 calories = total calories per day

Take total calories and multiple by 30 percent.

_____ calories per day × .30 = calories from fat per day

Take calories from fat per day and divide by 9 (there are 9 calories per gram of fat)

_____ calories per day ÷ by 9 = _____ fat grams per day

Now you can aim to keep your saturated fat to less than 7 percent of your total fat gram per day. So for example, if you eat 2,000 calories a day, 7 percent of that is 140 calories, or 16 grams of saturated fat per day.

Remember the more active you are, the more calories (and fat) you can eat, as long as you keep them both in balance!

Healthy Fish Recipes

Are you afraid to cook fish at home? Do you only order fish when at a restaurant? Seafood offers a bevy of versatile culinary opportunities. From paella to pasta, fish dresses up dishes with low-saturated fat, high-protein nutrition—not to mention healthy omega-3 fats. It's easy, simple, and delicious to cook with fish—whether fresh, frozen, or canned give it a try!

Rotate the following recipes to get your two fish meals per week. Remember fish can fit in at breakfast and/or dinner.

Ginger Sesame Salmon

Serve the salmon with sticky rice, soba noodles, or black bean salsa.

Yield:	Serving size:	Prep time:	Cook time:
2 servings	1 salmon fillet	5 minutes	25 minutes

Each serving has:			
603 calories	46 total fat	5 g saturated fat	0 g trans fat
94 mg cholesterol	343 mg sodium	14 g carbohydrates	1 g fiber
10 g sugars	35 g protein	11 percent iron	

¼ cup low-sodium soy sauce

¼ cup lemon juice

1 TB. rice wine vinegar

1 TB. agave nectar

1 TB. sesame oil

¼ cup canola oil

2 6-ounce Atlantic salmon filets, wild*

2-in. piece of fresh root ginger, peeled and cut into matchsticks

1. Preheat oven to 425°F. In medium bowl mix together soy sauce, lemon juice, rice wine vinegar, agave nectar, sesame oil, and canola oil.

2. Place the salmon (skin side down) in a foiled lined shallow baking dish and cover with a third of the sesame oil marinade.

3. Bake fish for 20 minutes and then baste with more marinade and top with ginger sticks. Turn the oven to broil setting on high. Broil for 5 minutes, checking the fish frequently to make sure it doesn't burn. Remove salmon from oven when golden brown and ginger is sizzling (about 5 minutes). Serve immediately with extra marinade on the side, if needed.

munch on This

Salmon offers 3,130 milligrams (3.13 grams) omega-3 fatty acids per 6-ounce serving.

Spicy Fish Tacos

Use firm-fleshed white fish, such as halibut, barramundi, or albacore tuna.

Yield:	Serving size:	Prep time:	Cook time:
10 tacos	1 taco	10 minutes	30 minutes

Each serving has:			
188 calories	5 g total fat	1 g saturated fat	0 g trans fat
19 mg cholesterol	57 mg sodium	20 g carbohydrates	4 g fiber
2 g sugars	16 g protein	7 percent iron	

⅓ cup low-fat plain yogurt

1 jalapeno, seeded

2 TB. fresh lime juice

2 TB. cilantro, chopped

Pinch of salt

½ cup cornmeal

1½ lbs. halibut*, cut into 1-in. strips

10 (6-in.) soft corn tortillas, warmed in the oven

1 semi-ripe avocado, peeled and cut into chunks

1 cup cherry tomatoes, chopped

¼ small red onion, thinly sliced

1. Heat oven to 400°F. In a food processor, purée yogurt, jalapeno, lime juice, cilantro, and salt. Set aside.

2. Spread cornmeal on a plate. Coat fish in cornmeal, place in a single layer in oven-safe baking dish. Bake until lightly browned, about 20 minutes.

3. To assemble tacos, top each tortilla with fish, yogurt sauce, avocado, tomato, and red onion, and then fold in half. Serve immediately and enjoy.

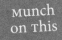

munch on This

Halibut offers 790 milligrams omega-3 fats per 6-ounce serving.

Rigatoni and Tuna with Pink Sauce

This creamy, yet light, pasta dish can be made with baked chicken breast, tofu, or sautéed shrimp. Aromatic herbs like basil add a fresh, clean accent.

Yield:	Serving size:	Prep time:	Cook time:
4 servings	1½ cups	20 minutes	10–12 minutes

Each serving has:			
426 calories	9 g total fat	2 g saturated fat	0 g trans fat
98 mg cholesterol	419 mg sodium	61 g carbohydrates	2 g fiber
8 g sugars	25 g protein	24 percent iron	

3½ cups dried rigatoni pasta (or any type of pasta you like)

2½ cups tomato sauce, no-salt added

2 tsp. fresh basil, chopped

¼ cup low-fat ricotta cheese

8–10 pitted black olives, cut into rings

6 oz. canned tuna, in water

Salt and ground black pepper

1 TB. extra-virgin olive oil

1. Cook pasta in a large pot of boiling water for 10 minutes or use instructions on the package. When pasta is done, reserve ½ cup of water and drain the rest. Place pasta in a large serving bowl and set aside.

2. Meanwhile, heat tomato sauce to a simmer in a separate pan and add basil, ricotta cheese, and olives. Remove from heat and cover.

3. Drain canned tuna and flake it with a fork. Add the tuna to sauce with about 4 tablespoons of hot water used for cooking pasta. Taste and season with salt and pepper accordingly.

4. Pour tuna sauce over pasta, add olive oil, and toss gently to mix. Serve immediately with a salad of mixed greens.

Munch on This

Canned chunk light tuna has 240 milligrams omega-3 fats per 3-ounce serving. For a different fish flavor, replace the tuna in this recipe with salmon or halibut.

Essential Takeaways

- Fat is one of the big three nutrients (along with proteins and carbohydrates) that are essential for overall health.

- The "good" fats are unsaturated fats, like those found in olive oil, canola oil, nuts, seeds, olives, and fish.

- The "bad" fats are saturated fats, such as those found in butter, beef, cheese, and chocolate.

- Omega-3 fats come from two sources: seafood and plants; each one plays a different role in maintaining optimal health.

- Be cautious with omega-3 supplements, as they may not offer any benefits (and may be dangerous) to your health.

- You need to balance omega-3s and omega-6s for optimum health. Aim for two servings of fish per week for omega-3s, and use vegetable oil, nuts, and seeds for natural sources of omega-6 fats.

chapter 11

Living with Food Allergies

Identifying eight major food allergens

Making simple substitutions

Shopping with food allergies

Knowing the difference between allergies and intolerances

Approximately 12 million Americans suffer from food allergies; you may have experienced a tingling sensation in your tongue after eating eggs or your neck may get itchy after drinking milk. These could be allergic reactions to food. Food allergies can range from life-threatening to mildly irritating. Although food allergies are most common in young children under the age of 3—with 1 in 17 diagnosed with a food allergy every year—they can flair up at any age.

The culprit in food allergies are the proteins in certain foods, such as milk, eggs, fish, and peanuts. It doesn't take eating a lot either—even teeny trace amounts of allergens in food can cause a severe reaction in some people. It happens fast, too! Reactions typically occur within minutes to two hours of eating an allergen-containing food. Heating or freezing the food will not take the protein-based allergens out of foods. So once a reaction has occurred, get tested for a food allergy and take medical precautions.

In this chapter, I discuss the gamut of food allergens, how to know if you have an allergy, and which foods are safe to eat. I also offer simple lifestyle changes to live allergy-free, happily.

The Food Allergy Phenomenon

Why do some foods pose a threat to your immune system? It's actually a case of mistaken identity: your body thinks a food's protein is a foreign invader and so the immune system attacks it by releasing chemicals, such as histamine, which initiates an allergic reaction. Reactions can be minor, such as rashes, hives, itching, and swelling; or very serious, life-threatening reactions called anaphylaxis. A food allergy is the number one cause of anaphylaxis (other causes are insect stings, medication, and latex) and requires a visit to the emergency room and injectable epinephrine (an EpiPen). Being prepared for any type of reaction is vital to living with food allergies.

> **food wise**
>
> It's important to note the difference between a food allergy and a food intolerance. Allergies involve the immune system's reaction to a certain food(s) and can be life-threatening. Intolerances are gastrointestinal (GI) tract sensitivities in which a certain food(s) causes gas, bloating, and/or diarrhea after eating it.

Let's get acquainted with some key terms:

- **Food allergies** occur when your body attacks a food protein releasing chemicals in defense.

- **Allergic reactions** are the body's response to the immune system's release of chemicals; symptoms include hives, rash, wheezing, trouble breathing, and eventual death.

- **Histamines** are chemicals released in the body that causes an allergic reaction.

- **Allergens** are proteins in certain foods that the immune system attacks.

- **Anaphylaxis** is a potentially fatal allergic reaction that progresses quickly from a rash, wheezing, and swollen lips to a drop in blood pressure and loss of consciousness.

Today, it's almost as if food allergies are in our water supply. They are so commonplace that many preschools and elementary schools do not allow peanuts or tree nuts, such as walnuts, almonds, and pistachios, in their doors to protect children with allergies. What about the other six major food allergens? Rarely do you hear of a school banning milk, eggs, or wheat—and although these allergies may not be fatal like a peanut or tree nut allergy can be, these pose a very serious concern for children (and adults) with allergies to them.

An allergy has to be tested for with a skin test and/or blood test prior to official diagnosis.

The Major Eight Food Allergens

According to the Food Allergy & Anaphylaxis Network, 90 percent of all food allergic reactions come from the following eight foods:

Milk	Fish
Eggs	Shellfish
Peanuts	Wheat
Tree nuts	Soy

Just because these are the most popular sources of allergens doesn't mean other foods never cause allergies. Any food can harbor a potential allergen if your immune system decides to strike!

Healing Hints

Next time you wheeze, sneeze, or break out in hives after eating a bagel or hummus, think about sesame seeds. Although the FDA does not recognize sesame seeds as one of the eight main allergens, allergic reactions to them is on the rise. Nonfood items like lipsticks and lotions may contain sesame seeds, so check those labels, too!

Got Milk Allergies?

Cow's milk allergies are more popular in children than adults. For infants and young children under 3 years old, an allergy to milk (or the proteins in milk) occurs in 2.5 percent of the population. The good news is children typically outgrow milk allergies within the first few years of life. There are two proteins in milk: casein from the solid (curd) part of milk and whey in the liquid part of milk. An allergy can exist for one or both of these proteins.

An allergy will rear its ugly head shortly after drinking milk with hives, wheezing, vomiting, and later diarrhea, abdominal cramps, runny nose, watery eyes, and colic (in babies). If any of these symptoms occur, seek medical attention as soon as possible.

The only treatment for a true milk allergy is to completely rid the diet of milk from cows, sheep, goat, and buffalo. People with milk allergies are often also allergic to soy. However, if there is no soy allergy, soymilk is a perfectly acceptable milk alternative.

FOOD wise — An allergy to milk looks very different than an intolerance to milk protein or lactose. With an allergy, the immune system reacts quickly after drinking milk with symptoms like a skin rash, swollen lips, hives, or difficulties breathing. (The good news is anaphylaxis is not typical with a milk allergy!) A milk intolerance affects the gastrointestinal tract with annoying and sometimes embarrassing gas, bloating, and/or diarrhea.

Is prevention possible for a milk allergy? Not really, but there are things you can do. Breastfeeding infants for the first four to six months or using hypoallergenic formulas may help fend off a milk allergy.

Healing Hints — If you or your child are on a milk-free diet be sure to consult a registered dietitian about ways to replace the nutrients found in milk such as calcium, vitamin D, phosphorus, and B-vitamins like riboflavin.

Reading food labels is a must with a milk allergy—or any food allergy. Some of the hidden sources of milk protein to watch out for are …

- Artificial butter flavor
- Artificial cheese flavor
- Casein
- Chocolate, nougat, and caramel
- Fat replacement products like simplesse
- Hydrosolate
- Lactose or lactate
- Protein powders
- Whey

When dining out be sure to let the wait staff and/or chef know that you cannot tolerate milk or anything made with dairy products, such as butter, yogurt, cheese, sour cream, or half-and-half.

Egg-Centric

Of all the food allergies, an egg allergy is the one that is most likely to go away over time. Both the egg whites and yolks contain allergy-inducing proteins; however, proteins in egg whites are the most common source of a reaction. Infants can have allergic reactions to egg proteins passed through breast milk. Allergic reactions to eggs stem from mild skin irritations, such as rash and hives, to vomiting to inflamed nasal passages. Anaphylaxis can occur, but it's rare; however, being prepared with an EpiPen is smart and can save a life.

Eliminating eggs totally from the diet is key to treating an egg allergy, but the widespread presence of eggs in food products makes this tricky. Check food product labels for the following terms that may indicate egg proteins are present:

- Albumin
- Globulin
- Lecithin
- Livetin
- Lysozyme
- Ovalbumin
- Ovoglobulin
- Simplesse
- Vitellin

Nonfood items like shampoo, medications, cosmetics, and finger paints may contain egg proteins, which can cause allergic reactions, too.

Foods to watch out for that do or may contain egg are marshmallows, mayonnaise, meringue, baked goods, mixes, batters, sauces, frostings, soft pretzels, processed meat, meatloaf, meatballs, pudding, salad dressing, pastas, root beer, and specialty coffee or alcoholic drinks topped with foam that may be made with egg.

Baking can be tricky when you have to go eggless. Here are some ingredients to replace eggs (in lieu of 1–3 eggs) in your baking recipes:

- 1 tsp. baking powder, 1 TB. water, 1 TB. vinegar
- 1 tsp. yeast dissolved in ¼ cup warm water
- 1½ TB. water, 1½ TB. oil, 1 tsp. baking powder
- 1 packet gelatin, 2 TB. warm water (mix just before using)

munch
on This
People with allergies to chicken eggs have been found to react to duck, turkey, quail, and goose eggs, too. Plus, people who are allergic to eggs are often allergic to chicken. This is called the "bird-egg syndrome."

The Peanut Deal

Once a childhood staple, peanut butter has been banned from most schools and many homes because of the rising rates of peanut allergies. According to the results of a recent survey of U.S. households, the incidence of peanut (and tree nut) allergies was reported by over 3 million subjects, or 1 percent of the U.S. population, and has increased significantly, especially among children, over the last 10 years. The good news is that 20 percent of children diagnosed with a peanut allergy will outgrow it.

Researchers still don't know exactly why peanut allergies occur. They may stem from a genetic predisposition for allergies. Peanuts are particularly dangerous as an allergen since their corresponding reactions are typically prone to anaphylaxis, which means they are much more severe and life-threatening. People with peanut allergies must carry an EpiPen at all times.

For your protection, the 2004 federal Food Allergen Labeling and Consumer Protection Act (FALCPA) requires that any packaged food product that contains peanuts as an ingredient must list the word "Peanut" on the label.

Be aware of the hidden food sources where peanuts may lurk, such as sauces (e.g., chili, mole, pesto, and gravy), salad dressing, pudding, hot chocolate, cookies, egg rolls, potato pancakes, pet food, specialty pizza, meat substitutes, foods with cold-pressed or expelled peanut oil, glazes, and marinades. Also, allergies for other nuts, particularly tree nuts, are common with a peanut allergy. So avoid all nuts and nut butters until you know if they are safe to eat or not. (Many nut butters become cross-contaminated with peanuts during processing.)

munch
on This
A number of clinical trials are underway to find a cure for peanut allergies, if you or a family member are interested in participating, take a look at this National Institutes of Health website: www.clinicaltrials.gov/ct2/results?term=peanut+allergy.

The Truth About Tree Nuts

Tree nuts are the hard-shelled fruit of a plant, not to be confused with legumes like peanuts or seeds like sesame seeds. Tree nuts include Brazil nuts, chestnuts, filberts/hazelnuts, macadamia nuts, pecans, pine nuts, walnuts, cashews, almonds, and pistachios. Other nut varieties that may fit into the tree nut classification are beech nut, ginkgo, shea nut, butternut, hickory, chinquapin, lychee nut, pili nut, and coconut. Remember an allergy to one of these typically means you have to banish all of them from your diet.

Like peanuts, the reaction to tree nut allergies is fast and furious (and can be life-threatening!). Tree nut allergies are common among young children, with the average age of a reaction at 36 months. Some 1.8 million Americans suffer from these allergies. According to the National Institutes of Health, 9 percent of children with tree nut allergies will outgrow them.

Healing Hints

People with tree nut and peanut allergies can eat nutmeg, butternut squash, and water chestnuts to their heart's content. Even though they have the word "nut" in their name, these foods are not considered nuts.

The same federal labeling law that applies to peanuts requires that labels name the specific tree nut used as an ingredient in a food product. Read labels every time you shop as ingredients can change in products! Also when dining out, especially at ethnic restaurants, such as Chinese, African, Indian, Thai, and Vietnamese, pay extra attention as these types of cuisine pose a high risk for nut contamination.

When at the grocery store check the labels in cereal, crackers, cookies, candy, chocolates, energy bars, flavored coffee, frozen desserts, marinades, barbeque sauces, and some deli meats (e.g., mortedella). Be aware of confections like nougat, gianduja (a creamy mixture of chocolate, chopped hazelnuts, and almonds), and marzipan (almond paste). Savory foods that often contain tree nuts include pesto, Nu-Nuts (artificial nuts), and nut meal.

Nut extracts are a no-no, too. Steer clear of natural extracts like pure almond extract and wintergreen extract (for a filbert and hazelnut allergy); use imitation varieties instead. Some alcoholic beverages are flavored with nut extracts, so check with manufacturers as the labels may not clearly reflect allergens (as alcohol is not regulated by the FDA).

Putting a Net on Shellfish

Who would think that enjoying lobster or shrimp could lead to a potentially life-threatening situation? Like tree nuts and peanuts, shellfish commonly ignite anaphylactic reactions. For 7 million Americans that's the reality—they are allergic to the proteins in shellfish. Shellfish allergies are more common in adults, although children with other allergies have been found to have reactions to shellfish as well. Management of an allergy to seafood is considered a life-long proposition, as people don't usually outgrow them.

Shellfish runs the gamut from crustaceans—such as shrimp, crab, crawfish, and lobster—to mollusks, such as abalone, clam, cockle, mussel, oyster, octopus, scallop, snail (escargot), and squid (calamari). Allergic reactions to crustaceans tend to be more severe than mollusk allergies, but if you're allergic to one type do not eat the other unless you consult your allergist or health-care provider first.

As with other food allergies, cross-contamination is a big concern with shellfish. FALCPA labeling laws do apply to shellfish, but you should always ensure food you eat from processing facilities, restaurants, and your own kitchen are shellfish free. It's easy to miss a site of contamination, such as the oil used to cook with or utensils passed from one dish to another. Even cooking vapors (that may contain seafood proteins) released from steam tables or stove tops can cause cross-contamination.

food wise

Marine algae, such as carrageen (used as a thickening agent in dairy foods) is safe to eat. But beware of bouillabaisse, fish stock, seafood flavoring, and surimi (an imitation crabmeat) as they typically have allergenic seafood and fish proteins.

Navigating Fishy Waters

The finned-fish family, such as salmon, tuna, and halibut, are the most likely to cause allergic reactions in people with fish allergies. Once again, the protein in the flesh of the fish is the culprit, but gelatin (from the skin and bones) and fish oils should be avoided, also. Fish allergies are common in adults—research shows that about 40 percent of people with a fish allergy had their first allergic response as an adult. Once a reaction occurs, it's usually a life-long allergy.

Finned fish on the "must-avoid" list include anchovies, bass, catfish, cod, flounder, grouper, haddock, hake, herring, mahi-mahi, perch, pike, pollock, salmon, scrod, sole, snapper, swordfish, tilapia, trout, and tuna.

The good news is canned tuna and salmon may be safe (as the canning process changes the proteins in the fish) for people with fish allergies. Check with your allergist or health-care provider because finned fish is not the same as shellfish and you may not be allergic to both.

Research on fish allergies has shown that people may be allergic to one type of fish, but not another. So it's tricky. A mixed skin prick test for both fish and seafood are available to test reactions to all types, or you can ask your allergist to test each fish (or shellfish) separately.

Fish labeling is also FDA-regulated under FALCPA laws. Be sure to check all labels for fish. Remember that cooking oil in fryers can be cross-contaminated, so even if you are eating fried chicken or fries you might be coming into contact with fish protein. Even invisible fish protein particles in the air where fish is being cooked can set off an allergic reaction in highly sensitive people. Carry an EpiPen or wear an allergy bracelet at all times, just in case.

Some additional food items that may contain fish proteins are Worcestershire sauce, Caesar salad, and/or Caesar dressing (usually contain anchovies or anchovy paste), Caponata (an Italian eggplant relish that may contain anchovies), and the imitation crab, surimi.

Watch Wheat

People with wheat allergies face a serious challenge because wheat is everywhere! Although a wheat allergy typically shows up in childhood and disappears before adulthood, it still has to be managed for its duration. Four proteins in wheat—albumin, globulin, gliadin, and gluten—can pose a threat to the immune system.

A wheat allergy is distinct from celiac disease, also called celiac sprue. The latter is an autoimmune disease in which the immune system abnormally reacts to gluten, causing poor absorption of nutrients in the small intestine. People with celiac disease have to steer clear of all grains containing gluten, such as wheat, rye, barley, and sometimes oats, for life! Be sure to rule out celiac disease by getting a simple blood test, as this disease can be associated with other serious diseases and conditions in the body. A wheat allergy occurs when your immune system attacks wheat proteins only, and you may be able to tolerate other grains. Reactions can be mild to very severe, but whatever the case, wheat and wheat products have to be eliminated from the diet.

Alternative grains for people with a wheat allergy (*not* celiac disease) are:

- Amaranth
- Barley
- Corn
- Oat

- Quinoa
- Rice
- Rye
- Tapioca

Grocery shopping can get tricky with a wheat allergy, so put your wheat-free cap on and shop smart. Read the fine print on food labels. The good news is that any food products must disclose all wheat ingredients on food labels under FALCPA, the federal labeling law.

Red flag foods for wheat include ale, baking mixes, batter-fried foods, beer, breadcrumbs, breakfast cereals, bulgur, candy, crackers, cereal extract, couscous, durum wheat and flour, frankfurters, emmer, einkorn, farina, all types of wheat flour (e.g., all-purpose, cake, enriched, high-protein, high-gluten, pastry), ice cream products, Kamut, processed meats, salad dressing, sauces, semolina, soups, soy sauces, spelt, sprouted wheat, surimi, triticale, vital wheat gluten, wheat (bran, germ, gluten, grass, malt, starch), and whole-wheat berries.

Food wise

In baking, substitute any of the following for 1 cup of wheat flour:

- ⅞ cup rice flour
- ⅝ cup potato starch flour
- 1 cup soy flour plus ¼ cup potato starch flour
- 1 cup corn flour

The Soy Story

Although soy protein is similar to peanut protein, as they are both in the legume family, it doesn't mean that an allergy to one indicates an allergy to the other. Usually a soy allergy is seen in young children, and about half of children outgrow the allergy by age 7. Unlike the other major allergens, soy protein can be tolerated in the diet in small amounts—the amount needed to spark a reaction may be 100 times more than other allergens! Reactions range from mild swelling of the lips to life-threatening anaphylaxis.

Infants allergic to milk may also be allergic to soymilk, but always test to be sure. Soybeans have become a large part of the American diet in processed food products. Many fast-food restaurants use soy flour in hamburger buns, as protein for hamburgers, or as thickening agent for sauces. Many brands of bread contain soy flour.

Soy-containing foods need to state "Soy" on the labels per FALCPA, the FDA law.

Here are some soy-based foods that you may want to watch out for: edamame (soybeans), miso, natto, shoyu sauce, soy (fiber, flour, grits, nuts, sprouts), soy (milk, yogurt, ice cream, cheese), soy protein (concentrate, hydrolyzed, isolate), soy sauce, tamari, tempeh, textured vegetable protein, and tofu. Soy oil and soy lecithin are safe to eat for people with soy allergies.

The Essential Takeaways

- Food allergies are your immune system's reaction to the proteins in certain foods.
- Reactions to allergens can be mild to life-threatening, so be prepared for any type of reaction.
- There are eight main food allergens: milk, eggs, peanuts, tree nuts, wheat, fish, seafood, and soy. But any food can cause an allergic reaction.
- The FDA regulates food labels to inform consumers about potential allergens in food products, so read labels carefully.
- There is a difference between allergy and intolerance. Allergies are an immune system response; intolerance generally leads to gastrointestinal discomfort, such as gas, bloating, and diarrhea.

chapter 12

Spice Up Your Health

Spicing up your health with herbs and spices

Getting a taste for the flavor sensations of herbs and spices

Swapping salt for spices

Sampling spice- and herb-filled recipes

Spices are the seeds, fruits, roots, and bark of plants. Herbs are the leaves and flowers of plants. These edible plant parts have played many important roles in human history. There is evidence that Egyptians used herbs for embalming the dead. World economies were fortified by the spice trade, which flourished throughout Asia, the Middle East, and Europe.

Spices and herbs have also long played a part in healing the body, mind, and spirit. There's a good chance that the cinnamon you sprinkle in your coffee, the nutmeg you shake over acorn squash, and the garlic cloves you crush into tomato sauce are contributing to your health.

The culinary world celebrates the broad spectrum of flavor sensations that spices and herbs offer. Dishes become fiery hot with capsaicin from chili or cayenne peppers; sweet and aromatic with yellow curry; and fresh and crisp with basil. Spices add a whole new dimension to cooking, but over the last two decades research has shown promise in their role in chronic disease prevention—including cancer, type 2 diabetes, heart, lung, cognitive, and autoimmune diseases. What's responsible for their health benefits? Plant-based antioxidants called polyphenols. It just so happens that these edible plants are one of the main sources of antioxidants in our diets today.

In this chapter, I delve into the intriguing and healing world of herbs and spices and some delicious ways to blend them into your everyday eating.

Prevent Disease, Improve Health

Early spice merchants were like traveling apothecaries or pharmacists, who sold and traded medicine in the form of spices and herbs. Medicinal herbs have been part of Chinese medicine for thousands of years, and Western medicine has only just begun to validate what the Chinese have known for ages: herbs and spices contain healing properties. Herbs and spices also provide a perfect antidote to calorie-laden foods by adding flavor without adding calories!

Spices and herbs come in different forms: fresh, whole, dried, or preground dried. The most commonly used are dried. Whole dried (not ground) spices store more easily, last longer, and are a bit less expensive than the ground variety. For the greatest flavor, grind the whole spice right before use. In general, the shelf life of a whole spice is two years, whereas the preground ones last only about 6 months. Store spices in a cool, dark place to maximize flavor and shelf life.

To grind spices, you can put some elbow grease into it with an old fashioned mortar and pestle or use a coffee grinder dedicated to spices (so you don't end up with coriander-flavored coffee or coffee-flavored peppercorns). Some spices, such as peppercorns and sea salts, come prepackaged in a mill.

Munch on This

Spices are jammed with antioxidants. One teaspoon of cinnamon has more antioxidants than ½ cup of fresh blueberries or 1 cup of pomegranate juice.

A recent study in *Nutrition Journal* examined more than 3,000 different foods, including herbs and spices, for their disease-fighting antioxidant content. Researchers found that herbs and spices topped the list for plant-based compounds. The spices with the highest levels were cloves, peppermint, allspice, cinnamon, oregano, thyme, sage, rosemary, and saffron. The following sections outline some healthy reasons to use these fabulous seasonings regularly.

Curing Stomach Upsets

Herbs and spices have long been used in teas, liquors, and nonalcoholic beverages (think root beer). They can work wonders for settling an overfull tummy, reducing gas, and relieving

Chapter 12: Spice Up Your Health

nervous stomachs. A wide variety of herbs and spices can calm these and other stomach ailments. I mention just a few.

Ginger

The pungent-smelling spice ginger, which looks like a knotty, thick root, but is actually the underground stem or "rhizome" of a plant, is a cure-all for stomach issues. Ginger has been used for ages as a panacea for gastrointestinal (GI) distress, such as stomachaches, nausea, vomiting, motion sickness, and morning sickness in pregnant women. You can use it fresh, pickled, dried, or crystallized. It doesn't take a lot to feel relief, try a teaspoon of powdered, fresh, or dried ginger in tea; dice up a teaspoon of the pickled variety in a salad; or just pop a crystallized ginger piece in your mouth.

FOOD wise

Eating too much ginger, particularly in powdered form, may backfire on your GI tract and cause belching, heartburn, bloating, gas, and even nausea—the very things it was supposed to clear up!

Coriander/Cilantro

Coriander seeds have been shown to help with digestion, too. It's considered a carminative, meaning it fends off gas formation in the GI tract. Coriander seeds are used in meat and poultry rubs and seasonings. It's the main ingredient in *garam masala,* a popular Indian spice blend, and it's commonly used in curries.

Definition

Garam masala is a popular blend of aromatic ground spices used in Indian and south Asian cooking. The spices can vary culturally, but the main spices in this mixture are peppercorns (black and white), cloves, cumin, cinnamon, cardamom, nutmeg, star anise, and coriander seeds. It may include garlic and ginger powder and dried red chili peppers among other spices and herbs.

Cilantro is coriander's leafy, herb sibling. It is a type of parsley common to Mexican and Chinese food. Store it by placing the stems in a glass of water (this is a great way to store many fresh herbs). You can also place herbs into a slightly dampened paper towel in the fridge to maximize freshness. Toss fresh cilantro into salads, onto tacos with lettuce, or atop your favorite Chinese dish. It adds a burst of fresh flavor as well as helping to quell digestive issues.

Anise

Anise, a licorice-tasting spice, has also been found to reduce gas, nausea, and sluggish digestion. A number of liquors are made from anise, including Greek Ouzo and Italian Sambuca. These liquors, called *digestifs* are often served as after dinner drinks because they are calming to the digestive system. Teas can be made from steeping anise seeds. If you go to authentic Indian restaurants, you'll likely see bowls with candy-coated seeds of anise and fennel (which also aids digestion). Guests chew on a few seeds after dinner to help them digest and to cleanse the breath.

Good for Your Blood

Herbs and spices can stave off heart disease by improving circulation. They do this by reducing the stickiness of blood, which also decreases the likelihood of blood clots. As you'll see, many herbs and spices help with a number of health issues.

Basil

Basil promotes good blood flow through its antiadhesion properties—preventing blood cells from sticking to the arterial walls. It's most common in Italian food and adds a fresh herbal boost to any pasta. It's also ground up with olive oil and pine nuts to make a delicious pesto, which goes well with pasta, seafood, and meats, or as a fresh alternative to butter when rubbed onto toasted bread.

In Chinese medicine, basil is used for kidney and circulatory problems. A type of basil called holy basil is sacred to those in India who practice the ancient healing art called Ayurvedic medicine. Holy basil has a more clovelike flavor than other basils and can be found in capsule form at most health food stores; people take it to reduce stress and for the heart-related issues that stress can cause.

Ginger

Ginger contains an active compound called gingerol, which may fend off inflammation, which can help with chronic diseases like heart disease. This spice's ability to increase circulation can also help with heart issues. Ginger brings blood to the surface, providing overall warmth as circulation increases. A little goes a long way when it comes to ginger. Just a pinch of powder in hot water makes a spicy hot tea. Or you can also shave off a bit of the fresh root and steep that in water as well.

Cinnamon

Cinnamon can prevent blood clotting and keep the heart supplied with a steady, smooth stream of blood 24/7. In addition, a 2006 study published in the *Journal of the American College of Nutrition* found that cinnamon reduced blood pressure in hypertensive rats. So sprinkle some cinnamon over oatmeal, peanut butter toast, and into soups—it may keep your blood pressure in check, too.

Fenugreek and Turmeric

Two medicinal herbs, fenugreek and turmeric (or its main antioxidant called curcumin), have been found to reduce high blood fats (e.g., high cholesterol and triglycerides) in obese rats. Turmeric leaves are used to wrap and cook food in some Indian cultures, and the dried, ground form is used in curry powders. Sprinkle turmeric into rice, tofu, and chicken dishes.

Fenugreek seeds have a bitter taste when eaten alone, so they are often ground into curry and mixed with other herbs and spices. Take a look at your curry bottle and you may find that fenugreek is one of the ingredients.

Bacteria Warriors

Among the benefits of many herbs and spices is their ability to fight off bacteria.

Munch on This

Humans aren't the only animals who use plants for healing. In fact, our ancestors may have first learned about medicinal plants from observing wild animals. For example, chimps have been known to eat Aspilia, a plant from the sunflower family, found to be a powerful antibiotic. They eat it very slowly and cautiously as if taking medicine.

Basil

Basil has been shown to contain natural oils, such as camphor, which act as an agent to fend off excess bacteria on foods. It's specifically helpful for doing so on produce, where bacteria levels can be high. Camphor also gives basil its distinct aromatic scent. So tossing basil into a vegetable salad not only adds fragrance and flavor, but can keep excess bacteria at bay.

Oregano

Oregano is extremely high in antioxidants among its dried herb peers. Rosmarinic acid is the active compound in oregano that boosts its antioxidant power. Research has shown that one of oregano's primary healing properties is its antimicrobial defense, which can make it a powerful player in fending off not-so-friendly bacteria.

Rosemary

Rosemary, a fragrant member of the mint family, contains a ton of beneficial antioxidants. One of the most noteworthy plant compounds is called carnosic acid, which fights off bacterial growth and explains why rosemary oil has been used as a preservative in foods for fending off bacteria, such as E. coli.

Thyme

Thyme's strong flavor is its main health asset. It reflects a key compound called thymol, an antiseptic that kills bacteria and fungus. Thymol is an active ingredient in mouth wash (e.g., Listerine), and is also used to prevent fungal infections and healing finger- and toenail fungus. You may also see thymol as one of the ingredients in alcohol-free hand sanitizers. In traditional folk medicines, thyme tea was prescribed to cure a variety of ailments from whooping cough to fevers.

On the culinary side, thyme is a popular meat seasoning.

Munch on This

The ancient Greeks used thyme as a fumigator to get rid of insects and pests. Today you'll find thyme oil as an ingredient in natural and organic insect repellants.

Feeling Fuller Faster

Herbs and spices pack a potent flavor punch without adding calories. Naturally flavored foods can be much more satisfying compared to bland foods, meaning you'll eat less. And peppery flavors can actually help us feel fuller on less food.

Capsaicin

The hot and spicy character of chili and cayenne peppers may play a role in satiety or feeling full. Because satiety is a target of weight management and/or loss, this can be very helpful in waistline control. Research suggests that seasoning foods with spicy capsaicin actually helped curb people's appetites. It's also been shown to boost metabolism. (I talk about that more in Chapter 17.) So turn up the heat with spicy peppers today!

Food wise
Be careful not to overdo capsaicin as the heat can cause a burning sensation in your nose, mouth, and throat. If your mouth is on fire from capsaicin, drink cold milk. A protein in milk called casein acts to neutralize the capsaicin and alleviate the burn.

The Spice-Salt Swap

We would be remiss if we didn't talk about one of the world's oldest food seasonings: salt. Table salt is an important mineral and electrolyte and is necessary for health. But we only need salt in small amounts, and large amounts can be harmful. The taste of saltiness is one of our five basic taste senses, which means that our palates are programmed to recognize and prefer salt from the moment of conception.

Munch on This
Along with salty, the other four known taste senses are sweet, bitter, sour, and savory (also known as umami). A sixth taste sense might be fat, which may explain why fat is so appealing to our palates!

Why do you need salt in your diet? Table salt is made up of two minerals, sodium and chloride, which are needed to balance fluids (water) in your body. Too much sodium, called hypernatremia, or too little sodium, called hyponatremia, can cause serious health problems, such as dizziness, muscle cramps, neurological problems, and even death. Balance is vital when it comes to sodium levels in your body.

The latest Dietary Guidelines for Americans advises that the average person eat no more than 2,300 milligrams of sodium per day. (The dietary guidelines drop sodium intake to 1,500 milligrams per day if you have high blood pressure or are at risk for it.) If you consume a lot of processed foods, you are likely way over that limit. Salt runs rampant in packaged baked goods, crackers, chips, processed meats like salami and hot dogs, and even soda.

Salt comes in several forms, colors, and varieties, including the following:

- **Refined salt** (a.k.a. table salt) is made up of 97 percent to 99 percent sodium chloride. It's iodized and used as a condiment in the West, but not in the East, where salty sauces replace it.

- **Sea salt** (a.k.a. "Fleur de sel") is naturally harvested from the sea. It contains varying amounts of iodine. It's the main ingredient in bath salts and can be grey or pink in color.

- **Kosher salt** has a much larger-size grain than table salt and is typically not iodized. The large grains easily draws the fluids out of foods such as meats.

Baking with Salt

Salt is an important ingredient in baking. If you are thinking of holding the salt in your cookies, cakes, and pies, think again. A recipe might only call for ½ to 1 teaspoon of salt, but baking experts contend that it intensifies the flavor of butter and flour, and brings out the other ingredients, especially chocolate. In bread, it lends the gluten (protein in flour) a hand by allowing it to hold more water and carbon dioxide for a tighter crumb.

When baking with kosher salt you must take into account its larger, coarse grain size. Large-grained kosher salt needs more liquid than table salt to dissolve, so if using coarse kosher salt in a recipe that calls for regular salt, use half the amount of kosher salt. If you are using fine grain kosher salt you don't need to make any adjustments.

Healing Hints

The average person should aim for consuming around 2,300 milligrams of salt per day. What does that look like? That's a mere teaspoon of salt. Most people eat over 4,000 milligrams per day, which is more than 2 teaspoons per day!

Flavor Creations to Savor

So what are some ways to swap out some salt for healthy herbs and spices in everyday cooking? Douse homemade tomato sauce with smoky paprika and dried basil; add crushed garlic or garlic powder to pizza; top salads and soups with a fresh sprig of rosemary; sprinkle fresh dill on fish and seafood; add fresh ginger to spring and sushi rolls. Here are some other spices and ways you can use them to boost your food's flavor:

- **Allspice:** Incorporate ground allspice into marinades and dressing for meat, chicken, and fish for an interesting Caribbean flavor.

- **Cinnamon:** Stir a cinnamon stick into your coffee or hot chocolate; sprinkle ground cinnamon over pancakes, waffles, or oatmeal.

- **Cloves:** Put dried cloves with some loose leaf tea into a tea ball and steep in hot water for some instant soothing chai tea. Add a drizzle of honey and steamed skim milk for a chai latte.

- **Mint:** Top your favorite ice cream with mint leaves (peppermint) or add peppermint oil into chocolate cake batter or frosting for a delicious flavor combination.

- **Oregano:** Give your tomato sauce a healthy boost with a couple of dashes of dried oregano or toss it over a Caprese salad for a refreshing flavor.

- **Rosemary:** Sprinkle fresh rosemary leaves into diced sweet potatoes with olive oil, garlic, paprika, and a dash of salt for a deliciously aromatic side dish.

- **Saffron:** Add a dash of golden yellow saffron to rice and quinoa dishes. It's pricey, so use sparingly to add a sweet flavor to foods. Saffron is one of the main ingredients in Spanish paella, a seafood rice dish.

- **Sage:** Rub meat or poultry with ground sage before roasting or add fresh sage leaves to gravy for an extra special flavor kick.

- **Thyme:** Pop a sprig of fresh thyme into tomato soup or a chunky stew; sprinkle dried thyme over pizza, scrambled eggs, or tomato and cucumber salad.

Spices for Life Recipes

Try any of these recipes to spice up your meals and give your health a boost.

Herbed Moroccan Couscous

You can add chopped grilled chicken breast, lean beef, or pork to this dish. The broth imparts a lot of flavor—you can also use low-sodium chicken or beef broth. Add or omit herb or spices as you wish, but they, too, add a lot of flavor without a lot of calories.

Yield:	Serving size:	Prep time:	Cook time:
4 servings	¾ cup	5 minutes	15 minutes

Each serving has:			
244 calories	1 g total fat	0 g saturated fat	0 g trans fat
0 mg cholesterol	215 mg sodium	43 g carbohydates	5 g fiber
4 g sugars	9 g protein	10 percent iron	

1½ cups low-sodium vegetable broth	1 TB. fresh mint, chopped
1 TB. olive oil	2 TB. fresh basil, chopped
1 cup whole-wheat couscous	1 TB. lemon zest, grated
1½ cups fresh or frozen peas	1 TB. lemon juice
2 TB. fresh parsley, chopped	Pinch black pepper

1. Bring broth and oil to a boil in a medium saucepan. Remove from heat and stir in couscous. Cover and let stand for 5 minutes.

2. Meanwhile cook peas in a medium saucepan of water just until tender (about 2 minutes) or microwave for a minute. Drain.

3. Add peas, parsley, mint, basil, lemon zest, and pepper to the couscous; toss lightly with a fork. Serve warm.

Roasted Garlic, Tomato, and Basil Pasta

This aromatic blend of garlic and basil ignites this pasta dish with wonderful sensory overload. Enjoy it with a side of greens and a glass of full-bodied red wine.

Yield:	Serving size:	Prep time:	Cook time:
4 servings	½ cup	10 minutes	50 minutes

Each serving has:			
409 calories	29 g total fat	5 g saturated fat	0 g trans fat
5 mg cholesterol	145 mg sodium	31 g carbohydrates	5 g fiber
2 g sugars	9 g protein	9 percent iron	

½ cup extra-virgin olive oil

1 whole bulb, garlic, top removed

Ground black pepper to taste

12 oz. spaghetti or angel hair pasta

1 cup cherry tomatoes, diced

1 TB. fresh basil, chopped

Fresh parmesan cheese, a few shavings

1. Preheat oven to 400°F. Drizzle 1 teaspoon of olive oil into open garlic bulb. Place the garlic in a pan and roast for 30 minutes and allow to cool.

2. Hold the garlic over a bowl and dig out the flesh from each clove with the point of the knife. When all the flesh has been removed, pour in the remaining olive oil and add plenty of black pepper. Place in food processor and mix well.

3. Cook the pasta as instructed on the package. Drain and return it to a clean pan. Pour in oil and garlic mixture and toss pasta over medium-high heat until all strands are well coated. Top with diced tomatoes and basil. Serve immediately with shaved parmesan.

Fire-Roasted Turmeric Eggplant Bake

You can serve this dish with grilled salmon, chicken breast, or baked tofu. A dollop of plain yogurt will cut the spice if the spiciness is too intense. You can also put all of these ingredients in a food processor and make a tasty dip.

Yield:	Serving size:	Prep time:	Cook time:
2 servings	½ cup	5 minutes	30 minutes

Each serving has:			
198 calories	14 g total fat	2 g saturated fat	0 g trans fat
0 mg cholesterol	19 mg sodium	18 g carbohydrates	10 g fiber
7 g sugars	3 g protein	8 percent iron	

1 medium eggplant, diced	1 TB. smoky paprika
3 garlic cloves, chopped	2 tsp. turmeric
2 TB. extra-virgin olive oil	A pinch of salt

1. Preheat oven to 400°F.

2. Place eggplant and garlic in a baking dish, toss with olive oil, paprika, turmeric, and salt. Bake until eggplant begins to brown and get crisp; check and toss every 10 minutes.

Essential Takeaways

- Herbs and spices are packed with beneficial plant-based compounds and antioxidants for overall wellness.
- Herbs are the leaves or flowers of edible plants; spices are the seeds, fruit, roots, and bark of plants.
- Herbs and spices have been shown to prevent chronic diseases including cancer, type 2 diabetes, heart, lung, cognitive, and some autoimmune diseases, such as rheumatoid arthritis.
- Culinary herbs and spices are a healthy alternative to salt and fat as they are sodium-free with zero calories and fat.

part 3

Drink to Your Good Health

You need to drink plenty of liquids for good health, but what type of liquid you drink matters. In a world full of designer drinks like gourmet coffee, juice, alcohol, and enhanced waters, how can you know what's good, what isn't, and what's just marketing hype? The chapters in this part offer deeper insight into the nature of liquid nutrition. For example, some designer drinks may offer health benefits, but they also can contain loads of extra calories. On the other hand, water, tea, coffee, and even alcohol, in moderation, can play a vital role in your health and wellness.

Balance is the key with liquids. Most people don't think about how many calories they drink, but this part helps you become fully aware of your drinking behaviors and find balance in your diet. I wrap up each chapter in this part with delicious recipes for healthy drinks.

chapter 13

Liquid Calories Add Up Fast

Calculating how liquids add up

Deciphering a good daily liquid dose

Getting the scoop on coffee, tea, and fruit drinks

Wetting your whistle with recipes

The beverage business is booming with everything from fancy coffee drinks to sugar-infused waters to juice concoctions. Beverages add variety to your diet and offer an alternate source of nutrition other than solid foods; however, research examining the last 20 to 30 years reveals that drinking has evolved into a high-calorie habit; the trend toward people drinking less water and more sugar-sweetened beverages is a global phenomenon.

The puzzling part of the equation is that drinking liquid calories does not stop us from eating just as much (if not more) solid food. In other words, we don't compensate by eating less food even after gulping down a 16-ounce regular soda. Studies have shown that beverages don't register in our brains (and stomachs) the same way food does. In a study performed in 2000, when people were given 450 additional calories from soda or jelly beans, the ones chewing the candy cut back on solid foods more than those drinking the carbonated beverage. What's not clear is whether the effect is because we chew solids or its because liquids leave the GI tract at a faster rate than solids. What is clear is that an overabundance of liquid calories eventually leads to weight gain and a whole host of related health problems.

On average, we drink 425 calories a day. Nutrition researchers have determined that since 1990, schools have replaced water fountains with vending machines filled with sugary beverages. Across the pond in the United Kingdom surveys have shown that 17 percent of calories of all age groups come from alcohol, sugar-sweetened beverages, and juice drinks, whereas adults in the United States have increased how much they drink by 21 ounces—and 100 percent of it is coming from sugary beverages! Mexican children, ages 2 and up, have doubled the number of calories they consume from liquids alone.

This chapter focuses on how to make smart beverage choices, be a conscious drinker, and balance liquids with solid food to maintain an ideal body weight and optimal health, while still occasionally enjoying a high-calorie beverage.

Daily Liquid Calculator

How much do you drink every day? You may never think about how much you imbibe on a regular basis, but the calories can add up fast! It's important that you take responsibility for how much and what you drink daily.

Munch on This

Experts project that adding a 10 percent tax to sugary beverages would reduce consumption by 8 to 10 percent!

The major sources of liquid calories in our diets are whole milk, fruit juice, soft drinks, and alcohol. To see where your beverage calories come in, record everything you drink for a single day. This is not only a great way to monitor caloric drinks, but you can also keep track of how much water you are drinking.

Sample Daily Liquid Calculator		
Time of Day	*Beverage*	*Calories*
Breakfast (8 A.M.)	Cafe Au Lait (Grande, whole milk)*	130
10 A.M.	Water	0
Lunch (12 noon)	16-oz. regular cola**	200
3 P.M.		

Time of Day	Beverage	Calories
Dinner (6:30 P.M.)		
8:30 P.M.		
Today's total beverage calories:	_____	

Switch to skim or nonfat milk and save 60 calories and boost the calcium a bit, too.

**If you swap diet for regular soda you'll significantly reduce the calories. However, you'll most likely replace some of the water in your day with needless chemicals from diet soda, so to drink clean, stick with unsweetened tea, coffee, and plain or mineral water as your go-to beverages.*

Try keeping a daily drink calculator for at least a week and then take a close look to see where you can cut back on the high-calorie, fatty and sugary beverages from your day. Remember, drinking 250 to 500 fewer calories a day will translate into losing ½ to 1 lb. in weight a week.

Smart Daily Drink Doses

Now that you know what you've been drinking, let's spend some time considering what you *should* be drinking. Your lifestyle, age, gender, and what you eat dictates your fluid needs. Are you active, sedentary, or in-between? This will affect your metabolism and how much fluid your body needs.

Water

Beverage experts recommend that water be your number one drink. Not only does water hydrate your body, but it fills you up with zero calories and so helps with appetite control. The more water you drink before a meal, the less hungry you will be. Take a look at your diet; if it's high in water-laden fruits and vegetables, then you may not need to drink as much water as someone who doesn't eat a lot of produce. Women should aim for at least four 8-ounce glasses of water a day and men should aim for six 8-ounce glasses a day. (See more on water and hydration in Chapter 14.)

Fruit Juice and Smoothies

In their natural state, whole fruits are nutrition powerhouses. And while juice may confer some nutrients from their parent fruit, when you drink juice, you don't eat any less to make up for those juice calories. And the calories can add up fast! A ½ cup serving of orange juice has 90 calories. That's not too bad, but most people drink way more than this small, 4-ounce serving. You should limit your juice intake to 1 cup a day.

Blended fruit smoothies are all the rage these days. And they are certainly delicious and can be nutritious, especially the ones just made from frozen whole fruit and juice. Beware of smoothies containing whole milk, soymilk, and sherbet as they can be higher in calories, fat, and added sugar!

Pure fruit smoothies contain a fair amount of vitamin C, antioxidants, and some fiber. Yet, the downside is the calories—they can range from 100 to almost 400 calories per serving. So before you order a fancy fruit concoction check the nutrition facts.

Healing Hints	If you want a juice fix, juice shops and natural grocery stores sell "shots"—or single gulp servings. Some shots blend juice with green tea for a refreshing burst of energy. A one-shot deal contains about 60 calories.

When you can't get the whole fruit or want something other than water, here are some smart fruit juice choices for less than 100 calories:

- Tomato juice—50 calories per 8 ounces. Watch the sodium—a small can of tomato juice can have almost 1,000 milligrams! Choose low-sodium varieties.

- Apple juice boxes (for kids)—50 calories per 6.75 fl. oz. box; some brands contain more water than juice.

- Light orange juice (50 calories per 8 ounces)

- Carrot juice (35 calories per 6 ounces)

- Apple juice (60 calories per 4 ounces)

- 100 percent cranberry juice (70 calories per 8 ounces)

- 100 percent white grape juice (80 calories per 4 ounces)

Coffee

According to the latest research, coffee is a fine beverage to drink, specifically unsweetened coffee. How much? Up to 4 cups a day—that's 32 ounces of coffee—is ok for a daily dose.

In its brewed, au natural state, coffee can be a replacement for some of the water in your diet. Although the caffine in coffee is a diuretic or a substance that causes dehydration, the latest science and consensus by the Institute of Medicine shows that coffee can be counted toward your total daily fluid consumption.

In addition, some research shows that 4 cups of coffee a day might protect against type 2 diabetes. Coffee drinkers have been shown to have less incidence of Parkinson's disease, gallstones, kidney stones, and liver cancer. Some people think that coffee's high-antioxidant content gives it these health benefits, but more research is needed in the area.

How much caffeine is in coffee? One heaping teaspoon of instant coffee contains 100 milligrams (mg) of caffeine. The typical brewed cup (8 ounces) of java has up to 150 milligrams; a shot (1 fluid ounce) of espresso has 75 milligrams, and Starbuck's coffee contains 20 milligrams of caffeine per fluid ounce, meaning that a cup of their Grande (16-ounce) brewed coffee has 320 milligrams of caffeine.

Pregnant women should not drink more than 300 milligrams of caffeine a day, as too much caffeine may cause low birth weight and miscarriages. Also, with age, a higher sensitivity to caffeine creeps up, thus jitters, headaches, and sleeplessness may ensue with too much caffeine. Even the average person may experience disturbances in mood, physical and mental sharpness, slower reaction time, and poor concentration with too much—over 400 milligrams—of caffeine per day.

Tea

Unsweetened tea is a good source of fluid with zero calories. After water, tea is the most common beverage in the United States; 127 million Americans drink it on any given day. From the leaves of the *Camellia sinensis* plant comes the green tea family: white, green, oolong, and black tea. The four tea types undergo different amounts of processing and fermentation.

Tea is not only a tasty low-calorie beverage that can replace sugary soft, sports, and energy drinks, but it contains powerful plant substances known as tannins (which give tea its astringent quality) and polyphenol antioxidants, such as epigallanocatechin (EGCG), which have the potential for a whole host of health benefits. There are only 30 to 50 milligrams of caffeine per cup in green or black tea, respectively.

Studies show that drinking four or more cups a day can lower the risk of heart disease, as tea dilates (widens) arteries keeping blood running smoothly to and from the heart. The effects of tea on health has been studied primarily in animals, thus more human studies are needed to determine tea's role in preventing chronic diseases, such as heart disease and cancer. Our advice to you is to drink anywhere from 2 to 4 cups of tea per day. It's soothing, low in calories and caffeine, and contains a whole host of powerful antioxidants, which can't hurt!

White and Green Tea

White and green tea leaves are not fermented after they are wilted (a process in which the excess water is removed), and thus they look very close to fresh tea leaves, especially white tea. White tea comes from the young, soft leaves of the tea plant; they are treated very tenderly and with great care. Green tea leaves are steamed and minimally processed. As a result, white and green teas are higher in antioxidants and contain less caffeine than black and oolong teas.

Black and Oolong Tea

Black tea leaves are wilted and then fermented, a process that determines their unique taste, color, aroma, and flavor profiles. Black has the highest caffeine content and is the lowest in antioxidants, whereas oolong is in the middle with moderate amounts of each.

Herbal Tea

Herbal teas are viewed as a form of medicine throughout Europe and are sold alongside prescription drugs in pharmacies. However, some herbal teas can cause allergic reactions and toxic affects if you are not aware of what's in the tea. Check the labels. Ingredients like comfrey and black cohosh may cause permanent liver damage if drunk daily, and lobelia contains toxins that are like nicotine in cigarettes. The herbs in herbal teas can interfere with the action of prescription drugs, so consult your health-care provider before regularly drinking an herbal tea.

munch on This

Herbal tea is caffeine-free and made from either dried fruit, fresh or dried flowers, herbs, leaves, seeds, and roots steeped with boiling hot water. Some popular varieties are hibiscus (made with rose hip or the fruit of the rose plant), rooibos a.k.a. red tea (made from a red plant in South Africa), and chamomile tea (made from the dried flowers of the chamomile plant).

Cow's Milk

Technically milk is the white, see-through substance that comes from the mammary glands of mammals, such as cows, goats, and sheep. Breast milk is the first nourishment for human infants before they can digest other foods. Breast milk is like liquid gold as far as nutrition, especially during infancy, as it passes on the mother's antibodies to the baby and helps fend off the risk of many diseases. Plus, breast milk contains fat, protein, calcium, and vitamin C—all essential nutrients for a developing infant. Humans are one of the only species in the world that drinks milk past infancy.

As far as cow's milk, the calories go up as the fat goes up. A cup of whole (full-fat) milk has 150 calories with 5 grams of saturated fat; 2 percent fat milk has 120 calories with 3 grams of saturated fat; 1 percent fat milk has 100 calories with 1.5 grams of saturated fat; and fat-free (skim) milk has 90 calories and 0.5 grams of saturated fat. The recommendation for milk is 2 cups a day of fat-free or 1 percent fat milk.

Plant Milk

Plant beverages such as soymilk, hazelnut milk, almond milk, rice milk, and oat milk have become very popular in the United States. Because these milks are from plants, they are naturally lower in saturated fat and cholesterol than cow's milk.

food wise

All milk, whether dairy or nondairy, contains calories. Dairy milk has saturated fat and cholesterol, and plant-based milks often contain added sugar. So read labels and portion out your daily milk dose. Try to stick with 2 to 3 cups a day of the plain, low-fat, or fat-free varieties.

Soymilk

Soymilk comes from soybeans and is actually a mixture of ground soybeans, oil, and water. Soymilk is comparable to cow's milk in protein and a bit more iron. Because it doesn't naturally contain a lot of calcium, soymilk is typically fortified with calcium. Soymilk is good for people with milk allergies or lactose intolerance, as it's lactose-free. It contains plant-based estrogens called isoflavones, which studies have shown to be beneficial for decreasing menopausal symptoms, fibroids, and endometriosis in women; they have also been shown to fend off hormone-related cancers, such as breast cancer, particularly in post-menopausal women. In men, isoflavones may reduce the risk of prostate cancer by acting as an antioxidant to keep cells healthy. Plus, isoflavones have shown promise in reducing LDL (bad) cholesterol levels and keeping arteries elastic. Soymilk comes in plain, vanilla, and chocolate flavors. Just like cow's milk, there's a light variety with less fat and calories. An 8-ounce cup of reduced-fat soymilk has 40 fewer calories and 2 grams less fat than regular soymilk.

Nut Milks

A number of nuts are processed into "milk" beverages. Vegans often use nut milks, such as almond milk, as a nondairy alternative to animal milk. The calories aren't bad, either, unless you go for the sweetened versions, which can be double the calories. Unsweetened, plain almond milk has a mere 40 calories and 200 milligrams of calcium per cup.

munch on This	You can also make nut milk easily in a Vita-Mix blender. Here's a simple method by The Raw Food Coach, Karen Knowler. Add 1 cup of nuts (almonds work well, but any nut works), 2 cups of purified water (use 3 cups for a thinner texture), and blend on high speed. Once blended, strain through a nylon mesh bag or cheesecloth. You can drink as is or sweeten with a couple of table-spoons of a natural sweetener like agave nectar or two to three dates; blend again until smooth and combined. For a hint of flavoring, add a splash of vanilla or almond extract.

Almond milk is just ground almonds and water. It's lactose-free, contains no casein (a milk protein that causes allergies in some people), is low in saturated fat, and contains no cholesterol. It's also a great alternative for soy.

Rice and Oat Milk

Both of these milk beverages are made from grains: rice milk from brown rice and oat milk from the whole oat grain. Rice milk is a great alternative for people who are allergic to milk; however, it typically does not contain as much protein or calcium as cow's milk. The calories in rice milk are moderate: 1 cup has 100 calories, the same as in a cup of 1 percent fat cow's milk. Some brands are fortified with calcium, protein, and vitamins and minerals. Rice milk comes in plain, chocolate, vanilla, and almond flavors.

Healing Hints Want a natural drink alternative? Try the Japanese rice drink called amazake. It's made from fermented rice and its natural sweetness comes from carbohydrates breaking down into sugar molecules over time. Amazake is a healthy beverage choice as it doesn't contain added sugar, salt, or preservatives. It's sold in natural grocery stores.

Oat milk is another nondairy alternative to cow's milk. It is made from oat groats (the hulled grain broken in pieces) mixed with filtered water and other grains and beans. It's used as an alternative to cow's milk as it's lactose-free. Oat milk has a natural sweet flavor that works well in hot or cold cereal, pudding, hot chocolate, and coffee. It contains a fair amount of calcium, iron, and vitamin A. Oat milk can have up to 150 calories per cup.

Alcohol

There are a few reasons to limit alcohol in your diet. It can be addictive for some people, the calories can stack up, and it can cause you to eat more (as alcohol decreases your inhibitions with food). However, when drunk in moderation, alcohol can be beneficial for health; we talk about this in depth in Chapter 15.

Here's how the alcohol calories stack up:

- A 12-ounce beer is about 150 calories

- A 5-ounce glass of wine is about 100 calories

- A 1.5-ounce glass of distilled liquor is about 100 calories

Awareness is the key. Drink alcoholic beverages in moderation by alternating a glass of water for each alcoholic drink and you will save calories, stay hydrated, and be less likely to overdrink. To keep your calories under control, you should limit your alcohol intake to no more than one drink a day.

Smart Drink Recipes

Here are some recipes for smart drinks that will liven up your palate without expanding your waistline.

All-Fruit Smoothie

Use any fruits you desire or whatever is in season.

Yield:	Serving size:	Prep time:	Cook time:
1 smoothie	1 smoothie	5 minutes	None
Each serving has:			
257 calories	1 g total fat	0 g saturated fat	0 g trans fat
0 mg cholesterol	12 mg sodium	64 g carbohydrates	7 g fiber
51 g sugars	3 g protein	5 percent iron	

Juice of a large orange (about ⅔ cup)

⅔ cup unsweetened apple juice

1 small ripe peach, pitted and quartered

2 large or 4 small strawberries, hulled

1. Put orange juice, apple juice, peach, and strawberries in a blender and mix well. You could also blend in ½ cup plain low-fat yogurt, but don't forget to account for those calories.

Raspberry Green Tea Shake

This frothy shake has refreshing hints of raspberry with the clean green tea taste.

Yield:	Serving size:	Prep time:	Cook time:
2 shakes	1 shake	5 minutes	None

Each serving has:			
145 calories	2 g total fat	1 g saturated fat	0 g trans fat
71 mg cholesterol	51 mg sodium	8 g carbohydrates	1 g fiber
4 g sugars	25 g protein	1 mg iron	

1 cup freshly brewed green tea, cooled

1 cup fresh or frozen raspberries

1 cup skim or fat-free milk

2 scoops vanilla whey protein powder

1. Steep the green tea for 3–4 minutes in boiling water; let cool.

2. Combine tea, raspberries, milk, and vanilla whey powder in a blender. Purée until blended well. Pour into a glass and enjoy.

Bubbly Fruity Mocktail

Cut the alcohol and try this bubbly festive mock-up to the traditional bubblini. Perfect for a weeknight or a staple for women during pregnancy.

Yield:	Serving size:	Prep time:	Cook time:
2 drinks	1 drink	5 minutes	None

Each serving has:			
65 calories	0 g total fat	0 g saturated fat	0 g trans fat
0 mg cholesterol	3 mg sodium	17 g carbohydrates	0 g fiber
17 g sugars	1 g protein	2 percent iron	

2 cups sparkling or mineral water

¼ cup 100 percent cranberry juice

¼ cup 100 percent apple juice

Zest of an orange

1. Pour the sparkling water into fluted champagne glasses or any other glass, add the cranberry juice, and zest a bit of orange into each glass; top with a twist of orange rind. Sip and celebrate the day.

Essential Takeaways

- Drinking calories is not the same as eating them. Our bodies are not as satisfied on high-calorie beverages, thus they can lead to weight gain and chronic diseases like obesity.
- Water should be your go-to beverage.
- Banish high-calorie, sugary beverages, such as regular soda, fruit drinks, and sports drinks.
- Coffee and tea can count toward your total daily fluid consumption.
- Limit caffeine, especially if you are pregnant or sensitive to it.

chapter 14

The Right Water Fix for You

Understanding the importance of water

Staying hydrated for health

Eating hydrating foods

Every cell, organ, tissue, and metabolic process in your body relies on water for proper function and health. Depending on your size, more than half of your body is made of water. The good news is Americans get plenty of water. A 2004 report from the Institute of Medicine revealed no signs of chronic dehydration in the U.S. population overall.

There is no set-in-stone requirement for how much water you should drink. Experts say to aim for about 2 quarts, that's 8 cups, per day for optimal hydration. However, your water needs depend on a number of factors, including how active you are, how much you lose with sweat or urine, and your environment. If you live or work in a hot climate and are under heat stress, you will need more water than someone who lives in a cooler, milder climate.

You can get the water you need from a variety of sources, including drinking water (tap or bottled), other beverages (i.e., coffee, tea, juice, etc.), and eating foods with high-water content. In this chapter, I explore the wonderful world of water—from getting enough to the signs of a water imbalance.

Water for Your Health

If your body is well-hydrated you will think clearly, feel alert, be happy, stand steady, and have clear or light yellow urine. On average, if you urinate 1 to 2 liters (that's 6–8 glasses) a day you are probably well-hydrated. Remember, how much you urinate depends on a number of things, such as how much you drink, how active you are, your body size, and your overall health.

Dark yellow or brownish urine is a classic sign of dehydration.

While *dehydration* is far more common than having too much water—called *water intoxication*—in the body, both conditions are life-threatening.

Thirst is the not the best indicator of hydration needs, as people are typically dehydrated long before they actually feel thirsty. Sipping water throughout the day is the best way to stay properly hydrated.

Definition

Dehydration is the extreme loss of body water; it's typically noticeable when 2 percent of the body's normal body water is lost. Symptoms include headache, dizziness, and fatigue.

Water intoxication is a life-threatening condition caused by drinking too much water, which leads to loss of electrolytes, abnormal brain function, and possible death.

Water is the only zero calorie nutrient on the planet. Getting enough water in your diet positively impacts your health in numerous ways, including the following:

- Helps keep your kidneys working properly and helps prevent kidney stones.

- May decrease the risk of some cancers, such as bladder cancer.

- May contribute to mineral intake (as tap water contains calcium, magnesium, and fluoride).

- Keeps your metabolism fine-tuned and in working order.

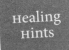

It's particularly important for people with diabetes to drink plenty of water, because high blood sugar levels can shrink cells and cause dehydration.

Tap Water

Tap water is one of the cheapest and most convenient ways to get drinking water. However, some people shun tap water for fear that it contains impurities. The Environmental Protection Agency (EPA), which sets the safety standards for contaminants in drinking water, is charged with ensuring that the 80 likely water contaminants stay below legal limits. Although tap water in some parts of the world is known to contain dangerous levels of impurities, most tap water in the United States is safe to drink.

That's not to say you shouldn't look into the safety of your tap water. Water can contain harmful substances, such as by-products from chlorination, minute disease-causing organisms, lead, arsenic, and parasites. Check with your local water company and ask for the latest Consumer Confidence Report—it may clear up questions or prompt you to ask more!

Bottled Water

Companies started selling water in recyclable plastic bottles in the 1980s, and the bottled water industry hasn't stopped growing since then. Whether it's spring water, carbonated (sparkling), mineral, distilled, purified, and/or flavored water—people are gulping it down. The bottled water industry is slated to make over $86 million in 2011, with purified water the top global seller.

Is Bottled Water Safe?

As far as the Centers for Disease Control and Prevention (CDC) is concerned, there is no reason to believe that bottled water is unsafe. The CDC reports no known cases of water-borne disease from bottled water. Approximately 75 percent of bottled water comes from springs or tap water from city water systems. Mineral and sparkling water come from spring water; the former contains minerals, like magnesium and calcium, and the latter has carbon dioxide gas added to it. Purified and distilled water come from city water that has undergone further purification.

Munch on This
Experts recommend buying water bottled by companies that are members of the International Bottled Water Association (IBWA), as they are randomly safety checked by independent certification agencies like NSF International. For more information, go to www.nsf.org.

Environmental Issues

But it's not just the water that poses a health concern—it's the environmental impact from all those bottles—about 200 billion a year—introduced into the environment. The bottled water industry is under fire for polluting the environment with excess plastic.

The majority of plastic water bottles are now made with polyethylene terephthalate (PET or PETE), which is easily recycled. If you look on a plastic water bottle that is made from PET plastic, it will have an identification code of 1 (that's the small symbol of three arrows in the shape of a triangle with a number in the middle of it on the bottom of plastic bottles and containers). There are pros and cons to PET plastic bottles. On the good news front, PET water bottles can be easily recycled into other materials.

The downside of PET bottles is that they may release phthalates (substances added to plastics to give it flexibility and durability) into the water that you drink. Studies have shown that phthalates could disrupt hormone levels, which can be particularly dangerous for pregnant women, as overexposure has shown that male babies may be born with abnormal testicular growth and stages of development if exposed to too many phthalates.

Companies are beginning to introduce more eco-friendly water bottles. For example, Dasani has a new bottle called PlantBottle, which is made from a combination of sugarcane and molasses turned into 100 percent recyclable plastic. Aquafina has an Eco-Fina Bottle, which is reported to have 35 percent less plastic than its previous bottle.

Flavored Water

People don't just want water, they want jazzy flavors and compelling health reasons to drink it—which many flavored water companies promise. You can find bottled water containing everything from added vitamin C to vitamin D to agave nectar to herb and spice blends. Some companies infuse real fruit flavors along with non-nutritive (zero calorie) sweeteners or variations of sugar and vitamins and minerals to appeal to health conscious, sports-minded, and/or active women and men.

| Healing Hints | Want to get purified water without the plastic waste? Grocery stores and retail outlets across the United States have vending machines that dispense purified water. Bring your own bottles and fill them up. You can buy purifiers for your house, too. A bottle of water averages $2 per bottle, whereas a home purification system costs about a dollar a day for up to 5 gallons. |

As far as calories, flavored waters range from 0 calories to 50 calories per 8-ounce serving—and some brands contain 2.5 servings in a bottle. As with any beverage, the additional calories and added sugar can add up—some brands have over 30 grams of sugar in a bottle!

Munch on This

It's easy to make your own flavored water. Fill a glass with mineral or plain water and add a splash of lemon, lime, or orange juice to create a delish low-calorie beverage that you can enjoy anytime.

Hydrating Foods

A recent national nutrition survey showed that men and women age 19 to 30 years get the majority (81 percent) of their fluids from water and other beverages (i.e., juice, coffee, tea, and soda), with the other 19 percent coming from water in food. Foods with high water content are unique in that they can help curb appetite and keep excess weight off—more so than drinking plain water before or during meals and snacks.

Eating water-rich foods, such as fruits, vegetables, and soup (mainly broth-based ones) can make you feel full on fewer calories, thus preventing overeating and weight gain. People eat significantly less when offered food with high volume (more on your plate), but less calories—think tons of veggies on pizza or in soup. It's filling and satisfying.

Healing Hints

You can eat 2 cups of water-filled grapes or ½ cup of dehydrated raisins for the same calories. What would satisfy you more? The grapes, of course.

Fruits and vegetables tend to have higher concentrations of water than other types of food. Here's how water stacks up in some common foods.

Amount of Water in Foods	
Food	*Water Content (percent)*
Fruits and vegetables	80–95
Soups	80–95
Hot cereal	85
Yogurt, low-fat, fruit	75

continues

Amount of Water in Foods (continued)

Food	Water Content (percent)
Egg, boiled	75
Pasta, cooked	65
Fish and seafood	60–85
Meats	45–65
Bread	35–40
Cheese	35
Nuts	2–5
Saltine crackers	3
Potato chips	2
Oil	0

Source: Rolls, B. The Volumetrics Eating Plan, HarperCollins, 2005.

The fruits and veggies that top the water list (consisting of more than 90 percent) are broccoli, cabbage, cauliflower, cucumber, eggplant, sweet peppers, spinach, zucchini, tomatoes, grapefruit, cantaloupe, strawberries, and watermelon.

Hydrating Recipes

Here are some simple and delicious hydrating recipes.

Artichoke-Inspired Salsa

Use this salsa on fish, chicken, lean beef, or baked potatoes; it makes a great appetizer with whole-grain crackers or pita chips.

Yield:	Serving size:	Prep time:	Cook time:
5 servings	½ cup	10 minutes	None
Each serving has:			
90 calories	4 g total fat	1 g saturated fat	0 g trans fat
0 mg cholesterol	254 mg sodium	13 g carbohydrates	6 g fiber
2 g sugars	4 g protein	10 percent iron	

2 cups marinated artichoke hearts, drained and chopped

3 Roma or plum tomatoes, chopped

2 TB. red onion, diced

¼ cup black olives, diced

1 TB. garlic, minced

1 TB. small capers

2 TB. fresh basil, chopped

Salt and pepper

1. In a medium bowl, mix together artichoke hearts, tomatoes, onion, olives, garlic, salt, and pepper.

2. Serve chilled or at room temperature.

Roasted Tomato, Three Bean, and Mushroom Soup

This is a quick, tasty, and hydrating meal. Use low-sodium tomatoes and beans to bring down the sodium in this dish.

Yield:	Serving size:	Prep time:	Cook time:
4 servings	1 cup	10 minutes	30 minutes

Each serving has:			
309 calories	11 g total fat	2 g saturated fat	0 g trans fat
0 mg cholesterol	601 mg sodium	42 g carbohydrates	12 g fiber
5 g sugars	14 g protein	24 percent iron	

3 TB. extra-virgin olive oil

2 garlic cloves, minced

½ cup onions, minced

1 cup white or baby bella mushrooms, sliced

2 (15–oz.) cans diced tomatoes, fire-roasted

2 cups cold water

3 to 4 leaves dark green cabbage or kale, shredded roughly

2 sprigs fresh rosemary, minced

1 cup cooked cannellini beans, rinsed and drained

1 cup cooked kidney beans, rinsed and drained

1 cup cooked black beans, rinsed and drained

Salt and pepper

1. Add 1 tablespoon of olive oil to a large stock pot over medium heat. Add garlic and stir for 1 minute. Add onions and heat through until translucent or clear.

2. Add mushrooms and sauté together. Add tomatoes and water. Bring to a boil and then reduce the heat to a simmer; add rosemary and stir.

3. Add shredded cabbage leaves to soup. Partially cover the pot and simmer gently for about 15 minutes, or until cabbage is tender.

4. Drain and rinse beans, add to soup, and warm through for a few minutes. Taste to see if you need salt and pepper.

5. Ladle soup into bowls and drizzle each with a touch of olive oil. Serve with crusty whole-grain bread, if desired.

Spicy Spaghetti with Garlic Broccoli

Simple and tasty, this pasta dish is flavored with a bit of red pepper and balanced with citrus and garlic notes.

Yield:	Serving size:	Prep time:	Cook time:
4 servings	½ cup	5 minutes	15 minutes

Each serving has:			
184 calories	7 g total fat	1 g saturated fat	0 g trans fat
0 mg cholesterol	19 mg sodium	27 g carbohydrates	5 g fiber
2 g sugars	6 g protein	7 percent iron	

12 ounces whole-grain spaghetti

1 medium crown of broccoli, chopped

1 large lemon, juiced

2 garlic cloves, minced

½ tsp. red pepper flakes

2 TB. extra-virgin olive oil

A pinch of salt

1. Cook pasta in a pot of boiling water according to instructions on the package (about 10 minutes), then drain well and return the pot.

2. Steam broccoli over boiling water (in a steamer pot, if you have one; otherwise, place a colander in the pot and cover). When broccoli is bright green and slightly tender, remove from heat. Overcooking the broccoli will make it mushy, so keep a close eye on it.

3. Toss broccoli into the pasta and add lemon juice, garlic cloves, red pepper flakes, and olive oil. Season with salt to taste.

Essential Takeaways

- It's necessary to get water every day; although everybody's needs vary, aim for about 8 cups.

- Water hydrates your cells and organs and enables proper breakdown of your food into energy.

- You get water from drinking water, other beverages, and foods containing water.

- Most foods contain water; fruits and vegetables top the list. They can help curb your appetite with less calories, which has proven to be an effective weight-management tool.

chapter 15

Cheers: A Case for Alcohol

Looking at the pros and cons of alcohol

Distinguishing between different types of drinks

Deciding whether or not to imbibe

Do you ever wonder if that glass of wine you enjoy with dinner or couple of beers after work is good for you? Alcohol's effect on health has been under the research microscope since the early 1970s. Experts believe that alcohol acts differently in people—what may be beneficial for some, is not good for others. Overall, however, occasional imbibing shows promise for heart health, type 2 diabetes, and dementia. It may not bode so well for people prone to certain types of cancer, particularly breast cancer. Alcohol is the most abused drug in the United States, with 7 percent of American adults afflicted with a dependency on alcohol. Surprisingly, though, our society drinks less than people did 50 to 100 years ago. This chapter takes a sobering look at alcohol—the good, the bad, and the uncertain side of drinking.

The Buzz Behind Alcohol

Ethanol, the chemical component of alcoholic beverages, such as beer, wine, and spirits, is the key player in the neurological buzz— and eventual depression of the central nervous system—that you get from drinking alcohol. This is why drinking a beer or glass of wine enables you to break out of your shell and become less inhibited or maybe even the life of the party! However, after a few drinks that buzz can turn into heightened emotions—typically depressive, which can lead to tears, fears, anger, and/or overly amorous interactions. Having a few drinks also affects physical performance by slowing reaction time, which explains why driving a car or operating any type of equipment can be dangerous even after just one drink.

Serving Up Alcohol

The size of a standard drink is a 12-ounce beer, 5-ounce glass of wine, or 1½-ounce (standard shot) glass of distilled spirits. If you enjoy the taste of alcoholic beverages, it's important to set limits based on the standard serving sizes. Men should strive to drink no more than one to two drinks a day, while women should drink no more than one drink per day. These limits enable you to harness the health benefits of alcohol without suffering from its detrimental effects.

Do not save up your daily drinks for one day of the week—that's called binge drinking, and it's unhealthy. If you are a nondrinker, do not start drinking alcohol to reap its health benefits. Healthful, balanced eating and regular exercise trump drinking alcohol any day.

Mind Your Alcohol Calories

With 7 calories per gram, alcohol contains less calories than fat (9 calories per gram) and more than carbs and protein (4 calories per gram). Alcohol is not needed for growth, development, and healthy survival, so it's considered to be a source of empty calories.

In addition to empty calories in alcoholic drinks themselves, alcohol can cause eating amnesia, in which you forget from one minute to the next what you've eaten and, before you know it, you've eaten twice the amount of calories you'd normally eat at that time if you weren't drinking. The best way to watch the calories and number of drinks is to stagger plain water or mineral water with a fruit twist in between alcoholic beverages—you'll stay hydrated and fend off a hangover the next day, too.

Alcohol Calories Add Up	
Drink	*Calories**
Regular domestic beer (12 oz.)	140–170
Regular imported beer (12 oz.)	160–295
Light beer (12 oz.)	95–110
Hard cider (12 oz.)	140–200

Drink	Calories*
Table wine (5 oz.)	90–140
Dessert wine (2 oz.)	65–110
Distilled spirits (1.5 oz.)	100
Hard lemonade (11.2 oz.)	240
Hard light lemonade (11.2 oz.)	100
Wine cooler (12 oz.)	200
Margarita (4 oz.)	210
Gin martini (2 oz. alcohol)	140
Vodka soda (1.5 oz. vodka)	100
Vodka tonic (1.5 oz. vodka)	165
Cosmopolitan martini	215

*Calorie ranges are used when various brands contain different calorie levels.

Source: The CalorieKing Calorie, Fat, & Carbohydrate Counter, 2010 edition.

Alcohol in Your Blood

Because your body can't store alcohol like other nutrients, it makes a priority of eliminating it from the digestive tract. There is an enzyme called dehydrogenase, which breaks down alcohol in the stomach. Women have less of this enzyme than men, so alcohol passes from the stomach and into the bloodstream more quickly in women.

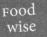

Food wise

Remember not to drink on an empty stomach; eating a sensible snack or meal while drinking slows the rate of alcohol absorption into the bloodstream.

The other thing that gets women tipsy faster than men is that alcohol likes to occupy water-filled spaces in the body (which also explains why it's dehydrating). On average, women are smaller and have more body fat than men, so there's less fluid space for it to occupy, and it stays in the bloodstream longer. It's believed that women only metabolize 10 percent of alcohol compared to 30 percent for men, so the *blood alcohol content (BAC)* varies quite a bit between genders. Plus, body weight, fat percentage, and age (the older you are the harder it is to process alcohol) affect BAC, also. That's why a single drink may not seem to affect a man but can make a woman drunk!

definition **Blood alcohol content (BAC)** measures the level of alcohol in your bloodstream. The legal BAC limit in the United States is 0.08 mL/L—that's the volume of alcohol in exhaled breath. BAC can also be measured by analyzing the urine and/or blood. It may only take five minutes after taking a sip of alcohol for your blood to register alcohol in it.

Alcohol and You

Alcohol is a bit of a mystery when it comes to health. The actual alcohol (or ethanol) appears to be the major beneficial component. As with all nutrition intervention, there is no one-size-fits-all answer when it comes to alcohol; you have to look at your unique set of health circumstances. A little alcohol can go a long way toward health, but decades of research has shown that you have to look at your genetic, medical, and gender-specific history to see whether it will have a positive or negative impact on your health.

For example, a 35-year-old woman with a family history of alcoholism, a cancerous lump removed from one of her breasts, and a sedentary lifestyle, would most likely not benefit from alcohol use—even in moderation. For her, the benefits of more fiber, fruits, vegetables, and regular physical activity would far exceed anything alcohol could do. However, a 50-year-old male with no family history of alcohol dependency, low HDL (good) cholesterol level, and fairly active lifestyle may benefit from a drink or two a day.

Even drinking reasonable amounts can lead to more drinking, especially if you have family history of alcohol addiction. As far as heart health, the research has shown that moderate alcohol consumption is particularly beneficial for increasing good, HDL-cholesterol levels. A drink or two a day has been shown to increase HDL by as much as 15 to 20 percent. This can reduce narrowing of the arteries (atherosclerosis) and risk for blood clots, two risk factors for heart attacks.

Alcohol and Cancer

On the flip side, even with alcohol's heart health benefits, moderate amounts (one or two drinks a day) can increase chances of cancer of the breast, liver, colon, throat, and/or mouth.

The likelihood of getting liver, colon, and oral cancers appears to increase with more than two drinks a day. Oral cancers are more prevalent in drinkers who smoke, as lowered inhibitions tend to make people light up. And breast tissue appears to be super sensitive to alcohol. With all cancers, aging (over age 50) causes your risk to go up. Although you can't stop the aging process, you can make lifestyle changes that will decrease your risk of cancer.

Even a drink a day puts women—young and old alike—at risk for being part of the one in eight women (12 to 13 percent of U.S. women) diagnosed with breast cancer over their lifetime. Men get breast cancer, too—but they comprise less than 1 percent of the cases. Even if you have no family history of breast cancer, you are not in the clear—70 to 80 percent of breast cancer occurs in women with no family links to the disease. Genetic abnormalities are believed to be the cancer culprit, and two of the biggest risk factors are being a woman and aging.

Alcohol and Your Weight

As we mentioned previously, your weight can be affected by even moderate drinking. Not only does drinking alcohol add empty calories to your diet, but alcohol is an appetite stimulant, meaning that it makes you want to eat. It also changes usual behaviors and can cause even the most disciplined eaters to throw in the towel and overindulge. Of course, the occasional episode of overconsumption (of both food and drink) is nothing to be alarmed about, but when it's a regular occurrence—twice a week or more—it should be addressed.

Strictly from a calorie standpoint, if you are drinking two regular beers a day, that's about 300 extra calories, which can lead to at least a half-pound of weight gain per week, unless you make up for those extra calories by eating less or exercising more. And if you eat less, then you might be replacing nutrient-rich calories with empty calories from alcohol, which is not a good choice for your health.

munch on This	Social, moderate drinking has proven to have healthful heart benefits than drinking solo. In a large study of middle-aged Japanese men, those who enjoyed a drink or two with friends, co-workers, or family members enjoyed better health from the social support—as well as a healthier lifestyle as they were found to be more active, too. So grab a drink with your cronies and toast to your good health!

Chronic heavy alcohol use can lead to weight loss and malnutrition. The notion of the "liquid lunch," in which one forgoes food for the sake of drinking alcohol, is a reality for some people. If you drink and don't eat well, this can lead to a calorie deficit and anorexic tendencies, which causes muscle wasting or loss, disruption of menstrual cycles in women, vitamin and mineral deficiencies, and damage to major organs such as the liver and heart.

Alcohol and Your Brain

Although alcohol can affect the brain in a variety of ways, moderate drinking has shown to protect the brain from cognitive decline or dementia. A French study showed that dementia and/or Alzheimer's disease was lower among moderate wine drinkers, thanks to the alcohol (or ethanol), which is believed to be the protective agent for keeping the brain sharp and healthy in older men and women. So feel free to enjoy a glass of red wine every day to prevent brain drain!

Alcohol and Blood Sugar

The dangers of drinking on an empty stomach, especially for someone with diabetes, is that alcohol can cause hypoglycemia (or a drop in blood sugar). It is vital to eat food along with your alcoholic beverage to avoid dangerously low blood sugar levels.

The good news is that moderate amounts (one to two drinks a day) of alcohol can cause insulin, the hormone the helps blood sugar get into your cells for energy, work better in the body. In a study of almost 3,000 healthy, middle-aged Japanese men, moderate drinking improved insulin sensitivity, therefore making it easier for sugar (glucose) to enter the cells and fend off type 2 diabetes. Results from a different study of 51 older, nondiabetic women found that after eight weeks of having two drinks per day (compared with the group that did not drink or abstained) their insulin sensitivity went up and fasting insulin levels went down—which is all good!

Uncorking the Health Benefits of Wine

Wine experienced a surge of popularity in the United States in the 1990s when news exploded about its potential heart health benefits. Certain cultures, such as the French, have less heart disease even though they eat high saturated fat foods, and researchers believe the answer, resveratrol *(rez-veer-AH-trahl),* could be in the wine they love to drink. Called "The French Paradox" the decades-old theory of eating high-fat foods but counteracting them with wine still needs more scientific explanation, yet a connecting observation is that wine drinkers typically lead a healthy lifestyle—they are typically more active, don't smoke, and eat a wide variety of nutritious foods.

What's in Wine

The skins, seeds, and stems of grapes are high in chemical compounds called polyphenols. More than a heart elixir, polyphenols affect the taste, color, and mouthfeel (how wine feels in your mouth). Polyphenols are divided into two groups, called flavonoids and nonflavonoids. Flavonoids called anthocynanins give wine its rich color; flavonoids called tannins provide the bulk of the feel in your mouth. The nonflavonoids contain the chemical resveratrol, a component in the skin of grapes. It's thought to be a powerful player in health, particularly heart health.

The Health Benefits of Resveratrol

Studies on insect and mice have shown that resveratrol may increase life span and counteract the detrimental effects of a high-fat diet. Mice fed a high-fat diet and given resveratrol had a lower mortality (death) rate—one similar to that of mice on a balanced, healthy diet—than mice just fed a diet high in saturated fat.

As for your heart, resveratrol may prevent cardiac disease by keeping the lining of the heart (endothelium) in working order and helping keep LDL (bad) cholesterol levels in check. It's also been shown to aid in lowering total cholesterol and blood sugar in diabetic rats and might also decrease diabetes symptoms like the desire to eat too much (polyphagia) and excessive thirst (polydipsia).

Resveratrol may also fend off viruses like the genital and oral versions of the herpes simplex virus. Studies have found that resveratrol stops the growth of herpes cells by impairing herpes genes and the production of viral DNA (genetic material). It's a complex process, in which many questions remain unanswersed, but resveratrol has proven to be beneficial in squelching the effects of the herpes virus.

Not only does resveratrol fend off plaque formation in the blood vessels, but it might keep away beta-amyloid plaques—a cause of Alzheimer's disease and other mind-eroding diseases—in your brain. To see these benefits, however, you'd have to drink more wine than anyone could reasonably drink on a daily basis. Researchers believe given in supplement form, it may prevent your brain from aging.

To Drink or Not?

Experts believe that abstinence from alcohol isn't necessary if you enjoy a drink or two with a meal, but you should steer clear of it if you fall into any of the following categories:

- You can't control the amount of alcohol you drink.

- You are pregnant or trying to conceive a child.

- You are taking prescription or nonprescription medications.

- You plan to drive or operate heavy equipment, such as a car, motorcycle, or even a bicycle.

- You plan to participate in physical activities or sports that require concentration and skill (e.g., swimming, ice skating, or skate boarding, etc.).

- You are at high risk for any type of cancer.

Wine and other alcoholic beverages are social and a culinary staple worldwide. Like any dietary substance, too much can be toxic and harmful to the body. Know your limits, understand the ramifications for your body, and drink responsibly. And cheers to your good health!

Essential Takeaways

- Drinking alcohol in moderation can be healthy for some, but harmful for others. Know your individual risk factors.

- In some people, alcohol can decrease the risk of heart disease, type 2 diabetes, and dementia; in others it can increase the risk of cancer.

- Drinking alcohol on a regular basis can lead to unwanted weight gain.

- Because alcohol relaxes people's inhibitions, people tend to eat more food when drinking, which can load on extra calories.

- Wine, beer, and distilled spirits all contain the same amount of alcohol per standard serving size: 5 ounces, 12 ounces, and 1.5 ounces, respectively.

- Avoid alcohol if you are prone to overdrinking; pregnant or trying to conceive a baby; operating heavy equipment; playing sports; or at risk for cancer.

Part 4

Real Food to the Rescue

How can real food play a role in revving up your metabolism or helping you sleep better? This part looks at overall wellness and how certain foods can come to your rescue with cutting-edge nutrition tips. The following chapters look at the latest science on fighting inflammation and boosting your immunity, too.

Plus, I delve into the wonderful world of sleep: enough of it is a good thing, but too much or too little and your health will pay the price. The good news is that good nutrition can affect your sleep positively and give you the overall wellness you need—without medication.

chapter 16

Inflammation Fighters

Understanding inflammation

Eating anti-inflammatory foods

Making inflammation-reducing recipes

Inflammation is your body's natural way of healing. We've all experienced acute inflammation at one time or another, whether you burned your tongue on hot food, got a splinter in your finger, or stubbed your toe, inflammation sets in fast. Some of the first signs are pain, redness, and swelling—you know exactly where the injury is straight away!

Chronic inflammation occurs when acute inflammation lasts for weeks, months, or even years. The site of inflammation is in a perpetual state of defense against foreign invaders produced by toxins, which can ultimately lead to irreversible tissue damage and a condition called fibrosis, in which the affected tissue can no longer perform its usual function.

Chronic inflammation can also travel deep in the body and silently attack the lining of blood vessels (endothelium) and organs such as the heart. This is called systemic inflammation and is the focus of this chapter.

What can you do to fend off systemic, silent inflammation? Cleaning up your lifestyle helps. Start with weight loss (if you need it) and make healthful food choices. Although more research may be needed to hone in on which foods work best for reducing inflammation, choosing high-fiber whole grains, vegetables, fruits, nuts, fish, olive oil, herbs, and spices are currently acknowledged as helpful choices.

This chapter dives deeply into inflammation and looks at the best ways to keep it at bay.

Inflammatory Markers

Weight gain is the most obvious indicator of inflammation that you can't see. Obesity can create changes internally that cause your immune system to mobilize the troops for inflammatory battle.

Why? Extra pounds on the scale and inches around your middle can cause a cascade of events: rising levels of LDL (bad) cholesterol, triglycerides (a blood fat), blood sugar, and blood pressure; while decreasing levels of beneficial HDL-cholesterol. This cluster of conditions is a sign of *metabolic syndrome,* a condition that puts you at risk for injury inside your arterial walls that you may not know about until it's too late. Your immune system steps in to save your arteries from injury, creating an inflammatory state in an attempt to heal the arterial walls. Basically, your immune system sends up a flair indicating that something is wrong inside of you!

Definition	**Metabolic syndrome** is a triad of disorders that includes high blood pressure, high blood sugar, and high cholesterol levels, which collectively lead to insulin resistance. It is primarily related to excess fat around your midsection.

Anti-Inflammatory Eating Patterns

Because inflammation may be a mirror on the wall into future heart attacks, stroke, and diseases, the medical and nutrition community has made strides in making the public aware of ways to cut inflammatory processes in your body. The first line of defense used to be medication for inflammatory diseases like rheumatoid and osteoarthritis. Recent research indicates that food can provide just as much relief, although it may take longer to see results. However, changing your overall pattern of eating can help with so much more than just inflammation!

Many of the foods that are believed to be anti-inflammatory are part of cultures that eat more plants, high-fiber carbohydrates (e.g., whole grains, beans, legumes), and oily fish, nuts, and olive oil; and consume less red meat and saturated and trans fats. Diets of the Mediterranean and Asian cultures naturally incorporate this style of eating. In addition, people who eat this way typically have a healthy body weight, get plenty of exercise, and are nonsmokers.

Healing Hints	Popping medications such as nonsteroidal anti-inflammatory drugs (NSAIDs), such as ibuprofen, on a daily basis is not the best bet from a health standpoint. NSAIDs may actually create a whole host of health problems, including indigestion (take the meds with a meal to alleviate this), nausea, vomiting, diarrhea, and more severe problems like heart attack, stroke, and intestinal bleeding. Use food as your anti-inflammatory agent instead of NSAIDs!

Trans fats are one of the primary food culprits that trigger inflammation. They are found in store-bought baked goods and some stick margarines. Check the nutrition facts on labels to make sure there are 0 grams of trans fat and avoid any foods that list "partially hydrogenated vegetable oils" in the ingredient listing.

Your overall pattern of eating or total diet has an impact on your body's inflammation levels. Healthful, balanced eating is anti-inflammatory eating, and vice versa.

Eat Fewer Calories

Less is more when it comes to eating to fend off inflammation. Evidence shows that calorie restriction and losing just 5 to 7 percent of your body weight (if you need to) can bring down the inflammatory fire in your body. Immune cells tend to go haywire as fat cells multiply, meaning that obesity is a hallmark of inflammation. In addition, obesity leads to higher levels of insulin—the hormone that regulates blood sugar—in the bloodstream, which also fires up the immune system.

munch on this
There are 3,500 calories in a pound of fat, so to lose a pound a week you need to eliminate 500 calories a day from your diet. Skip the Venti Frappaccino (with whip cream) or extras like butter, cream cheese, bacon, and mayonnaise, and you'll be amazed how easy it can be to lose a pound in a week.

Monitor Your Fat Intake

Although eating fat does not necessarily make you fat, the calories from fatty foods can add up fast. Because saturated fat and trans fat contribute to inflammatory diseases like atherosclerosis (plaque in the arteries) and obesity—which can lead to rheumatoid and osteoarthritis and diabetes—it's important to pay attention to these fats in your diet.

Unsaturated fats (monounsaturated and polyunsaturated fats—including omega-3 fats) have potential in fending off inflammation. This includes good fat foods like olive oil, canola oil, fish, walnuts, and avocados. Aim for at least 2 tablespoons of olive and/or canola oil per day; two 6-ounce servings of fatty fish (wild salmon, halibut, tuna, and sardines) per week and 1 ounce of walnuts per day for omega-3 fats; at least one fifth (1 ounce) of a medium avocado per day.

Take a close look at the types of fat you eat in a day and start replacing saturated and trans fats with unsaturated fats. Because fatty foods usually have a combination of saturated and unsaturated fat, we look at the main or primary fat in that food. The following table identifies the various types of fats in several common foods. Keep in mind that plant foods typically have unsaturated fat and meat usually contains saturated fat, which sets off the inflammatory response.

Anti-Inflammatory Fat Guide

Food	Primary fat	Anti-Inflammatory Potential
Avocado	Unsaturated	Yes
Bacon	Saturated	No
Butter	Saturated	No
Canola oil	Unsaturated	Yes
Cheese	Saturated	No
Coffee creamers	Trans fats	No
French fries	Saturated	No
Milk chocolate	Saturated	No
Oily fish	Unsaturated	Yes
Olive oil	Unsaturated	Yes
Nuts	Unsaturated	Yes
Red meat	Saturated	No
Seeds	Unsaturated	Yes
Store-baked goods	Trans fats	No

Use the information on this table to make wise choices about which fats to eat to fend off inflammation. This is not to say that you can never eat any saturated fats (however, you should try to avoid all trans fats), but you should try to limit them to 7 to 10 percent of your total daily caloric intake. Unsaturated fats should make up the other 15 to 20 percent of your daily fat intake.

Eat More Plants

Plant-based foods are low in fat and calories (except nuts); high in antioxidants like vitamins A, C, and E, and carotenoids like beta-carotene, lycopene, lutein, and zeaxanthin; and are high in dietary fiber. Fruits, vegetables, whole grains, nuts, seeds, beans, and legumes are all powerful players in weight loss and management. And you already know that losing weight is one of the most effective means of minimizing inflammation in your body.

Healing Hints	Because the average American falls far short of meeting the recommended daily amounts of whole grains, fruits, and vegetables, the 2010 Dietary Guidelines for Americans recommends we focus more on plant-based foods and less on animal products.

Plant-based foods also contain many immune-boosting compounds called phyto (plant) nutrients. They can do your body a whole host of good by helping to decrease the severity of cold symptoms, fend off disease, and keep energy levels up.

In addition, fruits, vegetables, and whole grains typically offer a lower glycemic load, which means they don't raise blood sugar as high as those that are more refined, higher glycemic carbohydrates, such as cakes, cookies, candy, soft drinks, and white bread. Although, it's not completely clear if these high glycemic foods play a role in inflammation, continually plying your body with refined sugar, which requires a lot of insulin, can place extra wear and tear on your blood vessels. This arterial damage can set the wheels in motion for your immune system to fix the damaged blood vessels, which triggers an inflammatory response.

Eat Less Red Meat

An occasional steak, burger, or slice of bacon isn't going to send your immune system into crisis mode, but a daily dose of high-fat red meat—which is full of saturated fat, cholesterol, sodium, and calories—may increase risk factors for inflammation, such as elevations in blood pressure, blood cholesterol, and weight. Try to replace most of the red meat in your diet with skinless chicken or turkey breast. Experts recommend cutting red meat to 18 ounces per week (that's 3.6 ounces over five days a week). In addition, they recommend avoiding meat with additives like nitrates or nitrites, such as lunch meats, hot dogs, bacon, and sausages, as these may aggravate chronic inflammation.

Try to go meatless at least two days per week. Instead, try these meat-free sources of protein:

- Add black, kidney, or white beans to chili, soups, and stews

- Enjoy falafels (chick pea balls) in pita bread

- Spread hummus on rice cakes

- Toss cubed, extra-firm tofu into pasta salads or stir-fries

- Add bean dips to sandwiches

- Fill peppers or cabbage rolls with a mixture of soy crumbles and rice

Spice Squelchers

Sprinkling certain spices in your food can slow the progression or fend off the slow, silent burn of chronic inflammation. Two spices that are believed to have both antioxidant and anti-inflammatory properties are turmeric (the active component is curcumin, which gives curry it's orange-yellow color) and ginger. These two spices appear to be able to regulate inflammatory cytokines—substances that are involved in many steps of the inflammatory response—just like pharmaceutical medications.

MUNCH ON THIS   A recent study found that turmeric and ginger decreased the number of cases and severity of rheumatoid arthritis in rats. Turmeric proved to be a bit more potent than ginger in acting on sites of inflammation.

Turmeric (Curcumin)

Turmeric has been revered for its anti-inflammatory properties since the onset of Ayurvedic medicine around 1900 B.C.E. Its active component, curcumin, has been used as a nontoxic drug for pain, swelling, and inflammatory diseases like arthritis in both Indian and Chinese medicine. Although curcumin doesn't appear to have any nutritional value, it's been found to regulate the immune system very well. Also, it's a highly tolerable spice with safe doses up to 12 grams (0.8 tablespoon) a day.

Ginger

Ginger has been used as a natural anti-inflammatory for centuries. Indonesian medicine uses red ginger—a type of ginger with a purplish peel that's high in anthocyanin pigments—as a remedy for arthritis pain. In the early 1970s researchers discovered ginger's powerful compounds, such as gingerols and shogaols, were on par with nonsteroidal anti-inflammatory drugs (NSAIDs).

So flavor your food and fend off inflammation at the same time in the following ways:

- Sprinkle turmeric or curry powder into soups, stews, chili, or over steamed vegetables with brown rice.

- Add fresh, minced ginger to salad dressings, homemade lemonade, noodle dishes, and tea. Bake it into muffins and quick breads.

- Sprinkle dry, powdered ginger into smoothies, over roasted new potatoes, and into mashed sweet potatoes.

- Chop crystallized ginger into homemade cookies, brownies, oatmeal, and cream of wheat or farina.

Soy and Tea

Studies have shown that Asian cultures have lower incidence of certain cancers, such as prostate cancer in men. One possible explanation is that certain components of their diet fend off inflammation. Inflammation of the prostate is a strong determinant of prostate cancer down the road. In particular, researchers have found that soy foods—such as tofu, tempeh, soymilk, and edamame—and green tea may have anti-inflammatory powers.

Asian men eat about 25 to 100 milligrams of soyfoods per day—that's 1 to 4 servings of tofu, soybeans, or soymilk. American-born Asians eat significantly less soy—only about 1 to 3 milligrams per day. Similarly, Asian men drink at least 2 cups of green tea a day, whereas American-born Asian men as a whole don't even average a cup a day. The inflammatory marker of prostate cancer is 50 percent higher in Asian men born in the United States than men born in Asia. The educated medical guess is that those with a higher consumption of soyfoods and green tea fend off inflammation in the prostate.

Why are soyfoods and green tea thought to defend against inflammation in men? Although further examination is required, one research review suggests that soy's anti-inflammatory action is due to its plant-based estrogens called isoflavones, which may affect the action of cancer-causing hormones. As for green tea, its powerful polyphenol called epigallocatechin-3-gallate (EGCG) is thought to be the prime anti-inflammatory agent.

So upping the soyfoods and green tea may prevent chronic inflammation of the prostate.

food wise

Women (or men) who are prone to breast cancer should consult their health-care provider before eating significant amounts of soyfoods, as their plant hormones might actually increase risk for breast cancer.

Inflammation-Reducing Recipes

Try these recipes to help reduce inflammation and fend off future diseases.

Simple Veggie Chow Mein

This is a fun way to incorporate more color and crunchiness (and anti-inflammation) into a meal. Feel free to add other veggies or tofu.

Yield:	Serving size:	Prep time:	Cook time:
2 servings	1 cup	10 minutes	20 minutes

Each serving has:			
557 calories	46 g total fat	4 g saturated fat	0 g trans fat
0 mg cholesterol	82 mg sodium	34 g carbohydrates	6 g fiber
13 g sugars	6 g protein	14 percent iron	

¼ lb. Chinese soba noodles or whole-grain linguini

¼ cup low-sodium soy sauce

¼ cup lemon juice

1 TB. rice wine vinegar

1 TB. *agave nectar*

2½ TB. sesame oil

¼ cup canola oil

1 garlic clove, peeled and crushed

1 cup shiitake mushrooms

1 cup sugar snap peas

½ small red pepper, cut into thin strips

4 green onions (scallion), finely sliced

1 cup zucchini, sliced

1. Cook noodles in lightly salted boiling water, following the cooking instructions on the package (about 10 minutes). Once cooked, drain them and set them aside.

2. Meanwhile, whisk together soy sauce, lemon juice, rice wine vinegar, agave nectar, and 1 TB. sesame oil, and canola oil. Set aside.

3. Heat 1½ TB. of sesame oil in a wok or large skillet. Add garlic and stir-fry for a few seconds. Add shiitake mushrooms, sugar snap peas, and red pepper; sauté for 4 to 5 minutes, stirring occasionally. Add green onions and zucchini and continue to cook for a few minutes, stirring occasionally.

4. Add noodles to the pan with vegetables and stir in marinade. Cook for 1 to 2 minutes, or until noodles are heated completely. Serve immediately.

Definition

Agave nectar is a syruplike sweetener made from the agave plant. You can purchase it at any grocery store, usually in the natural food section.

Curried Stuffed Peppers with Peas and Leeks

Feel free to add soy crumbles, lean ground beef or turkey to the stuffing mixture and substitute any vegetables that you like. Use the stuffing in large tomatoes instead of peppers, if you desire.

Yield:	Serving size:	Prep time:	Cook time:
2 servings	1 stuffed pepper	5 minutes	25 minutes

Each serving has:			
346 calories	9 g total fat	1 g saturated fat	0 g trans fat
1 mg cholesterol	444 mg sodium	59 g carbohydrates	14 g fiber
13 g sugars	11 g protein	23 percent iron	

1 leek, chopped

1 TB. extra-virgin olive oil

½ cup green peas

½ cup barley, uncooked (1 cup, cooked)

1¼ cups low-sodium vegetable broth

1 TB. tomato paste

¼ tsp. curry powder or turmeric

Pinch of salt and pepper

2 large bell peppers, top cut off and hollowed out

Dash of parmesan cheese, optional

1. Preheat oven to 400°F.

2. Put broth and barley in a saucepan over high heat, bring to a boil, and turn heat down to simmer. Cover and let cook until liquid is dissolved.

3. In a large skillet over medium heat, add oil and sauté leeks, peas, cooked barley, curry or turmeric, tomato paste, salt, and pepper.

4. Stuff peppers with the mixture, add a sprinkle of parmesan cheese on top, if desired, and bake for 20 minutes. When peppers have softened, they are done.

Edamame, Red Pepper, and Ginger Salad

Add any type of bean(s) that you like to this dish for a fiber-filled, plant-based meal or snack.

Yield:	Serving size:	Prep time:	Cook time:
4 servings	2 tablespoons	5 minutes	None

Each serving has:			
274 calories	14 g total fat	3 g saturated fat	0 g trans fat
6 mg cholesterol	130 mg sodium	18 g carbohydrates	5 g fiber
5 g sugars	19 g protein	43 percent iron	

1 cup edamame (soybeans), frozen and shelled	1 TB. fresh ginger, minced
1 cup red bell pepper, chopped	2 TB. extra-virgin olive oil
1 shallot, minced	1 TB. balsamic vinegar
2 TB. feta cheese, crumbled	1 TB. Dijon mustard
	Salt and pepper

1. Defrost edamame on the countertop for an hour (or heat in the microwave on high for 60 seconds).

2. Toss edamame, red pepper, shallot, feta cheese, and ginger in large mixing bowl.

3. In a separate bowl whisk together olive oil, vinegar, and mustard and pour mixture on top of vegetables. Toss to coat, and add salt and pepper as desired. Serve with whole-grain pita chips or as a filling in a small, whole-grain pita.

Essential Takeaways

- Inflammation is the body's natural way of healing. It's marked by pain, redness, immobility, swelling, and heat.

- Acute inflammation is felt immediately and lasts briefly; chronic inflammation can be silent and last for years, which can cause lasting damage.

- Anti-inflammatory eating is the same as a healthful diet: more fruits, vegetables, whole grains, fish, nuts, beans, legumes, and olive oil. Plus, adding spices like ginger and turmeric can help promote anti-inflammation efforts as well.

- Weight loss is the best way to decrease systemic and chronic inflammation.

chapter 17

Metabolism Boosters

- Making sense of your metabolism
- Firing up your energy engine with foods
- Making your own metabolism-boosting meals

Metabolism refers to the transformation of food into energy. Your metabolic rate is the rate at which you turn food into energy-giving fuel. It is partly dictated by your genes, but also partly by how much you move, your age, what you eat, and your overall health. Metabolism is where The Big Three nutrients—carbs, proteins, and fats—really come into play. Your body breaks down these nutrients for energy but also uses them to build up tissue and cells in your body.

The food you eat does affect your metabolism. Chewing, biting, swallowing, and moving foods along the digestive tract takes energy. In general, your body devotes about 10 percent of its energy to just digesting the food you eat. The energy required to eat and digest food is called the thermic effect of food. Certain foods are believed to require more energy to digest, which means that they have a higher thermic effect.

Some foods require more energy to digest than others. Protein-rich foods, such as low-fat dairy products, fish, eggs, and beans have the greatest thermic effect, using up to 30 percent more energy than fats, which use only 2 to 3 percent of your body's energy to digest. Carbohydrates fall in the middle of protein and fats when it comes to how much energy is required for digestion.

High-fiber foods are also effective at keeping your metabolism on its toes. Because they move so slowly through your system, they help stabilize blood sugar levels and keep you feeling full longer.

This keeps your metabolic rate steady, which means you're hungry less often and eat less! It's a fascinating process, and this chapter delves into the foods and behaviors that can remodel and reshape your metabolism for life.

Metabolism-Boosting Food and Drinks

The more you stoke your metabolic flame throughout the day, the more efficiently you'll burn calories and maintain a healthy body weight. After age 30, metabolism begins to decline by a rate of about 3 to 5 percent every year. To keep it moving, try eating 5 to 6 small meals throughout the day. And don't skip breakfast as this jumpstarts your metabolism for the day! If you go too long between meals without any healthy snacks, you will create a slow, less efficient metabolism.

Calorie-loading at any time of day, but especially at night (unless you work at night), can set you up for weight gain and a slow metabolism. The evening is typically wind-down mode for your metabolism as you prepare for sleep. Make it a habit to stop eating at least two hours before you go to bed. Getting enough sleep—at least seven hours—every night also does wonders for your metabolic rate. (I talk more about this in Chapter 19.)

Specific foods show promise in the metabolism department. They're like high-octane fuel to keep your body engine running in peak condition. Research in this area is abundant; we know that spices, protein-packed grains, green tea, coffee, and high-fiber foods like beans and legumes can improve your metabolic rate. Replacing some fat with fiber and carbs with protein can do wonders to fire up your calorie-burning power throughout the day. Of course, it doesn't hurt to go for a walk, run, or jog, as movement keeps your metabolism firing. And remember, the more muscle you have, the more calories you burn at rest, so try to squeeze in some strength-training, too.

Chili Peppers

Hot chili peppers do more than add fire to your taste buds; they can rev up the rate at which you burn calories. Research has shown the chemical compound in hot chili peppers called capsaicin is responsible for the metabolic boost that may help slim your waistline. It's the seeds and thin, white membranes inside chili peppers that create the heat.

Because not all heat in chili peppers is equal, the actual burn among hot chili pepper family members is quantified on a scale called the Scoville scale. The number of Scoville units assigned to a pepper tells you the amount of capsaicin present in a chili pepper; it indicates how much a pepper's heat would have to be diluted before the capsaicin is not detectable on the tongue. A sweet or bell pepper—with no heat—would rank zero on the Scoville scale as it contains no capsaicin. Pure capsaicin is 15 to 16 million Scoville units.

Food wise

Some people can handle the heat more than others—so know your tolerance. Some of the hottest peppers can cause severe gastrointestinal pain in sensitive people.

The following table lists some of the hottest peppers out there:

Chili Peppers Heat Power	
Pepper Name	*Heat Rating in Scoville Units*
Naga Viper/Naga Jolokia	855,000–1,359,000
Red Sabivia Bonnet	580,000
Scotch Bonnet/Habanero	100,000–350,000
Cayenne	30,000–50,000
Serrano	10,000–23,000
Jalapeño	2,500–8,000
Poblano	500–2,500

Use hot peppers strategically in cooking by adding cayenne pepper flakes to pasta sauce, pizza, meat rubs, and chili. Stuff the cooler peppers like poblanos with rice and cheese or dice them up into guacamole for a bit of a punch. Toss slices of jalapeño into a stir-fry. Studies found that even sweet and bell peppers can have some effect on metabolism as they contain nonpungent capsaicin compounds called capsinoids. These taste-neutral compounds have been shown to increase energy expenditure—without the irritating heat—by stimulating intestinal nerves. So something to think about when you want to add sweetness to an omelet, pasta sauce, chili, or salad.

Protein-Rich Foods

If hot peppers aren't your thing, remember, protein can give you a slight metabolic boost as it requires a bit more energy to digest and absorb into your muscles, thus more calories are expended just by eating high-protein foods. The proteins in milk, casein, and whey, have been shown to slightly raise thermogenesis, the energy needed to digest food. Whey protein is a favorite for body building enthusiasts because it has a lot of high-quality protein per ounce. So as we mentioned, protein raises your metabolism slightly more than carbs or fat. Plus, protein helps you feel more satiated and less hungry throughout the day by keeping blood sugar and insulin levels stable and keeping your metabolism moving at a steady rate.

Almonds

Nuts are a great source of protein. Almonds have shown specific promise as they boost energy with 6 grams of protein per serving (23 almonds). A study in which 20 healthy, overweight women consumed an extra 300 calories in almonds a day over a 10-week period found no increase in body weight as they compensated for the additional calories by not eating as much at the next meal as they weren't as hungry. Plus, the protein helped keep their metabolisms humming along.

Walnuts

Walnuts are another great protein source. They have 4 grams of protein per ounce (7 whole walnuts; 14 halves). In a study of 16 overweight people, the walnut-eating group was found to have greater fat loss and energy expenditure over the nonwalnut group. Thus, the metabolic rate was affected (for the better) in the people who ate walnuts.

Healing Hints

Some great ways to get almonds and walnuts is to chop them up and toss them into hot cereal, yogurt, salads, chili, quick breads, and over fresh fruit.

Quinoa

With 9 grams of protein per cup, quinoa is a great metabolism booster. Substitute some of the other grains in your diet with a higher protein option like quinoa to get an extra energy boost. Add quinoa to leafy green salads or toss a handful of dried fruit, nuts, and a dash of curry into it for a delish meal in no time.

Caffeine Kick

When it comes to metabolism, caffeine's role is questionable. Some research has shown that it promotes greater energy expenditure and weight loss; others show that it causes weight gain by increasing stress hormones. If you use caffeine to get an extra kick, watch the sugar-sweetened coffee and tea drinks as the calories can counteract any calorie-burning boost. And choose the lower-fat, dark chocolate; not only will you get a tad more caffeine, but less calories and fat, which can only bode well for stimulating your metabolic rate.

Cinnamon

Numerous studies have shown that cinnamon helps keep blood sugar levels in check. If blood sugar levels are stable, hunger and fullness are controlled at a steady rate, which is ideal for an efficient metabolism. Studies have shown that only ½ teaspoon a day of cinnamon can do wonders! Sprinkle cinnamon onto sliced apples or in applesauce, hot cereal, plain yogurt, pumpkin soup, creamed cauliflower, and rice pudding.

Munch on This

Chewing gum may give you a metabolic boost! One study found that people who chew sugarless gum burned 11 more calories per hour than those that did not chew gum. Be careful, though—sugarless gum that contains polyols (such as sorbitol and xylitol) can wreak havoc on your digestive tract causing diarrhea, gas, and bloating.

Beans

Not only are beans packed with protein as natural metabolic uppers, but they are high in fiber—which has been shown to regulate metabolism by keeping blood sugar steady and making you feel full with fewer calories for a longer period of time. In other words, fiber can help control how many calories you eat. Beans contain from 10 to 16 grams of fiber per cup, which is almost half of the fiber you should get in a day.

Here are the top five beans to fire up with fiber (1 cup, cooked):

Split peas, 16.3 grams

Lentils, 15.6 grams

Black beans, 15 grams

Lima beans, 13.2 grams

Baked beans, 10.4 grams

Simple ways to add beans to your life are to toss black beans into tacos or fajitas, add kidney beans to chili and stews, make split pea soup, or have a baked bean casserole as a main meal. Steam edamame over boiling water in its shell and sprinkle with a touch of kosher salt for a protein-packed appetizer or side dish.

---

munch on This

Research has shown that soy foods can affect how your body metabolizes sugar and fat, thus it's been shown to keep blood sugar levels steady and contribute to weight and fat loss. Although more research is needed to determine exactly what in soy foods creates the metabolic benefits, it can't hurt your metabolism to add some soybeans to your weekly meal plans.

Be aware that soy can affect metabolism for the better and worse. Like all foods, eat soy in moderation as raw soy products (e.g., tofu and soymilk) can be goitrogenic, meaning they can affect the thyroid gland, which is the gland that regulates metabolism. What can you do? Cook soy foods before eating them and stick to a serving or two a day—that's ½ cup of tofu or edamame and 1 cup of soymilk.

Chilled Water

The temperature of the water you drink may play a role in metabolic rate. Ice-cold water appears to tweak your metabolism as your body has to work a bit harder to heat the water up to absorb it.

So add a handful of ice cubes to water or choose iced tea or iced coffee over the hot stuff.

Food wise

The thyroid gland controls metabolism and hormone levels in your body. Raw cabbage, as well as other raw cruciferous veggies, may act as goitrogens, meaning they may block the thyroid from getting enough iodine, which is the mineral needed for proper thyroid function. This can lead to a low-functioning thyroid (hypothyroidism) or a goiter, an enlarged thyroid gland, which appears as a large lump in the throat. Cooking raw veggies can alleviate this problem, plus being aware of goitrogenic foods and eating them in moderation. For a list of goitrogenic foods visit thyroid.about.com/cs/drugdatabase/f/goitrogen.htm.

Rev Up Recipes

Here are some recipes to tweak your metabolism by using hot chili peppers, nuts, or beans.

Mushroom and Chili Pepper Crepes

These crepes are delicious served for brunch and dinner. They make a perfect presentation when hosting house guests. You can add other vegetables, too, such as spinach, red peppers, and/or zucchini.

Yield:	Serving size:	Prep time:	Cook time:
6–8 crepes	1 crepe	15 minutes	5 minutes

Each serving has:			
143 calories	0 g total fat	2 g saturated fat	0 g trans fat
42 mg cholesterol	109 mg sodium	12 g carbohydrates	2 g fiber
6 g sugars	5 g protein	5 percent iron	

½ cup onions, minced

2 TB. canola oil

2 garlic cloves, minced

1 cup tomatoes, chopped

1 small poblano pepper, chopped, seeds and membranes removed

1 cup water

1 tsp. cumin

¼ tsp. coriander seed, ground

¼ tsp. cayenne pepper

¼ tsp. black pepper

½ tsp. chili powder

2 TB. tomato paste

2 tsp. dry red wine (optional)

1 cup white whole-wheat flour

1 cup low-fat milk or soymilk

1 egg

1 TB. canola oil

Pinch of salt

½ cup mushrooms (any type you prefer), sliced

¼ cup low-fat Swiss cheese, diced

1 tsp. vegetable oil

1. Sauté onions and garlic in oil until onions are translucent. Add tomatoes, poblano peppers, water, cumin, coriander seed, cayenne pepper, black pepper, chili powder, tomato paste, and wine. Cover and simmer; the flavor of the spices will come out the longer they cook. Taste and add a pinch of salt if necessary prior to serving.

2. For crepes, combine flour, milk, egg, oil, and salt in a mixing bowl. Mix with a handheld blender or with a spoon until batter is smooth. Heat oil in a small, nonstick (10-in.) omelet pan. When pan is hot, pour in enough batter to thinly coat bottom of pan. When crepe appears to be solid, lift the edges gently and flip over with a small spatula. Turn out onto clean, dry surface.

3. For filling, heat small pan, add oil and mushrooms. Sauté until mushrooms are golden brown. Spoon mushrooms onto crepes and sprinkle with cheese; fold crepe over and drizzle with chili sauce. Crepes can be served hot, cold, or at room temperature.

Healing Hints

To store for later use, stack crepes on a large plate until you need to reheat them. They can be kept warm by wrapping them in a dishtowel and putting them on a plate set over a saucepan of simmering water. To freeze, stack them with sheets of waxed paper in-between; wrap in plastic wrap and then place in the freezer.

Sweet and Spicy Tofu Stir-Fry

This dish is fabulous over a dollop of brown rice or thin soba noodles.

Yield:	Serving size:	Prep time:	Cook time:
2 servings	1 cup	35 minutes	15 minutes

Each serving has:			
423 calories	23 g total fat	3 g saturated fat	0 g trans fat
0 mg cholesterol	445 mg sodium	38 g carbohydrates	10 g fiber
19 g sugars	21 g protein	41 percent iron	

1 cup extra-firm regular tofu	2 tsp. cayenne pepper
1 TB. low-sodium soy sauce	2 cups broccoli florets
1 TB. hoisin sauce (an Asian dipping sauce available in regular grocery stores or ethnic markets)	1 cup mushrooms, diced
	1 medium red pepper, sliced
	1 cup snow peas
2 TB. rice wine vinegar	½ cup water chestnuts, sliced
1 TB. peanut or canola oil	½ cup scallions, diced
1 TB. honey	¼ cup sesame seeds

1. Rinse and drain tofu; pat dry with paper towels. Cut into 1½-in. squares, place in a medium bowl. Combine soy sauce, hoisin sauce, rice wine, oil, honey, and cayenne pepper in a small bowl. Gently toss tofu with ¼ cup of the marinade, reserving the rest for later. Cover and let tofu marinate in the refrigerator for 30 minutes, gently turn the tofu after 15 minutes.

2. Heat oil in wok or sauté pan over medium heat. Place tofu and remaining marinade in the wok or pan, gently stirring it. Slowly add broccoli, mushrooms, red pepper, snow peas, water chestnuts, and scallions. Cover the pan to allow vegetables to steam (about 30 seconds). Stir until vegetables are coated with sauce, tender, and brightly colored. Sprinkle with sesame seeds; serve hot.

Bean and Nut Dumplings with Spicy Salsa

This appetizer is high in fiber and protein from the beans and walnuts, and the spicy salsa gives it an extra metabolic kick!

Yield:	Serving size:	Prep time:	Cook time:
8 dumplings	2 dumplings	5 minutes	20 minutes

Each serving has:			
257 calories	6 g total fat	1 g saturated fat	0 g trans fat
0 mg cholesterol	45 mg sodium	29 g carbohydrates	10 g fiber
2 g sugars	14 g protein	26 percent iron	

2 15-oz. cans black beans or any bean, drained and rinsed

1 tsp. cumin, ground

½ cup plain dry breadcrumbs

2 cups tomatoes, finely chopped

½ cup walnuts

1 shallot, minced

¼ cup chopped fresh cilantro

1 tsp. smoked paprika

Pinch of salt

1 TB. extra-virgin olive oil

1 avocado, diced

1. Preheat oven to 425°F. Line a baking sheet with foil. Set aside.

2. Blend black beans, cumin, and walnuts in a food processor until they form a paste-like consistency. Transfer to a mixing bowl and add ¼ cup of breadcrumbs (save the rest for later in the recipe) and mix.

3. Combine tomatoes, scallions, cilantro, ½ teaspoon paprika, and salt in a medium bowl. Stir 1 cup of tomato mixture into the black bean mixture.

4. Mix the remaining ⅓ cup breadcrumbs, oil, and the remaining ½ teaspoon paprika in a medium bowl until breadcrumbs are coated with oil. Divide the bean mixture into small balls (makes about 8 balls). Lightly press each bean ball into the breadcrumb mixture and coat. Place on the baking sheet.

5. Bake the bean dumplings until heated through and the breadcrumbs are golden brown, about 20 minutes. Add avocado to the remaining tomato mixture and stir to make a salsa. Serve the salsa with the dumplings.

Essential Takeaways

- Your metabolic rate is how fast (or slowly) you burn calories throughout the day.

- Genetics, activity level, age, and gender all affect your metabolic rate.

- Protein requires more energy than carbs and fat to digest; eating protein-rich foods can give you a slight metabolic boost.

- Fiber keeps the metabolism running smoothly by keeping blood sugar stable and allowing you to feel full longer, which means you eat less throughout the day.

- Metabolism declines with age. You can temper its decline by doing regular cardio and strength-training activities, and eating smaller meals more frequently.

chapter 18

Immunity Defenders

Identifying the three types of immunity and how they are acquired

Using food to boost your immunity

Understanding the role of probiotics and prebiotics for your health

Making immune-boosting recipes

We've come a long way since the theory that illness and disease were caused by poisonous, foul-smelling vapors in the air. Today, we know that microscopic organisms, germs, and potential disease-causing pathogens all around us can attack our immune system at any time. It's a test to see who can get in, invade your body, and wreak havoc.

The good news is we are born with a natural resistance, or innate immunity, which defends against foreign invaders by preventing them from entering, setting up shop, and spreading inside of you. In the case of immunity, the best offense is a good defense. Food can offer extra defense to boost your natural immunity.

This chapter delves into foods that work hard to build a strong, reliable, immune system for life.

Immunity Explained

Before delving into the foods that help boost your body's immunity, let's take a look at the three different types of immunity:

- **Innate immunity** is the natural resistance you are born with; it provides fast-response, short-term defense against general infections.

- **Artificially acquired immunity** is temporary protection against disease or illness due to vaccinations, in which you are given a small dose of the disease to build *antibodies.*

- **Naturally acquired immunity** is when you "catch" a disease, cold, or the flu due to contact with an infected agent. Your body's response to the disease helps you develop a natural immunity so you may not be hit as hard with it next time.

definition

Antibodies are proteins produced by your body's immune system in response to foreign invaders (e.g., bacteria and viruses), which bind with the invaders, neutralize them, and block them from harming your body.

Let's take a look at eight powerful immune-boosting foods.

Eating for Strong Immunity

Foods play a natural role in boosting your immune system. Fruits and vegetables contain plant compounds in their skins, seeds, and flesh that can assist your body in fending off diseases. Shellfish contains minerals that can support the immune system. Fermented dairy products like yogurt, kefir, and some cheese contain friendly bacteria. And nuts contain antioxidants that can decrease cell damage and subsequent illnesses.

Yogurt

A cup or two of low-fat yogurt can help keep your immune system—not to mention your bones!—strong. Yogurt is beneficial for immune health for a couple of reasons. Some yogurt brands contain vitamin D. (Check the nutrition facts on the container.) Research has shown vitamin D from sunlight can play an antimicrobial role and boost your natural innate immune system. Thus, it may fend off the common cold, flu, and autoimmune diseases like type 1 diabetes, multiple sclerosis, lupus, and rheumatoid arthritis.

Yogurt is made from fermented milk, which contains powerful players in immune health called *probiotics.* These are "friendly bacteria" that naturally reside in your gut and provide health benefits. Our intestinal tracts naturally have large amounts—100 trillion colonies of microscopic bacteria—that live in ever-changing interaction. Experts believe that 80 to 90 percent of bacteria in the colon have never been cultured. These armies of good bugs rally to combat the ill-effects of bad ones in your gastrointestinal tract, working to maintain proper digestion and boost immunity. The key is to keep the disease-causing bacteria outnumbered by the do-gooder bacteria!

> **definition**
>
> **Probiotics** are live microorganisms that can confer a health benefit. The majority of cultured probiotics in foods are similar to the natural bacteria in our guts. So when you eat them, it feels like home!

Probiotics like the species Lactobacillus and Bifidobacterium, as well as the starter culture for yogurt and other fermented milk products such as kefir and some cheeses, Saccharomyces Thermophilis, are the most widely used varieties or strains. Dietary supplements also contain strains of probiotics such as Enterococcus, Bacillus, and Escherichia for digestive health and immune support.

Most yogurt containers claim to contain live active cultures to denote the presence of live beneficial bacteria. However, be aware that this claim doesn't always let you know what type or how much additional bacteria is in the product. Plus, the amount that is still "alive" is debatable as the starter culture—called lactic acid bacteria—which ferments raw foods like yogurt, may not always survive processing, transport, and shelf time before you actually eat it. Call the manufacturer or check out their website for the finer probiotic details. You want to ensure that the cultures are live when consumed, have a documented health benefit, and contain enough to actually confer that benefit.

Probiotics thrive in the presence of prebiotics, which are nondigestible carbohydrates (sugars) that feed friendly bacteria already in the gut, encouraging it to grow, multiply, and become more active. The main prebiotics in the United States are called fructo-oligosaccharides (FOS), which are found in foods like onions, bananas, honey, wheat, artichokes, garlic, and leeks. Prebiotics are also sold in powder and supplement form.

Berries

Compounds called anthocynanins, primarily found in the dark blue, purplish pigment of the berry's skin, are believed to be responsible for their powerful defense against immunity-busting invaders. So colds, flu, and even normal aging processes may be thwarted by adding berries to your daily diet.

Broccoli

Broccoli packs a punch against colds, flu, and more chronic diseases like cancer, heart, and eye diseases. Broccoli's immune system benefits come from its high levels of an antiviral and antibacterial compound called diindolylmethane, which also fends off cancer. Broccoli also contains more carotenoids like lutein than other crucifer veggies. These two compounds are known for fending off free radical damage, which can cause illness and weaken the immune system.

Oysters

Oysters contain high amounts of zinc, which is an essential immune-boosting mineral. A Boston-based study of 578 people age 80 + years who were residents in nursing homes found that those with normal zinc levels had fewer cases of pneumonia, used fewer antibiotics, and had lower death rates compared to people with lower zinc levels.

Food wise

Too much zinc can actually weaken the immune system and also interfere with the levels of minerals like copper and iron in your body. Plus, overdoing zinc can damage nerves in your nose and render your sniffer unable to smell odors.

Other food sources of zinc include wheat germ, sesame paste (tahini), low-fat roast beef, roasted pumpkin seeds, and unsweetened cocoa powder.

Mushrooms

The white button mushroom contains many immune-boosting properties, thanks to significant levels of selenium and B-vitamins, niacin, and riboflavin. Selenium is instrumental in fending off viral infections; and low levels of niacin and riboflavin has been found to make the body susceptible to infections.

Some brands of white button mushrooms are exposed to ultraviolet rays to increase their vitamin D content—which adds to their immunity benefits.

Munch on This

A 3-ounce serving of white button mushrooms contains 400 IU of vitamin D—that's as much as 20 minutes of sun exposure and almost 100 percent RDA for adults.

Spinach

Spinach's rich green leaves are packed with antioxidants, such as vitamins A, C, and E as well as selenium; plus it contains a significant amount of the B-vitamin, folic acid, which is good for repairing DNA and promotes healthy cell growth and division. Folic acid also plays a role in defending against many chronic diseases including obesity, type 2 diabetes, heart disease, osteoporosis, age-related macular degeneration, renal disease, rheumatoid arthritis, and infertility.

Almonds

The vitamin E content in almonds provides its immune-boosting kick. Vitamin E is a powerful antioxidant that defends cells from damage, but it's also shown to play a big role in immune function. Foods like almonds that contain high amounts of this fat-soluble vitamin can play a healthy role in fending off chronic disease and illness.

Healing Hints

Almonds can also defend your skin health and improve your complexion. Facial scrubs, masks, and lotions are made from almonds. To make your own mask at home, mix 2 tablespoons of crushed almonds with 1 tablespoon of honey; apply to your face for five minutes and rinse with cool water.

Watermelon

This fruit often gets dismissed because of its high water content, but it contains a lot of nutritional value. Its deep red flesh and white part closest to the rind (which many people discard) contain numerous antioxidants, such as glutathione and the carotenoid lycopene. Lycopene is a big player in preventing cancer, specifically prostate cancer in men. It's also an antioxidant that prevents disease and illness from oxidant-related damage to your cells.

As far as immune response and function, glutathione is a powerful assistant that enables the immune system to spring into action at the first sign of attack; it regulates the cascade of events by the immune system army. Watermelon also contains immune-boosting nutrients, vitamins A, C, and B_6.

Immune-Boosting Recipes

Choose a variety of whole fruits, vegetables, nuts, and low-fat dairy products to fend off future colds, flus, and diseases. Here are some delicious recipes to support your natural immunity.

Mushroom, Brown Rice, and Vegetable Paella

Mushrooms add a wonderful meaty flavor and texture—plus an immunity-boost!—to this vegetarian dish. Add a dozen oysters, which are rich in zinc, for some extra defense.

Yield:	Serving size:	Prep time:	Cook time:
4 servings	1 cup	10 minutes	25 minutes

Each serving has:			
150 calories	6 g total fat	2 g saturated fat	0 g trans fat
6 mg cholesterol	331 mg sodium	41 g carbohydrates	3 g fiber
3 g sugars	7 g protein	5 percent iron	

1 TB. extra-virgin olive oil	½ cup frozen peas, thawed
2 garlic cloves, minced	½ cup cherry tomatoes, halved
1 cup white button mushrooms, chopped	¼ cup goat cheese, softened
2¼ cups low-sodium vegetable broth	1 TB. jalapeño pepper, seeded and minced
1¼ cups brown rice	Pinch of cinnamon
	Salt and pepper

1. Add olive oil to a deep skillet and heat over medium-high heat for 1 minute.

2. Add garlic and mushrooms and sauté for about 2 minutes, or until mushrooms soften.

3. Add broth and rice and bring to a boil. Reduce heat, cover, and simmer until all the liquid is absorbed and the rice is soft and tender.

4. Remove from heat and, while still hot, mix in peas, tomatoes, goat cheese, jalapeño, and cinnamon.

5. Add salt and pepper to taste. Serve warm.

Munch on This

If you prefer, use instant brown rice to save time as some brands cook in 90 seconds in the microwave. Just heat it up and throw into the broth; you will need to decrease the liquid by as much as 1½ to 2 cups as the instant rice might not absorb as much water.

Nutty Couscous, Watermelon, and Spinach Salad

Feel free to replace the edamame with any other kind of bean; all beans contain immunity-boosting folate.

Yield:	Serving size:	Prep time:	Cook time:
6 servings	½ cup	10 minutes	20 minutes

Each serving has:			
279 calories	14 g total fat	2 g saturated fat	0 g trans fat
0 mg cholesterol	168 mg sodium	32 g carbohydrates	5 g fiber
4 g sugars	9 g protein	14 percent iron	

1 cup whole-grain couscous

1½ cups vegetable broth, low-sodium

¼ cup plus 1 TB. extra-virgin olive oil

2 scallions, chopped

1 cup edamame (soybeans)

6 cherry tomatoes, halved

¼ cup raw almonds, chopped

1 cup watermelon, diced

2 TB. lemon juice

¼ cup extra-virgin olive oil

1 tsp. cumin, ground

1 tsp. fresh garlic, minced

Pinch of salt and pepper

6 cups spinach, rinsed and drained

1. Add broth and oil to a pot over medium heat and bring to a boil. Add couscous to boiling broth and remove from heat. Cover and let sit for 5 minutes while the couscous absorbs the liquid. Fluff with a fork.

2. Mix scallions, edamame, tomatoes, almonds, and watermelon with couscous.

3. Whisk together lemon juice, ¼ cup olive oil, cumin, garlic, salt, and pepper.

4. Place spinach in a shallow salad bowl, top with couscous mixture, and drizzle with dressing. Toss together and serve.

Berry Melon Yogurt Parfaits

Jammed with powerful immune-boosting power, these parfaits make a delicious breakfast, brunch, or after-dinner dessert. Feel free to substitute any fresh berry or use a combination of berries for a colorful treat.

Yield:	Serving size:	Prep time:	Cook time:
4 parfaits	1 parfait	10 minutes	45 minutes

Each serving has:			
366 calories	11 g total fat	1 g saturated fat	0 g trans fat
2 mg cholesterol	168 mg sodium	32 g carbohydrates	5 g fiber
4 g sugars	9 g protein	14 percent iron	

1 cup rolled oats	Pinch of salt
¼ cup raisins	½ tsp. cinnamon
2 TB. slivered almonds	¼ tsp. nutmeg
1 TB. flaxseed, ground	2 cups low-fat yogurt, plain
1 TB. vegetable oil	½ cup blueberries
1 TB. agave nectar	½ cup watermelon, chopped

1. Preheat oven to 350°F. In a medium bowl combine oats, raisins, almonds, and flaxseed.

2. In a small bowl mix together oil, agave nectar, salt, cinnamon, and nutmeg. Drizzle into the oat mixture and stir together.

3. Spread oat mixture onto a cookie sheet and bake for 45 minutes to one hour. Remove from oven and let cool.

4. For the parfaits, use long fluted dessert glasses. Layer a dollop of yogurt, a sprinkle of berries, watermelon, and granola. Repeat until filled to the top. Serve chilled.

Essential Takeaways

- We are born with a natural, innate immunity to fend off potential pathogens.
- We can also acquire immunity through vaccinations or by inadvertently coming in contact with disease-causing agents.
- Certain foods contain immunity-boosting agents such as probiotics, prebiotics, vitamins, minerals, and antioxidants.

Sleep Rules

Sleep is as important to good health as exercise and healthy eating. Although some people appear to function better on less sleep than others, the fact is we all need it. Adults need between seven and nine hours of sleep per night; infants, children, and teens need even more for proper growth and development.

Getting good-quality sleep fends off a number of health problems, including mood disorders like depression, anxiety, and attention deficit hyperactivity disorder (ADHD); obesity; high blood pressure; high blood sugar; and insulin resistance.

One of the biggest indicators of lack of sleep—in everyone from young children to older adults—is weight gain. Your appetite is regulated by circadian rhythms or your inner biological clock, plus the sleep hormone melatonin. Low levels of melatonin can disrupt sleep. So if you don't get enough ZZZZs, your hormones—especially the ones that control hunger and fullness, as well as your calorie-burning capacity—will be out of whack. That's why regular sleep deprivation causes intense cravings for high-calorie, high-carb foods, such as salty, fatty, and sweet foods.

What you eat—and when—is a big part of getting a restful sleep. In this chapter, I delve into the optimal foods and eating behaviors to ensure good beauty sleep.

Sleep Empowering Eats

Sleep is directly affected by what you eat. Recent research has shown the timing of meals, portion sizes, and the composition of your diet plays a role in getting a good night's sleep.

When fueling your brain and body well for the day and for the overnight fast, you need a proper combination of the right types of carbs, protein, and favorable fats in order to relax the body and rejuvenate the brain. Drinking too many liquids before bed, particularly caffeinated beverages, will stimulate your body and disturb sleep with the need for frequent urination and/or insomnia.

Here's a sample timetable and meal plan for a good night's sleep:

Eating for Restful Night's Sleep

Time	Meal/Snack	Foods
7:00 A.M.	Breakfast	1 cup of oatmeal with 1 cup skim milk + mixed berries (½ cup)
10:00 A.M.	Snack	6 whole-grain crackers + ¼ cup walnuts
12:30 P.M.	Lunch	2 cups mixed greens + 4 oz. chicken breast, chopped
3:00 P.M.	Snack	Low-fat cottage cheese (½ cup) + 1 small piece of fruit
6:00 P.M.	Dinner	1 cup veggie chili with beans + 1 cup brown rice
8:30 P.M.	Snack	Chamomile tea + 1 whole-grain tea biscuit

Healing Hints

Aim for eating breakfast within an hour of waking. This gets your metabolism going plus regulates your hormones and your natural circadian rhythm.

The following sections outline some surefire ways to fuel your body for some good power sleep.

High-Fiber Carbs

Sleep is another good excuse to get more fiber into your day. If you want to promote slower digestion and a steady stream of energy during the day and overnight, eat whole grains, fruits, lightly steamed vegetables, beans, and legumes. Carbohydrates play a vital role in feelings of well-being and getting a good night's sleep by starting a chemical cascade of events: the carbs boost levels of the amino acid tryptophan, which promotes the production of the feel-good brain chemical serotonin, which in turns ignites the hormone melatonin, which helps induce sleep. This is why people crave more carbs when they aren't sleeping well.

Sleep experts believe that you should ideally give your body anywhere from two to four hours to digest foods before lying down to sleep. Because we digest food better when upright, going to bed on a full-stomach is not a good idea from a purely digestive perspective, plus it can disrupt sleep and lead to uncomfortable acid reflux or heartburn.

munch on This	If you have to have a snack before bed, include a complex, high-fiber carb, such as whole-grain bread, whole-grain pasta, brown rice, or a handful of whole-grain crackers. These whole-grain carbs signal the brain to release serotonin (a feel-good hormone) that induces sleep.

Protein Power Foods

Include some protein for nutritional balance and satiety (feeling fullness) to your evening meal or snack. The protein will also help rebuild and repair muscles that you used during the day.

In studies comparing protein sources, whey protein (such as that found in cow's milk, cottage cheese, and protein powders) versus protein found in tuna fish, turkey, and eggs. The whey protein was found to be more satiating and therefore more effective for managing and losing weight. When eaten with a carbohydrate-rich food, whey protein was found to help decrease the total amount of food eaten, and kept blood sugar in better control, which also aids in sleep by keeping you feeling satisfied longer.

Spread a tablespoon of almond butter on whole-grain toast, a slice of low-fat cheese on a rice cake, or put a slice or two of turkey in a whole-grain pita.

food wise Lack of sleep causes the body's two main appetite hormones—leptin, which signals fullness and ghrelin, which gauges hunger—to go haywire. When these hormones are out of whack, you will experience hunger and fullness differently than when you are well-rested. There's a double whammy: low leptin causes overeating (as you never feel full) *and* the brain thinks your starving, so your body burns calories more slowly.

Favorable Fats

Too much fat before bed can render you sleepless. A few drizzles of olive or canola oil, a handful of nuts on salad, or slices of avocado on a turkey, lettuce, and tomato wrap will balance your nighttime meal with "good" unsaturated fat. However, a deep dish cheese pizza, cheeseburger and fries, or a loaded beef burrito can wreak havoc on your circadian rhythms. Fat, particularly saturated fat, slows down digestion.

Too many fatty foods before bedtime can also lead to indigestion and/or acid reflux (heartburn). So choose and time your fats wisely. If you want pizza, lasagna, or fried mozzarella sticks, have a sensible serving midday instead of midnight.

Cutting the Caffeine and Alcohol

Caffeine and alcohol can have a dramatic effect on your ability to sleep at night. Although people's sensitivity to caffeine varies, it is a stimulant that will rev up your heart, brain, and metabolism. Give your body at least four hours without caffeine before retreating to the bedroom.

Alcohol can have a sedative effect—which means it can make you sleepy—but it will not keep you there. Drinking alcohol as much as six hours before bed can disturb sleep throughout the night. Alcoholic beverages can affect the brain's chemical messengers that influence sleep. Thus, you may be able to fall asleep easily after a few beers, but you'll wake up periodically throughout the night from dreams and not be able to fall back to sleep. You'll pay for it the next day with fatigue, lack of concentration, and sleepiness!

Elderly people are particularly susceptible, as alcohol affects them more intensely. After a poor night's sleep an older person may walk less steady and be at greater risk for falls and injuries.

Mid-Night Munching

Have you ever gotten up in the middle of the night and raided the refrigerator? If this happens regularly over the course of two months, than you may have a serious eating and/or sleep disorder called Night Eating Syndrome (NES). A similar, but less known, disorder is called Nocturnal Sleep-Related Eating Disorder (NSRED), a.k.a. sleep eating. These sleep-related conditions affect 1 to 5 percent of adults, primarily young women.

Nocturnal Sleep-Related Eating Disorder

People with NSRED eat while asleep and are not conscious of their nighttime binges. They wake up in the morning with crumbs on the table and empty packages on the counter, but don't remember eating during the night. NSRED has been found to be prominently a sleep disorder associated with insomnia and is common in people with binge-eating tendencies. People with NSRED often experience weight gain because of all the extra calories they consume.

Night Eating Syndrome

People suffering from NES wake from sleep several times during the night to eat. They are fully conscious during the nighttime binge-eating. Research has shown that NES occurs primarily in people with low-self esteem, depression, and lower levels of the hormones melatonin (the hormone that regulates sleep-wake cycles) and leptin, the fullness regulator.

Many people with NES respond well to medications which elevate serotonin (the feel-good hormone) levels in the brain.

Be on the lookout for NES or NSRED. The following may reveal cause for concern:

- Calorie-loading at night; eating one quarter of the day's calories—especially carbohydrates—after 9 P.M.

- Experiencing several episodes of waking up to binge eat overnight.

- Skipping breakfast the next day or most days; eating a few hours after waking.

- Generally feeling depressed or anxious; eating behaviors magnify those feelings.

- Experiencing guilt associated with nighttime eating.

- Difficulty sleeping (insomnia) and have had bouts of sleepwalking.

Nighttime eating, whether it's done while awake or asleep, requires professional help from a health psychologist and/or registered dietitian specializing in sleep-related eating disorders.

Natural Sleep Aids

If you need help falling asleep and staying there for at least seven hours, the following natural food-based remedies may help—and the best part is they're drug-free.

Warm Milk

Warm milk works best as a sleep aid when its accompanied by some carbs, as insulin, the hormone that is released when carbs are eaten, helps get the tryptophan from the milk into your brain to make you sleepy. If you're having trouble sleeping, try drinking a cup of warm skim milk with one or two small whole-grain cookies or a handful of whole-grain crackers.

Herbal Tea

Relaxation is one of the keys to good sleep. Chamomile tea is an herbal tea with a calming, relaxing effect. It's caffeine free, thus promoting a nonstimulatory effect and is used as a gentle sedative all over the world.

Studies on sleep-challenged mice have shown chamomile to decrease sleep latency—how long it actually takes to fall asleep. Keep in mind that with any natural remedy, your environment counts. Drinking chamomile tea in a quiet, serene nook of your house will relax you more than grabbing sips while listening to your children argue over a toy with the television blasting in the background. Sip in peace and quiet, and before you know it the sandman will be knocking.

munch on This	It turns out beauty rest is a real phenomenon. A good night's sleep can improve your looks. A study in the British Medical Journal of 23 young healthy people in Sweden, found that those who were sleep deprived (awake for 31 hours) were rated as less attractive and "less healthy-looking" as those who had a good night's sleep (8 hours).

Sleepy-Time Recipes

The following recipes are intended for meals or snacks to help promote a good night's sleep.

Fruity Whey Protein Shake

This makes a delicious breakfast or evening snack at least two hours before going to bed.

Yield:	Serving size:	Prep time:	Cook time:
2 servings	1 cup	5 minutes	None

Each serving has:			
189 calories	4 g total fat	0.5 g saturated fat	0 g trans fat
25 mg cholesterol	53 mg sodium	28 g carbohydrates	4 g fiber
16 g sugars	15 g protein	5 percent iron	

4 ice cubes

½ scoop whey protein powder

½ cup plain soymilk

½ cup water

1 small banana

½ cup fresh or frozen strawberries, chopped

½ cup fresh pineapple, chopped

1 TB. flaxseed, ground

1. Add ice cubes, protein powder, soymilk, water, banana, strawberries, pineapple, and flaxseed to a blender.

2. Mix until well blended and thick. Add more ice if needed. Serve chilled.

Mozzarella, Tomato, and Basil Lentil Salad

This salad is great to eat for dinner. Add your favorite vegetables, beans, or cheese. Add a dash of curry powder for a unique twist and delicious flavor.

Yield:	Serving size:	Prep time:	Cook time:
2 servings	1½ cups	5 minutes	30 minutes

Each serving has:			
281 calories	11 g total fat	3 g saturated fat	0 g trans fat
9 mg cholesterol	139 mg sodium	30 g carbohydrates	15 g fiber
1 g sugars	17 g protein	21 percent iron	

½ cup lentils, washed and drained

2 cups water

1 TB. olive oil

1 garlic clove, minced

5 basil leaves, chopped

¼ cup fresh part-skim mozzarella cheese

Pinch of salt and pepper

Mixed greens (optional)

1. Add lentils and water to medium saucepan, bring to a boil, then cover and simmer until water is absorbed and lentils are softened (about 20 minutes). If lentils are not soft, add more water (2–3 tablespoons).

2. In a saucepan heat oil over medium heat, add garlic, and sauté for 30 seconds.

3. Toss garlic with lentils, add basil leaves and fresh mozzarella. Season with salt and pepper to taste. Serve cold or warm on a bed of mixed greens.

Soothing Chamomile Tea

Make your own calming chamomile tea from scratch with fresh or dried chamomile flowers.

Yield:	Serving size:	Prep time:	Cook time:
1 cup	1 cup	5 minutes	15 minutes

Each serving has:			
0 calories	0 g total fat	0 g saturated fat	0 g trans fat
0 mg cholesterol	0 mg sodium	0 g carbohydrates	0 g fiber
0 sugars	0 g protein	0 percent iron	

1 TB. chamomile flowers, stems removed and washed

1 single serve tea pot of purified water

1 tsp. honey or a lemon wedge (optional)

1. Heat water in a tea kettle until boiling.

2. Pour water into the tea pot and place chamomile flowers into water. Let flowers steep in the water for 10 minutes.

3. Place a tea strainer in your tea cup to strain flowers and pour tea into a cup. Add honey and/or lemon, if desired. Enjoy during the day to relax or in the evening as part of your bedtime ritual.

This is a zero calorie beverage. If you add honey, a teaspoon of honey has 20 calories.

Munch on This

If you don't have chamomile flowers growing in your garden, you can buy them fresh or dried at a spice/tea shop. Blend them with dried rose petals for a beautifully relaxing flavor combination.

Essential Takeaways

- Getting a good night's sleep is a vital part of overall health, along with eating well and regular activity.
- Adults need between seven and nine hours of good-quality sleep every night. Infants, children, and teens need more for normal growth and development.
- Lack of sleep can cause weight gain, mood disorders, type 2 diabetes, high blood pressure, and accidents.
- Eating disorders, such as binge-eating, coupled with sleep problems like insomnia can lead to serious sleep-related eating disorders.
- Eating well for sleep includes getting high-fiber carbs, quality protein, and "good" fats; alcohol and caffeine can disturb sleep.

Part 5

Foods to Fight Disease

These chapters show you how food and healthful living can fend off diseases such as diabetes, heart disease, cancer, and osteoporosis. Armed with nutrition know-how, you can better tackle and defend against illnesses and chronic diseases to live a longer, healthier life.

This part is peppered with practical tips and recipes for using healthy and healing foods in your own kitchen. By getting comfortable cooking with a wide variety of foods, you will not only defend against disease but build a healthy relationship with food that will last a lifetime.

chapter 20

Heart Health for Life

Using food to help your heart

Creating a diet that's low in cholesterol

Choosing foods that help lower blood pressure

Making heart-healthy recipes

Every 36 seconds someone dies from heart disease. It's the number one killer in the United States. It makes sense when you consider that two out of three people are overweight and obese, and blood pressure and cholesterol levels are rising. All these chronic problems stress the heart, making it work harder.

Poor eating habits are literally feeding heart attacks. The average person consumes too many unhealthy solid fats, added sugars (SoFAS), refined grains, and sodium. On top of that, they eat too little heart-healthy foods such as whole grains, fruits, vegetables, low-fat dairy products, and fiber.

In this chapter, I help you swing the pendulum in the heart-healthy direction by highlighting foods that improve blood pressure, blood flow to the arteries, and the pliability of your arteries to stay young at heart forever.

The Cholesterol Connection

Almost 50 percent of American adults have high cholesterol levels (over 200 mg/dL) a major risk for heart disease, so it's important to identify foods that can keep cholesterol levels in check. Cholesterol comes from food (dietary cholesterol) and is also produced in your body (blood cholesterol). No matter where it comes from, high levels of total and LDL (bad) cholesterol in your body are an indicator of heart disease risk; whereas high HDL (good) cholesterol is a cardio-protective indicator. Food, lifestyle factors, and genetics play a significant role in your cholesterol levels.

Munch on This	The average person in the United States doesn't get the nutrition they need. Studies show that on average, we consume less than 20 percent of recommended whole grains and less than 60 percent of recommended vegetables, fruits, milk, and milk products. If we are not eating nutrient-dense foods, what are we eating?

Cholesterol is a factor in heart health because too much of the "bad" stuff—low-density lipoproteins (LDL)—can build up in your arteries and cause blockages, which lead to a heart attack and/or stroke. On the other hand, increasing the "good" or high-density lipoproteins (HDL) cholesterol can keep your heart beating smoothly. So the goal of a heart-healthy eating plan is to lower the LDL-cholesterol and bring up the HDL-cholesterol.

Here's what works for cholesterol lowering as far as the National Heart, Lung, and Blood Institute (NHLBI) is concerned. NHLBI advises healthy eating and living as part of an approach called therapeutic lifestyle changes (TLCs). The number one TLC goal is to lower the LDL-cholesterol to less than 100 mg/dL or less than 70 mg/dL (if you have a family history of heart disease). The TLC diet is based on eating more fiber, plant-based foods, and healthy fats. This translates into cutting back on saturated fat, refined and processed foods, animal foods, and sodium. Incorporating the TLCs for three to six months can help lower cholesterol, aid in weight loss (more on that later), and keep your heart healthy for life. For more on NHLBI's TLCs take a look at www.nhlbi.nih.gov/health/public/heart/chol/chol_tlc.pdf.

Another major area of concern for heart health is blood pressure. With age, blood pressure typically increases. Experts predict that 9 out of 10 people will develop high blood pressure if they live long enough. Because having high blood pressure (over 140/90) is a major risk factor for heart attack and stroke, the 2010 Dietary Guidelines for Americans emphasizes lowering daily sodium intake to less than 2,300 milligrams per day for healthy people, but less to 1,500 milligrams per day for those with high blood pressure or other risk factors for heart disease. (Most Americans eat over 4,000 milligrams every day!)

Healing Hints	Two large clinical trials showed that eating more fruits, vegetables, low-fat dairy products, whole grains, nuts, and beans brought down blood pressure significantly, without restricting sodium too much (although the best results were seen in those with a lower salt intake, too).

Healing Foods for the Heart

Because you're probably not thinking about your heart every time you eat, it's important to shape changes in your eating habits that become permanent fixtures instead of temporary fixes. New research shows that it takes one high-saturated fat, high-cholesterol meal to cause damage to your arteries!

So let's make some healthy changes to a typical food order that's high in artery-clogging saturated fat. Instead of always ordering a bacon double cheeseburger, why not ask for a single cheeseburger with lower fat cheese like part-skim mozzarella, Swiss, or provolone? Better yet, swap the beef burger for a veggie burger. You're not only saving fat grams, but hundreds of excess calories (and feeding your veins beneficial plant-based fuel). Whether you are at a fast-food joint or fancy restaurant, ask for extra lettuce, tomatoes, and pickles—it's an easy way to get more vegetables on your plate. In that same meal, if you want fries, order the smallest size and share them (opt for the sweet potato version, if available), or order a side of broccoli instead. Adding a small cup of broth-based soup and side salad adds heart-healthy nutrients into your day.

Keep in mind it's not only about what you don't eat, but what you *do* eat that helps your heart health. All of the following foods help keep both your blood pressure and cholesterol in a healthy range. In addition, these foods can help relax your arteries so they keep your blood flowing smoothly.

Here are 10 foods to eat to keep your heart happily humming along for life:

- Avocados
- Beans
- Brown rice
- Fish
- Leafy greens

- Oats
- Olive oil
- Soy
- Walnuts
- Yogurt

> **Healing Hints**
>
> Food is not the only factor in heart health. Getting regular physical activity (at least 150 minutes per week) and, if you are overweight, losing 5 to 10 percent of your body weight in 6 months will do your heart good!

munch
on This
Try some of these oat-enhancing culinary ideas: add whole oats to pancake batter, turkey meat-loaf, chili, homemade hamburgers, cookies, banana bread, muffins, and yogurt.

Avocados

Don't be afraid to eat avocados. Jammed-packed with vitamins, minerals, and plant-based goodness, avocados contain the "good" fats—monounsaturated fat (MUFA) and polyunsaturated fat (PUFA)—which help keep your total and LDL (bad) cholesterol in a healthy range. Avocados fit into the American Heart Association guidelines of eating less saturated fat, trans fat, cholesterol, and sodium every day.

A serving of avocado (1 ounce, which is about one fifth of an avocado) has a mere 50 calories, 0.5 grams of saturated fat, 0 grams of cholesterol and trans fat, 3 grams of MUFAs, and 0.5 grams of PUFAs. Avocados help swing your eating pendulum in a healthy direction by giving you
140 milligrams of potassium and no sodium, which is great for blood pressure control!

Avocados can easily be added to salads, dips, sandwiches, and wraps. Avocados are best served cold or room temperature, but you can certainly use a few avocado slices as a garnish on top of a soup, stew, or casserole.

Beans

Beans are a powerful player in heart health. Not only do they offer tons of fiber, particularly the cholesterol-lowering soluble type, but they fill you up on fewer calories. Beans are a delicious low-saturated fat form of protein. Thus, beans can feed you well at no cost to your health and very little cost to your wallet!

Beans are one of the best sources of dietary fiber, which plays a major role in fending off heart disease by ridding the body of excess cholesterol. Women should strive for at least 25 grams per day and men 38 grams per day (or 14 grams per 1,000 calories).

A single cup of kidney beans is 9 grams of fiber, 1 cup of black beans is 15 grams of fiber, and 1 cup of lima beans is 13.5 grams—that's almost half the fiber you need in a day. So add beans to salads, soups, chili, and pasta. They are a great replacement for meat and they fill you up.

Brown Rice

Brown rice is a whole grain that is particularly high in niacin (vitamin B_3), which has been shown to be very heart-healthy. Niacin has been shown to reverse atherosclerosis or hardening of the arteries by bringing down total cholesterol and LDL-cholesterol, and raising the "good" HDL-cholesterol.

There are 3.5 grams of fiber per half cup of cooked brown rice. The calories can add up fast, though: 3.5 ounces (less than $\frac{1}{2}$ cup) of uncooked brown rice has 370 calories! So when preparing meals at home limit brown rice to $\frac{1}{2}$ cup to 1 cup cooked.

Fatty Fish

Fish is your go-to source for omega-3 fats, specifically eicosapentaenoic acid (EPA) and docosahexaenoic acid (DHA), two rock stars as far as heart health goes! Fish is also low in saturated fat and a great source of protein. Although some research has shown omega-3 fats work for relaxing arteries for better function, you would have to eat a lot of fish (7 ounces) to get enough DHA and 15 ounces to get enough EPA—that's a lot in one sitting.

Set a goal of eating at least two, 6-ounce servings a week of fatty fish, such as salmon, halibut, and mackerel. Research has shown a strong link to DHA and EPA in keeping your heart beating regularly, thus fending off what's called arrhythmias which can lead to sudden death. Fish oil can also lower triglycerides, another blood fat, and it can be great for weight management. A 4-ounce serving of Atlantic Sockeye salmon makes a low-calorie protein source with a mere 230 calories!

Leafy Greens

There are nearly 1,000 species of plants with edible leaves. When was the last time you thought of spinach, romaine lettuce, or kale as being good for your blood pressure? Well, the bevy of mixed greens available to us today are great for lowering blood pressure and losing weight—both good for your heart. Not only are they packed with nutrients, like vitamins A, C, K, and potassium, but they are low in calories: a cup of spinach has 14 calories and $\frac{1}{2}$ cup of cooked collard greens has 38 calories! They contain no saturated fat, trans fat, or cholesterol.

Leafy greens can be stir-fried, stewed, or steamed to make heart-healthy meals. Leafy greens can be served with meat, grains, or used as a wrap for vegetable, rice, and/or meat filling. Of course, leafy greens are delicious raw in sandwiches and salads. Blend them into smoothies for a nutrient-packed beverage.

Some popular leafy greens are arugula, beet greens, Belgian endive, broccoli, bok choy, cabbage, collards, curly endive, dandelion greens, escarole, kale, lettuces, mustard greens, radicchio, rapini, spinach, Swiss chard, turnip greens, and watercress.

Healing Hints

Plants naturally contain compounds called plant stanols and sterols, which have been shown to block the absorption of cholesterol from the digestive tract. Studies show that 2 grams of stanols or sterols per day can lower "bad" LDL-cholesterol up to 14 percent within weeks. Although plant foods only contain small amounts of stanols and sterols, get a good mix of at least 2½ cups of colorful and leafy veggies, 2 cups of fruit, and 3 servings of whole grains every day to increase your chances of getting the cholesterol-lowering benefits of stanols and sterols.

Oats

Infamous for its fiber content, oats contain soluble (viscous) fiber, which dissolves in water to form a gel that sweeps through your arteries, taking some cholesterol with it as it goes. Whole oats have been shown to reduce LDL (bad) cholesterol and blood pressure, two major risk factors for heart disease.

The evidence behind oats to reduce the risk of heart disease is so strong that they are supported by a health claim. You may have seen this statement on product labels: "Three grams of soluble fiber daily from oatmeal, in a diet low in saturated fat and cholesterol, may reduce the risk of heart disease." What does 3 grams of soluble fiber look like? It's 3 packets of instant oatmeal or 4 servings of a ready-to-eat whole-grain oat cereal.

Oats are a versatile and delicious way to add fiber, flavor, and satisfaction to your day.

Olive Oil

Studies have shown that olive oil, particularly extra-virgin olive oil, contains powerful antioxidants (not only fats!) that help keep the walls of the arteries soft and pliable—more youthful, if you will. An international study looked at two groups of people for two days. One day they were given extra-virgin olive oil with high amounts of antioxidants and the other day they were given a lower-antioxidant olive oil. Upon examination of their arterial walls after eating each of the oils, the extra-virgin olive oil consumption produced greater elasticity in the subjects' arteries. The theory is that the greater the arterial elasticity (or less stiff), the less vascular stress and risk for heart disease and stroke. So go for the extra-virgin olive oil whenever possible!

As far as olive oil's heart-healthy fat properties, it's important to get a daily dose; the FDA supports the use of a total of 2 tablespoons of olive oil per day as part of an overall healthy diet. Evidence has shown that olive oil's heart-healthy MUFAs decrease the risk of coronary heart disease. Keep in mind, however, that you must replace MUFAs for the same amount of saturated fat in your diet and not increase your total number of calories in a day. Yes, weight control is a big factor in the heart health equation, too.

Food wise	Keep in mind that 2 tablespoons of olive oil adds up to 240 calories! Even though it's heart-healthy, watch the drizzles, dips, and spoonfuls. Measure out olive oil to avoid using too much.

Extra-virgin olive oil is perfect drizzled over mixed greens; tossed into pasta; and stirred into soups, chili, dips, and steamed veggies.

Soy Foods

Whole soy foods like tofu (soybean curd) and soybeans (edamame) are a great source of plant-based proteins, and they are low in saturated fat, making them a great alternative to animal proteins. Because animal proteins have been shown to raise cholesterol levels and may also increase weight, eating soy proteins in place of red meat in some meals is a positive step toward a healthy heart. Researchers continue to examine the specific heart health benefits of soy protein. The FDA calls soy protein a "complete" protein, which means it contains all essential amino acids that your body cannot make on its own.

Soy protein is found in many foods including tofu, soymilk, tempeh (ground soy beans mixed with grains to form a solid cake), textured vegetable protein or TVP (a ground meat substitute), and soy flour.

Walnuts

This tree nut is not only delicious and flavorful, but has shown promise in lowering total and LDL (bad) cholesterol levels, especially in people that already have high cholesterol levels. Walnuts contain the most omega-3 fats (alpha-linolenic acid or ALA) than any other nut (2.5 grams per ounce). Walnuts were the first food to have an FDA-approved health claim attached to it. You should strive to eat 1.5 ounces of walnuts a day to maximize your heart health!

Walnuts have shown promise in keeping the arteries to your heart more flexible, which keeps blood flowing smoothly. The effects become apparent when you look at the research. An Australian study of 40 middle-aged men and women were fed four different diets: one high in PUFAs, such as walnuts; one high in MUFAs from almonds and canola oil; one high in sugars from jam and marmalade; and the last one was high in saturated fat from butter. Among the four diets, the one high in walnuts showed less wear and tear on the lining of the arteries. As you might have guessed, the higher saturated fat diet had the opposite effect by lowering arterial function by 50 percent!

Compared to other "good" fat sources, here's how walnuts stack up.

Omega-3 Fats (ALA) Comparison	
Food	*Omega-3 Fats*
Walnuts (1 oz.)	2.5 grams
Canola oil (1 tsp.)	0.4 grams
Flaxseed oil (1 tsp.)	2.4 grams
Soy beans (½ cup)	1.2 grams

Courtesy of California Walnuts at www.walnuts.org

Remember, the calories add up fast with walnuts (as with all nuts), so portion out 1 ounce—that's 7 whole walnuts (14 halves or ¼ cup of pieces). One ounce is 190 calories!

munch on This	One 3.5 ounce serving of tofu (made with calcium sulfate) can have up to 350 milligrams of calcium. That's a great plant-based (vegan) source of calcium. So swap chicken or beef for tofu in stir-fries or marinade extra-firm tofu for grilling. Tofu itself is rather tasteless, but it absorbs flavor from the added sauces and spices.

Yogurt

Most people equate the mineral calcium with bone health, but it's also linked to lowering blood pressure. Of course, you could take a supplement, but high calcium foods like yogurt also contain other nutrients, such as vitamin D (in some brands), protein, and probiotics, the friendly bugs that we talked about in Chapter 18.

Calcium has been found to be effective in lowering the systolic (top number) blood pressure, which is the number to watch, especially in people over 50. For a 2,100 calorie diet, people watching their blood pressure should get 1,250 milligrams of calcium every day—that's 2 to 3 cups of yogurt per day. For adults (under 50 years), 1,000 milligrams is a good goal; if you're over 50 years old, you should shoot for 1,200 milligrams.

Healing
Hints

It's easy to decipher food label information about calcium. If the label says 25 percent calcium, it equals 250 milligrams of calcium. Just drop the percent sign and add a 0.

Make smoothies with fruit and yogurt. Dollop low-fat plain yogurt instead of sour cream in fajitas and over chili and soups. Mix it with fruit and add it to puddings, cakes, and pies.

Heart-Healthy Recipes

Wild Rice and Squash Risotto

Creamy like a typical risotto, but with less fat and calories, this nutty rendition of the Italian classic will keep your heart happy, too.

Yield:	Serving size:	Prep time:	Cook time:
4 servings	½ cup	10 minutes	30 minutes

Each serving has:			
176 calories	7 g total fat	2 g saturated fat	0 g trans fat
8 mg cholesterol	429 mg sodium	24 g carbohydrates	3 g fiber
4 g sugars	6 g protein	6 percent iron	

2 cups butternut squash, peeled and cut into bite-size pieces

1 TB. olive oil

1 onion, peeled and finely chopped

1 garlic clove, peeled and crushed

1 cup wild rice

2½ cups vegetable broth (low-sodium)

2 rosemary sprigs, needles removed

½ cup goat cheese

Pinch of salt and freshly ground black pepper

1. Steam the squash in a steamer pot over boiling water for 10 minutes or until tender. Mash with a hand blender (immersion blender) or a fork.

2. Heat olive oil in a heavy-bottomed pan and sauté onion and garlic over a low heat until soft, but not browned.

3. Add rice and stir until well-coated. Add broth and cook over medium heat for about 25 minutes, stirring frequently. Once rice has fully absorbed the liquid and is softening, add squash and rosemary. Stir to combine.

4. Stir in cheese and season with salt and pepper to taste. The risotto should be thick and creamy, and the rice should be soft on the outside, but firm in the middle.

Spicy Turkey and Greens Wrap

Simple and tasty, these lettuce wraps are jammed with lean protein and the goodness of leafy greens. Feel free to add any filling as lettuce offers a great envelope to satisfy a savory or sweet taste.

Yield:	Serving size:	Prep time:	Cook time:
4 servings	1 wrap	10 minutes	15 minutes

Each serving has:			
297 calories	17 g total fat	4 g saturated fat	0 g trans fat
90 mg cholesterol	269 mg sodium	15 g carbohydrates	3 g fiber
10 g sugars	23 g protein	16 percent iron	

1 garlic clove, minced	2 tsp. agave nectar
1 TB. extra-virgin olive oil	8 to 10 Bibb lettuce leaves
2 TB. red onion, finely diced	2 TB. cilantro, chopped
8 ounces lean ground turkey	1 medium carrot, shredded
¼ tsp. Chinese five-spice powder (or cayenne pepper)	1 cucumber, peeled and julienned
2 TB. low-sodium soy sauce	1 TB. chopped peanuts (optional)

1. In a sauté pan over medium-high heat, cook garlic in oil until fragrant, about 3 minutes.

2. Add turkey, five-spice powder or cayenne, soy sauce, and agave nectar and cook until turkey is browned (7–10 minutes).

3. Scoop turkey mixture into lettuce leaves. Garnish with carrots, cucumber, and peanuts (if using).

Marinated Tofu Veggie Kebobs

Use extra-firm tofu with the veggies in these kabobs. Chicken or shrimp works well, too.

Yield:	Serving size:	Prep time:	Cook time:
4 kabobs	2 kabobs	15 minutes	10 minutes

Each serving has:			
419 calories	21 g total fat	2 g saturated fat	0 g trans fat
0 mg cholesterol	572 mg sodium	45 g carbohydrates	7 g fiber
20 g sugars	18 g protein	22 percent iron	

1½ TB. soy sauce, low-sodium

1 TB. honey

1½ TB. lemon juice

1 TB. vegetable oil

1 green onion, finely chopped

8 oz. tofu, extra-firm, cubed

1 cup baby bella mushrooms, quartered

1 zucchini, trimmed and sliced into round chunks

8 cherry tomatoes

4 mini pita breads, split in half

1. Combine soy sauce, honey, lemon juice, vegetable oil, and green onion in a small bowl.

2. Put tofu in a shallow bowl and pour over marinade. Cover and let soak for an hour.

3. While tofu marinates, soak four skewers in water to stop them from burning under the broiler.

4. Thread tofu cubes and vegetable pieces alternatively onto the skewers. Brush with some of the marinade. Cook under a hot broiler or on the grill for about 3 minutes on each side, basting occasionally, or until vegetables are tender and tofu is browned.

5. To serve, slide kebobs off the skewers, arrange in the pita pockets, and garnish with salad leaves.

munch on this

For this recipe, you can substitute other vegetables and/or chicken, fish, or lean beef.

Essential Takeaways

- Heart-healthy foods help you maintain proper blood pressure and cholesterol levels and also help keep your arteries soft and pliable to keep your blood circulating well.

- The magic nutrients for heart health are fiber, calcium, magnesium, potassium, and "good" fats.

- Aim for lowering sodium intake to less than 2,300 milligrams (1 teaspoon); if you have high blood pressure or other risk factors aim for 1,500 milligrams or less per day.

- Maintaining a healthy body weight and exercising regularly should accompany healthful eating.

chapter 21

The Best Diabetes Defense

Understanding diabetes

Making food choices to keep diabetes in check

Cooking delicious diabetes-friendly recipes

Most of us will be touched by diabetes in our lifetime. Diabetes affects one in three people, and the National Centers for Disease Control predicts that diabetes cases may double or even triple by 2050. Millions of people go about their lives without even knowing they have this disease. And it's important to know if you have it, because it can negatively affect many of your vital organs. It's equally important to know if you're on the edge of getting diabetes (or prediabetes, as it's called) because you can take steps to prevent it.

Eating the right mix of foods and changing your lifestyle are keys to diabetes prevention. In this chapter, you learn more about the disease and discover how you can optimize your nutrition in ways that are delicious and easy.

The Types of Diabetes

There are three types of diabetes: type 1 (insulin-dependent), type 2 (lifestyle-related), and gestational diabetes (pregnancy-induced). Type 1 is with you for life, type 2 however, is preventable and controllable with healthy food and lifestyle choices.

Prediabetes is a warning phase, when blood sugar levels are higher than normal. This is a pivotal time to incorporate healthy foods into your lifestyle, pronto!

To better understand this disease, it's useful to know a few key terms:

- **Glucose/blood sugar:** Sugar and starches, which give the brain and body energy and growth.

- **Insulin:** The hormone that enables glucose to get into the body's cells for energy.

- **Insulin sensitivity:** The body's ability to use insulin, the higher the sensitivity the better.

- **Insulin resistance:** Occurs when the body's cells can no longer use insulin effectively (resists it), thus glucose cannot get into the cells.

- **Autoimmune disease:** Occurs when the body's immune system attacks itself, causing illness and diseases. Type 1 diabetes is considered an autoimmune disease.

Many people associate diabetes with being overweight, and that certainly is a major contributing factor. But diabetes is a complex disease: genetics, environment, and lifestyle all play a role. Even though the majority of people with diabetes, especially type 2, are overweight or obese, normal-weight and thin people get diabetes, too.

Some people are skinny-fat, particularly people with a rare genetic illness called lipodystrophy—they are thin but deposit fat in dangerous places like the liver, where fat is particularly harmful. These thin people develop severe insulin resistance and type 2 diabetes. Likewise, a person can be fit-fat, meaning they are overweight or even obese but their fat is on the surface of the body and not near vital organs. Though overweight, they might not necessarily get diabetes. If however, that excess fat is primarily around the belly, that's a diabetes situation in the making.

Food wise

The danger with diabetes is that excess glucose (sugar) in your blood can permanently damage your eyes, nerves, kidneys, heart, blood vessels, and cause foot ulcers, impotence, and gangrene (which can lead to amputations).

Diabetes Risk Checker

According to the National Diabetes Education Program, if you have prediabetes or have not had your blood sugar tested recently, it's time to get tested if you are:

- Age 45 or older (you should be tested every three years)

- Overweight or obese (Body Mass Index (BMI)$\geq$ 24.9)

- African American, Hispanic/Latino-American, Asian-American, Pacific Islander, or American Indian

- Have a parent, brother, or sister with diabetes

- Have high blood pressure (above 140/90)

- Have low HDL or "good" cholesterol (less than 40 for men; less than 50 for women)

- Have high triglycerides (250 or higher)

- Had diabetes when pregnant or gave birth to a baby over 9 pounds

- Are active less than three times a week

Foods to Fight Diabetes

What you eat and drink today can make a big difference in whether or not you get diabetes down the road. But don't think you'll be subject to a bland cardboard diet for life! No foods are "off limits" to people with diabetes. Even sweets are okay. What's key is portion size.

Munch on This
Contrary to popular belief, sugar does not cause diabetes. You can have sweets! It's a matter of portion size.

Think creatively. Think geometrically. Divide your plate in half and then one of the halves into two smaller sections. You now have three sections, as follows on the next page.

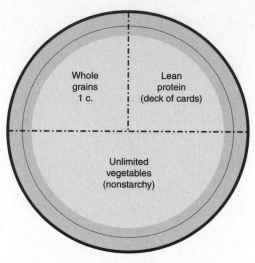

Setting your plate up in this manner is not only useful for monitoring your blood sugar, but for watching your waistline, too.

On the half of your plate devoted to vegetables, load your plate with colorful, nonstarchy veggies.

On the quarter of your plate devoted to protein, add 3.5 to 4 ounces (about the size of a deck of cards) of lean protein, such as tofu, chicken or turkey breast, fish, seafood, or loin cuts of beef or pork.

On the quarter of your plate devoted to grains and starches, add one cup of whole grains such as whole-grain bread, brown rice, cooked beans, or pasta.

Fill Up on Fiber

Plant foods—such as whole fruits, vegetables, grains, legumes, nuts, and seeds—contain a good amount of fiber, which is the nondigestible part of plants. Fiber is fantastic for stabilizing blood sugar levels, helping smooth out the peaks (ups) and valleys (downs). High-fiber foods are also very satisfying; they keep you full on fewer calories, which can help keep your waistline in check, too.

Two large research studies found that the participants who ate the most whole grains from breads, cereals, and pastas reduced their risk of diabetes by 40 percent over those who didn't eat as many whole-grain foods.

FOOD wise Just because a food product claims to be high fiber, it doesn't mean it is! Always check food labels for at least 3 grams or more of dietary fiber and aim for half of your grains to be "whole" every day.

How much fiber should you eat in a day? Try to get 14 grams per 1,000 calories—that's around 28 grams per day for the average person.

Here's how you can fit more fiber into your day:

- Dip baby carrots, cucumber slices, and/or whole-grain crackers in a couple of tablespoons of a bean dip like hummus, white bean, or edamame (soybean) purée for a fiber-filled snack.

- Sprinkle raw oats into yogurt or stuff a whole-grain pita with colorful red, green, and yellow peppers; add ripe avocado and a sprinkle of low-fat cheese.

- Roll a whole-grain wrap with lean turkey breast, low-fat cheese, sliced tomato, and mixed greens for a fiber fest at lunch.

Delight in Vitamin D

Also known as the sunshine nutrient, vitamin D is receiving a lot of scientific attention for its healing properties. Preliminary research shows that vitamin D may play a role in blood glucose control and insulin action, thus fending off diabetes.

Unfortunately, vitamin D is not naturally abundant in food. That makes getting at least 600 International Units (IU) of vitamin D foods a challenge. Among the foods that have vitamin D are egg yolks, fatty fish, and vitamin D–fortified milk and dairy products, such as cheese and yogurt. Mushrooms are the only vegan source of vitamin D.

One cup of vitamin D–fortified milk contains only 100 IU. One tablespoon of fortified margarine has a mere 60 IU; 3 ounces of mushrooms, exposed to UV light, contain 400 IU; and 3 ounces of cooked red salmon contains 800 IU. Given these low vitamin D levels in foods, it's smart to take vitamin D supplements (800–1,000 IU) especially if you fit any of these characteristics:

- Have very dark skin (as you may not be producing as much vitamin D from sunlight)

- Do not get enough sunlight (at least 10 to 15 minutes twice a week without sunscreen)

- Do not eat enough vitamin D–rich foods

Healing
Hints

Bask in the sunlight—without sunscreen—for 10 to 15 minutes at least twice a week to boost your vitamin D levels.

Be Selective with Fat

Fat plays a pivotal role in diabetes prevention. Although your body relies on daily doses of all types of fat, there are "good" fats and "bad" fats.

The bad fats are the saturated fats found in animal products, and trans fats (partially hydrogenated oils) typically found in fried foods and commercially baked sweets. Bad fats can lead to health problems associated with diabetes, including obesity, high cholesterol, and heart disease. You can start to rid your life of these bad boys by decreasing your intake of butter, bacon, fried foods, full-fat cheeses, heavy cream, and the partially hydrogenated oils found in store-baked muffins, cookies, and cakes.

Good fats are in vegetable oils, nuts, seeds, and avocados—all of which are better for heart health, maintaining healthy cholesterol levels, and fending off inflammation. Good fats are unsaturated fats and should be incorporated into your diet.

Food
wise

Beware that some commercial brands of nut butters are made with a lot of sugar and added hydrogenated oils. Look for "natural" peanut butter or almond butter made from the nuts only.

A 2002 study published in the *Journal of the American Medical Association* found that women who ate nuts or peanut butter, which are jam-packed with "good" polyunsaturated fats, at least five times a week had a 20 to 30 percent lower risk of diabetes. Be careful, though: nuts and nut butters are high-calorie foods, so watch your portions. Here's the caloric breakdown of one serving size of healthy fats:

- 1 tablespoon of vegetable oil (olive, canola) = 120 calories

- 1 ounce almonds (23 nuts) = 163 calories

- 1 ounce walnuts (14 halves) = 185 calories

- 1 ounce pistachios (49 nuts) = 162 calories

- 1 tablespoon nut butter (almond or peanut) = 100 calories

- 1 slice (⅕) of avocado = 50 calories

Finally, there are some simple ways to reduce the fat in your diet that can help you trim inches from your waistline and keep diabetes at bay. Switch from full-fat dairy to low-fat milk, yogurt, and cheese; ditch the full-fat mayonnaise for friendly fat avocado as a spread on sandwiches and wraps; toss the fried chips for baked ones; and use olive oil or canola oil instead of butter. Do that daily and you've made some wise choices to lower your dietary fat!

Sprinkle on Cinnamon

Antioxidants called polyphenols in cinnamon have been found to help insulin act more efficiently in the body by increasing the cells sensitivity to insulin. Although the research is mixed, there is some science behind cinnamon's relationship to lowering blood sugar levels.

How can you include cinnamon in your daily diet? You can sprinkle it on toast with almond butter, skim milk café au lait, steel cut oatmeal, yogurt, or fresh fruit. It also gives an exotic flavor to hearty soups and chili.

> **Food wise**
>
> Even moderate amounts (a teaspoon or two a day) of Cassia cinnamon or Chinese cinnamon can be dangerous for people with liver problems. Cassia cinnamon contains a flavoring agent, coumarin, which can be toxic to the liver. To be safe, get your daily dose from Ceylon cinnamon or true cinnamon, which is low in coumarin. Be sure to check your labels or ask your spice merchant: Ceylon is the species *Cinnamomum verum* and Cassia is *C. aromaticum*.

Mind Your Magnesium

Magnesium is an important mineral for metabolizing carbohydrates and regulating your blood sugar. Even though this nutrient doesn't make news headlines, magnesium is a powerful player in the game of diabetes prevention. Low levels of magnesium (hypomagnesemia) are believed to be related to insulin resistance, which can lead to diabetes. Magnesium helps balance blood sugar by assisting in the release and activity of insulin.

Magnesium stood out in two large, long-term studies of women and men. Both studies found that participants with high intakes of magnesium (375 milligrams a day for women; 450 milligrams a day for men) were at lower risk for type 2 diabetes. Keep in mind the Daily Value (DV) for magnesium is 400 milligrams.

What foods are high in magnesium? Chlorophyll-containing foods, such as leafy greens like spinach, kale, collard greens, and Swiss chard. In addition, eating legumes (peas and beans), nuts, seeds, and whole, unrefined grains can build up your magnesium stores.

Drinking tap water can boost your magnesium levels, too, depending on your water supply. So-called "hard" water contains more minerals such as magnesium, than does "soft" water.

Munch on This

Five fabulous food sources of magnesium are halibut, almonds, soybeans, spinach, and oatmeal.

Cater to Chromium

Not sure when you last ate chromium? It's not as if you can add a spoonful of chromium to your coffee or stir it into your soup. But to those with diabetes, this is one especially valuable trace mineral. Studies have shown that chromium helps the body maintain normal blood sugar levels.

You can find chromium in egg yolks, whole grain, bran cereal, green beans, broccoli, meat, brewer's yeast, wine, and beer. Practice caution with alcoholic beverages, as they can cause hypoglycemia, in which blood sugar levels fall to dangerously low levels.

Food wise

The jury is still out on using chromium supplements to fend off diabetes. The best bet is to stick with chromium-rich foods.

Control Your Carbohydrates

Carbohydrates offer vital fuel for your brain and cells. The type of carbohydrate you eat does matter from a blood sugar standpoint. Choosing more whole grains, fresh vegetables, and fruits can help manage blood sugar levels better than regularly eating the highly processed, refined grains. The system that ranks carbs based on their effect on blood sugar is called the Glycemic Index (GI).

GI ranks carbohydrates on a scale of 0 to 100. Those foods with a higher GI number, such as white rice, potatoes, and white bread raise blood sugar faster and increase the need for insulin. Lower GI foods, such as dried beans, peas, and lentils raise blood sugar more slowly and require less insulin output, hence less stress on the pancreas. Overstressing the pancreas can lead to diabetes.

For weight management, several studies have shown that people on low-carb diets (less than 130 grams per day of carbohydrates) lost more weight at 6 months than subjects on low-fat diets. Put less white bread, potatoes, rice, pasta, and couscous on your plate—it can help you maintain weight and keep your blood sugar in check.

Keep in mind, though, that food deprivation is pointless; in fact it may make matters worse. Some people binge when they feel deprived. Foods should not be considered good or bad based on GI; it is the portion of carbohydrates that matter most. According to an extensive review of the literature, the 2010 *Dietary Guidelines for Americans* Committee concluded that although a high-glycemic diet of white rice, potatoes, and baked goods is not good for blood sugar control, these types of foods do not cause diabetes. Balance is the key: choose starchy, refined carbohydrates, if you like, in smaller portions and combine with lean protein and nonstarchy vegetables for better blood sugar control.

Alcohol and Diabetes

Although some research has shown that alcohol can have a positive effect on insulin sensitivity, alcohol should always be consumed responsibly. You already know that weight gain is a primary cause of type 2 diabetes, and alcohol's high-calorie content can wreak havoc on your waistline in more ways than one.

Alcohol is an appetite stimulant, making you want to eat more during and after drinking, which leads to weight gain.

Alcoholic beverages not only contain additional calories, but it is believed to promote fat storage in the body, particularly around the belly. And as we said, research shows that fat around the middle makes people more susceptible to insulin resistance and diabetes.

Alcohol's Effects on Blood Sugar

Limit alcohol to no more than one drink per day for women and two drinks per day for men. Even after just a drink or two, your blood sugar can take a nose dive, if you are not careful. Hypoglycemia or low blood sugar can occur during and up to 12 hours after drinking. Hypoglycemia may cause confusion, blurred vision, tremor, heart palpitations, anxiety, sweating, and/or hunger.

You mitigate the risk of hypoglycemia by having a healthy snack with your drink. Eating when consuming alcohol can make all the difference between dropping into hypoglycemia or not.

> **Healing Hints**
>
> Avoid binge drinking by not saving up all of your daily drinks for one occasion. It can be very harmful, especially if you are at risk for diabetes, because it can cause hypoglycemic reactions, weight gain, and elevations in blood pressure, which compounds the heart risks associated with diabetes. Binge drinking equates to four alcoholic drinks for men and three alcoholic drinks for women within a two-hour period.

Foods to Drink With

As you undoubtedly know, it's not a good idea to drink alcohol on an empty stomach. Here are some tips to reduce how much you drink and keep your wits about you, too:

- Do not avoid carbs: Eat a portion-controlled snack, such as pretzels, popcorn, crackers, baked chips, raw vegetables and hummus, or low-fat yogurt dip.

- Eat a balanced meal with complex carbs: Whole-grain bread, brown rice, whole-grain pasta plus lean protein and nonstarchy vegetables, and "good" fat (avocado, olive oil, raw almonds, or pistachios).

- Sip your beverages, don't gulp: The longer you take to drink alcohol, the slower the effects on blood sugar.

- Alternate between drinking alcoholic drinks and mineral water, club soda, or plain water. For example, drink one beer and follow that up with one glass of water. The added bonus is you'll reduce your chance of a hangover by staying better hydrated, too!

- Enjoy a wine spritzer to dilute the amount of alcohol.

Movement Works

For good health, our bodies need to move. Sitting in cubicles, driving in cars, playing video games, watching television, and working on computers puts us at greater risk of diabetes. But how much exercise is enough? The Diabetes Prevention Program study found that regular exercise of at least 150 minutes per week (or about 20 minutes 7 days a week) remains a key prevention strategy. An active lifestyle improves the body's ability to use insulin and effectively escort glucose from the bloodstream into the cells for energy.

Know that you don't have to join a gym to get and stay in shape. You just need to be active. You can walk, jog, run, dance, take stairs, clean house, and do yard work. The strategy is consistent, daily activity. For example, take a brisk walk at lunch and after dinner and you've got it covered.

Recipes for Diabetes Control

Try any of the following recipes to help keep diabetes in check while enjoying a tasty meal.

Savory Roasted Root Vegetables

Roasted root vegetables are a delicious accompaniment to baked tofu, chicken breast, or salmon.

Yield:	Serving size:	Prep time:	Cook time:
4 servings	½ cup each	10 minutes	35 minutes

Each serving has:			
430 calories	14 g total fat	2 g saturated fat	0 g trans fat
0 mg cholesterol	233 mg sodium	74 g carbohydrates	12 g fiber
21 g sugars	7 g protein	24 percent iron	

1 whole pumpkin, sliced, peeled, and cut into chunks	1 tsp. ground cumin
6 fingerling potatoes, unpeeled, cut into chunks	1 tsp. fresh rosemary, finely chopped
2 small yellow onions, cut into wedges	¼ cup extra-virgin olive oil
2 fennel bulbs, sliced	¼ cup lemon juice
2 beet roots, diced	2 TB. brown sugar
4 garlic cloves, peeled and minced	½ tsp. paprika
	Salt and ground black pepper

1. Preheat oven to 400°F. Spread pumpkin, potatoes, onion, and fennel on a baking sheet. Put the beets on a smaller, separate baking sheet so as not to color the other vegetables.

2. In a small mixing bowl whisk together garlic, cumin, rosemary, olive oil, lemon juice, brown sugar, paprika, salt, and pepper. Drizzle mixture on top of vegetables, including the beets, tossing to fully coat.

3. Roast for 25 to 35 minutes, until vegetables are soft but not mushy. Let cool for a few minutes, and add beets to other vegetables before serving.

Munch on This

Fresh rosemary is more fragrant than dried rosemary. To substitute dried rosemary for fresh rosemary in a recipe, use 1 teaspoon dried rosemary for every 2 teaspoons chopped fresh rosemary.

Nutty Turkey Meatloaf

This hearty meatloaf can be made with lean ground beef, pork, or chicken. It tastes great accompanied by roasted vegetables.

Yield:	Serving size:	Prep time:	Cook time:
4 servings	4-ounce slice	10 minutes	30 minutes

Each serving has:			
391 calories	19 g total fat	5 g saturated fat	0 g trans fat
179 mg cholesterol	596 mg sodium	10 g carbohydrates	1 g fiber
3 g sugars	42 g protein	21 percent iron	

1 lb. ground turkey breast (93 percent lean)	¼ cup plain, whole-grain breadcrumbs
3 cloves garlic, minced	¼ cup walnuts, chopped
½ small yellow onion, chopped	2 TB. Worcestershire sauce
1 small red bell pepper, chopped	2 to 3 TB. tomato paste
3 basil leaves, finely chopped	

1. Preheat oven to 350°F. In a medium bowl, combine turkey, garlic, onion, pepper, basil, breadcrumbs, walnuts, and Worcestershire sauce. When completely mixed, transfer the mixture to a nonstick loaf pan and spread tomato paste on top.

2. Bake for about 30 minutes until nicely browned on top and the juices run clear inside.

Spicy Tomato and Olive Quinoa

This zippy quinoa, a Mediterranean grain, is delicious with tofu, shrimp, chicken, fish, and lean beef.

Yield:	Serving size:	Prep time:	Cook time:
6 servings	½ cup	5 minutes	15 minutes

Each serving has:			
174 calories	8 g total fat	1 g saturated fat	0 g trans fat
0 mg cholesterol	324 mg sodium	21 g carbohydrates	3 g fiber
2 g sugars	4 g protein	8 percent iron	

1 cup quinoa

1 cup low-sodium vegetable broth

1 cup water

2 TB. extra-virgin olive oil

3 green onions (scallions), chopped

1 cup cherry tomatoes, halved

½ cup black olives, pitted and sliced

1 tsp. smoked paprika

Salt to taste

1. Rinse quinoa and add to a medium pot over medium heat with broth and water. Bring to a boil, cover, reduce heat, and simmer until liquid is absorbed. Remove from heat and fluff quinoa with a fork.

2. Add oil, green onions, cherry tomatoes, black olives, paprika, and a dash of salt. Stir gently to mix. Serve warm on a bed of leafy greens.

Essential Takeaways

- Your risk of diabetes can be lowered with healthy foods and lifestyle changes.
- While there are no "bad" foods, some foods are more helpful in controlling diabetes than others.
- Fiber from whole grains, vegetables, and fruits is a diabetes defense.
- Minerals like magnesium and chromium play a role in blood sugar control.
- Sprinkling cinnamon in small doses can help prevent diabetes.
- Alcohol is not off limits, but limiting its consumption and not drinking on an empty stomach make a good plan for diabetes prevention.

chapter 22

Combating Cancer

Understanding common cancers and causes

Fending off certain cancers with food

Making cancer-combating recipes

Cancer encompasses hundreds of diseases with one common cause—abnormal cells go haywire and grow out of control. Cancerous cells are unique in that they infiltrate other tissues. Cancer cells are relentless and have no boundaries; if not treated, cancer can lead to grave illness and death.

In the United States, half of all men and one third of all women will get some form of cancer in their lifetime. Most cancers can be attributed to lifestyle and environmental factors, such as smoking, unhealthy eating, obesity, lack of physical activity, infections, stress, and pollutants. Genetics do play a role, but to a lesser degree.

What and how much you eat can play a vital role in squelching cancerous cells. For instance, increasing the amount of plant-based foods (e.g., fruits and vegetables) you eat and decreasing your intake of animal foods (e.g., red and processed meat) are two eating behaviors that could decrease your overall risk of getting some cancers. Losing weight is another powerful way to fend off cancers.

In this chapter, I delve into certain cancers and how your eating choices and lifestyle can make a difference in preventing this life-threatening group of diseases.

Breast Cancer

After skin cancer, breast cancer is the most common cancer in women; it's the second leading cause of cancer death in women after lung cancer. Genetics plays a role—your chances of getting breast cancer double if your mother, sister, or daughter have been diagnosed with it; however the majority of women diagnosed with breast cancer do not have a close blood relative with breast cancer.

Weight Gain Counts

Carrying excess body weight increases a woman's risk of breast cancer by 30 to 50 percent. The danger is particularly high for postmenopausal women because once a woman stops her menstrual cycle, the body relies on fat, rather than the ovaries, to produce estrogen. The more body fat, the higher the levels of the hormone estrogen, the main culprit in breast cancer.

The more weight a woman gains in adulthood (after age 18), the greater her chances of developing breast cancer later in life. Studies have shown that women who gain in the range of 21 to 40 pounds in adulthood have a 68 percent higher risk for breast cancer than women who gain less than 20 pounds. After that the risk keeps getting higher: those who gain between 41 and 60 pounds double their chances of getting breast cancer, and those who gain more than 60 pounds triple their breast cancer risk.

Plant-Based Plate

Eating an abundance of colorful fruits and vegetables is vital for overall health and weight management. Fruits and vegetables are jammed packed with disease-fighting antioxidants, plant compounds that rid the body of damaging cells. In particular, broccoli, spinach, and apples are low in calories, saturated fat, and sodium, and high in fiber—all good things for keeping your weight in check. The American Cancer Society recommends five or more servings of fruits and vegetables every day.

> **Munch on This**
>
> What does five servings (or 5 cups) of fruits and vegetables look like? That's 1 cup spinach + 1 cup broccoli florets + 1 large sweet potato + 1 large banana + 1 large peach.

Soy and Breast Cancer

Soy has been under the research radar for decades for its potential role in breast health. Soyfoods contain phyto (plant) estrogens called isoflavones. These weak estrogens can either help or hinder cancerous cells from growing and spreading. In test tubes studies they have done both. However, studies looking at women of Asian descent (as soyfoods are an Asian food staple), have found that women who started eating soyfoods during adolescence showed less of a risk for breast cancer later in life. The good news is the benefits were seen with only a serving a day of soyfoods.

Researchers think that in younger women with higher estrogen levels, soy's plant-estrogen may compete for cell receptors with the body's natural estrogen, keeping natural estrogen levels in a healthy, lower range, thus fending off breast cancer. However, after menopause soy estrogen may pose more of a threat—as feeding your body excess estrogen, even if it is a weak form of estrogen, may increase the risk for estrogen-sensitive breast cancer, particularly in overweight or obese women.

It's important to weigh your risk, but in moderation, soyfoods are a great source of low saturated fat and cholesterol-free protein. Research has shown that switching from animal proteins to plant proteins like beans and legumes stopped the destructive course of potential cancer cells. However, since soyfoods contain estrogen, experts recommend that women practice moderation at any age. That's not to say you can't enjoy a serving or two a day!

Alcohol and Breast Cancer

Although alcohol may benefit your heart health, numerous studies have found that alcohol—even a drink a day—can pose a risk for breast cancer (and other cancers). Although the risk is fairly low, it's nevertheless real. A large study of 300,000 women found each daily alcoholic drink increased breast cancer risk by 9 percent. Risk goes up with every drink, so if you have two drinks per day, your risk could go up by 25 percent!

One of the possible reasons is that alcohol depletes the body of nutrients, particularly folic acid. Folic acid is the B-vitamin that helps make and repair DNA, thus low levels can give rise to abnormal cell and tumor growth in the breast.

> **food wise**
>
> A sedentary lifestyle can pose a risk for breast cancer and other cancers. The American Cancer Society recommends at least 45 to 60 minutes of "intentional" physical activity at least five days a week for adults and children. That means making some time to speed walk, run, jog, do Pilates, or hop on the treadmill or elliptical machine.

Ovarian Cancer

Named "the silent killer," ovarian cancer typically has no or subtle symptoms such as bloating, abdominal pain, pain in back of legs, diarrhea, gas, nausea, pain during sex, abnormal vaginal bleeding, and trouble breathing. Cancerous tumors can grow in one or both the ovaries. During the reproductive years this dynamic duo takes turns releasing a single egg every month. Ovaries also provide women with the hormones estrogen and progesterone.

Ovarian cancer appears to be linked to genes. According to the National Cancer Institute, family history is the leading risk factor for ovarian cancer, so if your mother, sister, or daughter were diagnosed with it, there's a greater chance of getting it. Other factors include late menopause (as the longer your ovaries secrete hormones the greater risk), never having a baby or breastfeeding, and using hormone replacement therapy.

Eating Well for Ovaries

There is limited information on the ovaries and diet, but unlike breast cancer, drinking alcohol in moderation does not seem to affect your ovarian health. Intake of nonstarchy vegetables are suggested to play a role in decreasing risk for ovarian cancer. So now you have yet another reason to eat two or more servings of leafy greens, broccoli, cauliflower, carrots, zucchini, onions, and mushrooms every day.

Balancing calories in with calories out can help keep your ovaries healthy. Keeping your weight in check or losing weight (as little as 5 to 10 percent of body weight) can greatly reduce your risk of hormone-dependent cancers like ovarian cancer. Getting physical activity helps, too—at least 45 to 60 minutes five days a week, if not more.

Vitamin D and Ovarian Cancer

Vitamin D, the sunshine nutrient, may play a role in whether or not you get ovarian cancer. Ovarian cancer rates appear to be higher in cooler, northern climates versus sunnier, southern parts of the world. Researchers believe vitamin D plays a role in this geographic disparity.

A study in the *International Journal of Epidemiology* which looked at women who lived in 100 of the largest southern (and sunny) U.S. cities found lower incidences and death rates associated with ovarian cancer. This could have big dietary implications—so be sure to get at least your Recommended Daily Allowance (RDA) of vitamin D, which is 400 to 600 IU per day, if not more.

Sunlight is your best source of vitamin D, but if you live in the North, particularly during the winter months, try to drink two to three glasses of fat-free milk, which is fortified with vitamin D. Some cheeses and yogurts are fortified with vitamin D, too—so check the labels. White button mushrooms that have been exposed to ultraviolet rays have a daily dose of vitamin D in a 3-ounce serving. Also, fatty fish like salmon, halibut, and tuna contains significant levels of vitamin D—aim for at least two 6-ounce servings per week.

Colorectal Cancer

The colon is a powerful player in your digestive health. It's the largest part of the gastrointestinal tract; it absorbs water, maintains water balance, absorbs vitamin K, and is teaming with *microflora*. Over a lifetime, there's a 7 percent chance of developing this type of cancer. When cancerous polyps or fleshy growths develop in the colon, large intestine, rectum (opening of the colon), and in some cases the appendix, it's called colorectal cancer. In the United States colon cancer is the fourth most common cancer and the third leading cause of cancer-related deaths.

Definition	**Microflora** are microscopic bacteria living in the gastrointestinal tract that fend off disease-causing invaders.

Healing Hints	Fruits and vegetables have shown preventive benefit for cancers of the mouth, pharynx, larynx, stomach, and lung, as well as the prostate, colon, and pancreas. So aim for at least 2 cups of fruits and 2 ½ cups of veggies every day; go for the colorful, dark green and orange fruits and veggies, as these have shown the most benefit.

Plants Can Do Your Colon Good

The colon thrives when it gets a good dose of fruits and vegetables. Researchers aren't sure whether the benefits are due to the extra work put on the colon from the rigors of pushing through this plant roughage or the dose of additional plant-based nutrients that are in plants. They do know that plant foods contribute to colon health, whereas animal proteins do not.

For over 30 years, the Melbourne Colorectal Cancer Study has looked at the causes of colorectal cancer, and findings have revealed that diets high in vegetables, particularly cruciferous vegetables (e.g., broccoli, cauliflower, kale, cabbage, etc.) may protect the colon from cancer. Part of the reason could be that vegetables and fruit are low in saturated fat and they fill you up on fewer calories. Aim for at least five servings of richly colored dark leafy greens and orange veggies (2½ cups) and fruits (2 cups) every day.

Push Plant Protein

As far as protein, choose plant sources of protein over red and processed meat. Instead go for beans and legumes. A great source of low-calorie and filling fiber, beans and legumes can promote a healthy colon.

People who don't eat meat or eat it less often, have been found to have a lower body mass index (BMI), which can decrease your colorectal cancer risk. Although fiber's role in fending off colon cancer is not clear, there's a good chance that fibrous foods can indirectly affect colon health by decreasing your overall calorie intake and keeping weight gain at bay.

If you are going to eat red meat, limit it to less than 18 ounces a week, and avoid the processed meats such as ham, bacon, pastrami, salami, sausage, and hot dogs. Sodium nitrates or nitrites are preservatives in processed meats that have been linked to colorectal cancer, so check labels in processed meat products and purchase nitrate-free varieties. These products may be hard to find at your local grocer, but many natural food stores carry them.

food wise	Grilling or charbroiling meat, including red meat, pork, poultry, and fish, causes the formation of cancer-causing compounds called heterocyclic amines on the meat's flesh. Over time, eating too much charred, well-done meat may damage blood vessels leading to cancers, including colorectal cancer. Marinating meats may help prevent the formation of heterocyclic amines, but the best defense is to eat less red and processed meat overall.

Body Weight and Colon Health

Obesity promotes colorectal cancer. Even people who are just a couple of extra pounds overweight can be at higher risk. Because body weight—especially the amount of body fat around your midsection, can increase your risk for colon cancer—it's important to choose low-calorie foods.

Your body weight is something that you can control. Focus on a few things: eat nutrient-packed, healthy foods in moderate amounts and get a significant amount of physical activity. This will ensure energy (caloric) balance and lead to a healthy body weight for life.

Munch
on This

Men's waists should be under 40 inches in circumference and women's should be below 35 inches. Here are some simple steps for measuring your waist circumference:

1. To find your natural waistline, stand straight with shirt lifted and bend to one side; the crease in the side you're bending toward indicates your waistline. It should be above your belly button, but below your ribcage. Put your finger there as a placeholder.

2. Stand back up straight. Using a measuring tape, place it above your belly button at "0" and wrap it straight around your middle. Not too tight or too loose. Measure your waist.

3. Write down your current waist measurement and date it, so that you can note future body composition changes. Repeat this at least once a year to keep your waistline in check!

Calcium Helps the Colon

The mineral calcium—both from food sources and calcium supplements—has been shown to play a role in fending off colorectal cancer. Calcium supplements were found to work better for colorectal cancer, whereas milk specifically abated cancer in the colon (not including the rectum).

So what does this mean? For overall colorectal health a combination of calcium supplements and low-fat/fat-free milk can do your colon and rectum good.

Prostate Cancer

The prostate is a small gland that makes and stores the fluid that carries semen. Cancer of the prostate is the second most common form of cancer in men.

Certain foods have been shown to slow the onset and prevent prostate cancer. The key findings in this area points to eating less red meat and reducing total fat intake; eating more fruits—especially tomato products, vegetables, and fish (at least two 6-ounce servings a week); and consuming more plant-based proteins such as beans, legumes, and soy.

Tomatoes contain large amounts of lycopene, a plant-based carotenoid that has shown to play a role in keeping the prostate healthy. The protective effect appears to be greatest in cooked tomatoes—not raw ones, as the lycopene levels are much higher when tomatoes are heated.

Although the role of lycopene and prostate cancer prevention is still under investigation, studies have shown prostate specific antigen (PSA), a clinical red flag for prostate inflammation and possible cancer, goes down when more tomato products, such as tomato-based pasta sauce, are eaten. Lycopene supplements have proven to lower prostate cancer risk, too; however, eating the whole tomato offers so many more benefits, including antioxidants, vitamins C and E, soluble fiber, and other plant compounds (e.g., carotenoids and polyphenols).

Skin Cancer

Skin cancer is the number one form of cancer in both men and women in the United States. Approximately 120,000 new cases of melanomas—the most serious form of skin cancer—are diagnosed annually. More men than women are diagnosed with melanomas. Skin cancer stems from a few factors—the most common one is exposure to the sun over your lifetime—90 percent of skin cancers are related to too much fun in the sun. However, skin cancer can also occur in unexposed areas. Other factors are excessive moles on your body, fair-skinned with light eyes, a family history, burns or wounds that take a long time to heal, smoking tobacco (it's been shown to double your risk of skin cancer), and viral infections (e.g., human papilloma virus).

Food and Fun for Skin

Skin cancer is the one form of cancer in which an active lifestyle can pose a threat. Whether it's cold-weather or warm-weather sports or activities, when skin is exposed to UV rays from the sun, there's an increased risk for skin cancer. If you are going to go out in the sun, wear sunglasses, a hat, clothing with UV protection, and sunscreen with at least a sun protection factor (SPF) of 30 (depending on your skin tone; check with your dermatologist).

Strong Immunity Foods

Because skin cancer can strike when your immune system is weak, you should strive to maintain a stellar immune system by increasing antioxidant-rich fruits and vegetables, B-vitamin–packed whole grains, vitamin C foods like oranges, lemons, limes, guavas, and kiwi as well as herbs and spices like curry and ginger. (See Chapter 18 for details.)

Vitamin D can boost immunity and keep your skin cells healthy, but since sun exposure (without sunscreen) must be kept to a minimum, your vitamin D levels may drop. Supplement with at least 400 to 600 IU of vitamin D, especially if don't eat oily fish at least twice a week, drink milk daily, or eat other fortified foods like yogurt, eggs, cheeses, and white button mushrooms. (Check labels for vitamin D content on all these foods.)

Medications for diabetes, cholesterol, blood pressure, and inflammation may make your skin more sensitive to the sun's rays. So keep your diet healthy and fend off other disease states with a balance of whole foods. It will do your skin good!

Healing Hints

The number one cause of cancer-related death is lung cancer. To prevent lung cancer, quit smoking tobacco and avoid exposure to secondhand smoke. As far as nutrients, don't rely on supplements of vitamins A (beta-carotene), C, E, or folate, as they won't necessarily help your lung health. What works is more fruits and nonstarchy veggies and regular physical activity. For more information, visit www.dietandcancerreport.org.

Cancer-Combating Recipes

From fish to whole grains to vegetables, try these fresh recipes to keep your healthy cells growing for life.

Salmon with Curried Mustard Sauce

What better way to end a day than with healthy fats and protein from salmon. Feel free to substitute halibut, tuna, barramundi, or Arctic char.

Yield:	Serving size:	Prep time:	Cook time:
4 servings	1 filet	5 minutes	20 minutes

Each serving has:			
215 calories	11 g total fat	2 g saturated fat	0.3 g trans fat
62 mg cholesterol	183 mg sodium	4 g carbohydrates	0 g fiber
3 g sugars	24 g protein	6 percent iron	

1 lb. wild salmon filets, cut into 4 portions

1 TB. extra-virgin olive oil

½ cup yogurt, plain, low-fat

2 TB. Dijon mustard

1 tsp. curry powder

2 tsp. fresh lemon juice

Pinch of salt and pepper

1. Preheat oven to 425°F. Place salmon, skin side down, in an oven-safe baking dish.

2. Rub each filet with olive oil and a dash of salt and pepper.

3. In a small bowl, combine yogurt, mustard, curry powder, and lemon juice. Spread mixture evenly over salmon.

4. Bake salmon for 20 minutes. Check with a fork for flakiness and golden-color on top. Serve immediately with extra sauce for dipping.

food wise

Wild salmon contains less mercury and other contaminants than farm-raised salmon, plus it is an eco-friendly, sustainable choice. You can purchase wild salmon fresh or frozen at most grocery stores or ask your local fishmonger for it.

Fusilli with Spicy Tomato Sauce

Spicy and savory, this dish is perfect for an evening dinner party or weekend brunch. It's packed with lycopene-rich tomatoes!

Yield:	Serving size:	Prep time:	Cook time:
4 servings	1 cup	50 minutes	40 minutes

Each serving has:			
516 calories	11 g total fat	2 g saturated fat	0 g trans fat
82 mg cholesterol	596 mg sodium	89 g carbohydrates	7 g fiber
16 g sugars	20 g protein	49 percent iron	

2 cups whole-wheat fusilli	2 TB. balsamic vinegar
2 TB. extra-virgin olive oil	1 cup tomatoes, chopped
1 cup yellow onions, chopped	1 TB. fresh basil, minced
1 garlic clove, minced	1 tsp. oregano
2 tsp. crushed red pepper	1 bay leaf
1 cup green bell pepper, chopped	⅛ tsp. ground black pepper
1 cup white button mushrooms	Salt
2 cups crushed tomatoes	2 cups arugula, washed
6 oz. (1 small can) tomato paste	

1. Put a large pot of water on the stove at high heat to boil. When water is boiling, add pasta and cook about 10 minutes (until tender), drain, and set aside.

2. Add oil to a deep sauce pan. Add garlic and onions, sautéing until translucent or clear. Incorporate crushed pepper, green bell peppers, and mushrooms. Cook together for a few minutes.

3. Add tomato purée, tomato paste, vinegar, tomatoes, basil, oregano, bay leaf, and black pepper. Turn the heat down, cover, and simmer at least 30 minutes, stirring occasionally. Taste and add a pinch of salt, if desired.

4. Divide pasta into four shallow bowls, top generously with tomato sauce, and garnish with a handful of arugula. Serve immediately.

Citrus Couscous with Garden Vegetables

Feel free to add any vegetables or fresh herbs to this quick, colorful meal.

Yield:	Serving size:	Prep time:	Cook time:
6 servings	½ cup	10 minutes	20 minutes

Each serving has:			
216 calories	9 g total fat	1 g saturated fat	0 g trans fat
0 mg cholesterol	29 mg sodium	29 g carbohydrates	3 g fiber
3 g sugars	3 g protein	6 percent iron	

1 cup whole-grain couscous

2 cups water

¼ cup fresh lemon juice

¼ cup extra-virgin olive oil

2 cups plum tomatoes, halved, seeded, and coarsely chopped

2 cups zucchini, sliced

1 red bell pepper, chopped

2 scallions, thinly sliced

¼ cup flat-leaf parsley, finely chopped

2 TB. fresh mint, finely chopped

Pinch salt and freshly ground pepper

1. Place couscous and water in a medium pot over medium-high heat and bring to a boil. Turn heat off, cover, and let sit for 5 minutes.

2. In a large bowl, whisk lemon juice and olive oil. Add couscous, tomatoes, zucchini, red peppers, scallions, chopped parsley, and mint. Toss together.

3. Taste and season with salt and pepper, if desired. Let stand for 10 minutes before serving to let flavors blend together.

Essential Takeaways

- Eating healthful, plant-based foods and fewer animal products helps fend off many types of cancer.
- Weight gain and abdominal fat are major causes of most cancers. Keep your weight in check for life to keep your cancer risk low.
- Even one alcoholic drink a day increases your risk of breast cancer.

chapter 23

Gut Health from Top to Bottom

Making sense of your digestive system

Feeding your gut right

Identifying foods that promote and prevent gas

Making gut-friendly recipes

Your digestive system, or gut, keeps everything running and functioning in order. Your gut begins with the mouth and ends with the anus, but everything in between—from the esophagus to the stomach to the small intestine to the large intestine (large bowel)— keeps it moving like clockwork.

Your gut can be affected by your diet, diseases, and emotional stress. Your gut is connected to the emotional centers of your brain, and serves as a strong fortress of immune-fighting defense, shielding you from the plague of disease-promoting pathogens or germs trying to wage war inside you at any time. The lining of your gut consists of mucosa, or mucous membranes, that are home to trillions of microscopic bacteria, including friendly probiotics that promote good health and fight harmful bacteria that threaten it.

Nutrient-rich food plays a role in fortifying your good bacteria, keeping your intestines in good working order, and enabling smooth transit time (how long it takes food to get through the digestive system). On the flip side, fueling your body with nutrient-poor foods or irritants can further the progression of heartburn; inflammatory bowel disorders and diseases like colitis and Crohn's disease; and autoimmune diseases, like celiac disease, which effects the small intestine.

This chapter examines the conditions and diseases that can get you in the gut—from mild disturbances to severe autoimmune diseases that can affect the absorption of nutrients and lead to a host of other health problems down the line.

Acid Reflux

On occasion, most people eat spicy foods or too much food and experience heartburn or indigestion—that burning sensation in the chest or throat. About 15 million people in the United States complain about heartburn every day. The lower esophageal sphincter is a valvelike structure that opens to let food into the stomach and closes off the esophagus so that food doesn't come back up. The sphincter can malfunction by opening at random times or not fully closing, leaving an opening for acid in the stomach to back up into the esophagus which causes the burn. This burn is a symptom of acid reflux or gastroesophageal reflux (GER).

Gastroesophageal Reflux Disease (GERD)

If the acid backup continues to occur more than twice a week, you might have gastroesophageal reflux disease (GERD). A serious condition that can lead to changes in the cell wall of the esophagus, which can develop into cancer if it's not treated. The good news is you can often treat the disease by making eating and lifestyle changes. However, if the symptoms persist even after you've made changes, make an appointment with your health-care provider and/or a registered dietitian for an individualized eating plan.

Healing Hints

Your GI tract has a stress threshold. Because stress is known to play a role in heartburn, your eating environment is important to whether you get it or not. Try not to eat near loud music, loud talking, yelling, or stressful work situations. Family spats are not meant for the dinner table—or you'll feel the burn later. Relax when you're eating and your digestion will thank you!

Avoid the Burn with Food

You can avoid heartburn by making simple changes to what you eat and your overall eating habits. Foods that disrupt the natural flow of things and cause a backup are acidic foods like vinegar, coffee, orange juice, tomato sauce, ketchup, and mustard; caffeinated food and beverages like chocolate, coffee, soft drinks, and tea; alcoholic beverages like wine and beer; fatty and fried foods like French fries, batter-fried fish, mozzarella sticks, and nachos; and spicy foods, too.

Some eating behaviors that may prevent heartburn include the following:

- Not eating right before bed; wait a couple of hours at least before lying down to go to bed.

- Eating smaller meals. Too much food at one sitting can cause partially digested food to come back up.

- Avoiding the foods that you know trigger your heartburn. For some people it may be caffeine and for others it's alcohol.

- Maintaining a healthy weight. Even modest amounts of weight gain—5 to 7 pounds— can trigger heartburn as it's your body's way of saying, "it's too much," "I am not happy at this weight."

Listen to your heartburn, it may be telling you something! Know your own heartburn buttons and have an eating strategy to combat it.

Celiac Disease

Celiac disease affects 1 out of 100 people in the United States; it's a serious, genetic autoimmune intestinal disorder, in which the immune system is extremely sensitive to gluten—the protein in wheat, rye, and barley—and it attacks the surface of the small intestine, specifically the villi or the fingerlike projections on the lining of the small intestines. The villi are vital to getting good nutrition as they absorb nutrients from food. The nutrients most affected by celiac disease are calcium, iron, and folate, but more severe cases affect the absorption of lactose and fat-soluble vitamins (A, D, E, and K). One of the major risks with celiac disease is that many people with it live a long time before getting an actual diagnosis; by then, a lot of intestinal damage is done and malnutrition ensues.

Celiac disease often goes undiagnosed for so long because several of its symptoms are affiliated with other diseases. People with celiac disease might experience iron-deficiency anemia, folate or B_{12} deficiency, bone or joint pain, bone density loss, seizures, missed menstrual periods, infertility, and/or dermatitis herpetiformis (an itchy skin rash). In children, symptoms include irritability and behavior changes, failure to grow and develop, delayed puberty, dental issues, and lack of concentration.

People with other autoimmune diseases—such as type 1 diabetes, thyroid disease, liver disease, rheumatoid arthritis, Sjogren's Syndrome (a disease in which the tears and salivary glands are destroyed), and Addison's disease (a disease in which the glands that produce critical hormones are destroyed)—should be screened for celiac disease. This disease can rear its head at any age as a result of a viral infection, severe stress, surgery, or pregnancy.

Food and Gluten Intolerance

As far as food is concerned, the only bona fide nutrition treatment for celiac disease is ridding the diet of gluten completely. Gluten can be found in many food products and other grains related to wheat, rye, and barley; even oats can be cross-contaminated with wheat or barley. The good news is the food industry recognizes the growing number of people being diagnosed with celiac disease and offers a wide range of gluten-free foods. The following table lists foods that people with celiac disease should avoid.

Gluten Watch: Avoid These Foods & Ingredients	
Related Grain	*Food or Ingredient*
Wheat	Atta (chapatti flour)
	Bulgur
	Couscous
	Spelt (dinkel)
	Durum
	Einkorn
	Emmer
	Farina
	Farro or Faro
	Fu
	Graham flour
	Hydrolyzed wheat flour
	Kamut
	Matzoh
	Modified wheat starch
	Seitan ("wheat meat")
	Semolina
	Triticale

Related Grain	Food or Ingredient
	Wheat bran
	Wheat flour
	Wheat germ
	Wheat starch
Barley	Ale
	Barley flakes, flour, pearl
	Beer
	Brewer's yeast
	Lager
	Malt
	Malt extract/malt syrup
	Malt flavoring
	Malt milk
	Malt vinegar
Rye	Rye bread
	Rye flour
Oats*	Oatmeal
	Oat bran
	Oat flour
	Oats

*Be aware that oats can be cross-contaminated with wheat and/or barley. Watch out for commercially available oat products. You can buy pure and uncontaminated oats, but follow-up with your physicians as some people with celiac disease cannot tolerate even the pure oats.

Source: Gluten-Free Diet, A Comprehensive Resource Guide by Shelley Case, BSc, RD. Visit www.glutenfreediet.ca for more details on gluten-free living.

Gluten-Free Smarts

Gluten-free living has become a fad as celebrities are boasting the benefits of weight loss and improved energy after banishing gluten from their diets. Although it may be tempting to join the gluten-free bandwagon, practice caution—it can be detrimental to your health. Gluten-free products can be made from refined grains, which lack fiber and essential vitamins and minerals.

If you're going without gluten, be sure to incorporate whole grains that are naturally gluten-free like corn, millet, brown rice, buckwheat, quinoa, and wild rice.

The bottom line is if you suspect gluten-sensitivity or full-blown celiac disease, experts recommend a diagnostic blood test that looks for antibodies for the disease. If you deplete your body of gluten before you are tested, the results may not be accurate. Consult a gastroenterologist, if you would like to be tested for celiac disease or gluten-sensitivity.

Irritable Bowel Syndrome

No one likes to feel bloated, gassy, have chronic abdominal pain, constipation, or diarrhea, but these are some of the symptoms you may be experiencing if you have irritable bowel syndrome (IBS). Somewhat of a puzzling intestinal disorder, IBS is considered a "diagnosis of exclusion," which means that a definite diagnosis is difficult to make as the symptoms can resemble other intestinal disorders. Dietary detective work is needed! Dietary components are eliminated one-by-one until a diagnostic determination can be made. Even still, IBS sometimes remains a mystery. There's no real cure, but there are ways to alleviate symptoms.

IBS is classified based on the predominant chronic condition, whether it's diarrhea, constipation, or a combination of the two. IBS is believed to be related to the brain or psychological disorders—60 percent of people with IBS have depression or anxiety. This is why low doses of antidepressants are often prescribed for people with IBS. (Unfortunately, some of these medications can cause diarrhea, bloating, and gas!)

Food and IBS

Eating can be tricky with IBS. Because IBS symptoms are personal, you should keep a food journal and jot down symptoms after you eat. This can help you map out an eating plan that works for you. The foods you can eat (or not eat) depend upon your IBS symptoms. Try not to restrict your diet too much, however, as this can play even more into depression and anxiety, which may be the root of the IBS. Try to eliminate only the foods that seem to cause a flair up.

Carbohydrates can be the culprit in IBS, particularly the group of fermentable carbs called FODMAPs, which stands for **F**ermentable **O**ligosaccharides, **D**isaccharides, **M**onosaccharides, and **P**olyols. These carbs are poorly absorbed in the intestines and create gas, bloating, and diarrhea in people who have sensitive guts. Foods that are high in FODMAPs include dairy products, certain fruits, vegetables, beans, and products sweetened with high-fructose corn syrup and natural sugar substitutes (such as sorbitol, xylitol, and mannitol). To find out more about FODMAP-friendly foods, go to www.fodmap.com.

IBS with Constipation

If you have constipation—three or fewer bowel movements per week—adding dietary fiber can help. Lack of fiber can make it hard to pass stools, so try getting at least 14 grams of fiber for every 1,000 calories you eat. For women that's about 25 grams a day; for men it's 38 grams a day, which would be an improvement from the mere 15 grams of fiber that the typical American eats daily.

High-fiber foods that have been found to be natural laxatives include cabbage, whole-grain bread, oatmeal, fruits, seeds, honey, figs, prunes, raspberries, strawberries, and stewed apples.

Food wise

Add fiber to your diet gradually, because an overload can worsen IBS, especially bloating, gas, and intestinal pain. Also be sure to drink enough water throughout the day, which can help your body tolerate more fiber and alleviate constipation.

IBS with Diarrhea

On the other side of the spectrum, IBS can cause the need for frequent visits to the bathroom, which can disrupt work and life in general. Chronic diarrhea (three or more bowel movements in a day) or watery stools is a sign that the large intestine is not properly absorbing water. This is dangerous, as excess loss of fluids and electrolytes (e.g., sodium and potassium) can cause severe dehydration, fatigue, dizziness, and weight loss. If you experience IBS with diarrhea, try to go on a bland diet for a while. Avoid high-fat, high insoluble-fiber foods, spicy foods, and milk. To replenish electrolytes and get additional calories, drink clear broths and juices during bouts of diarrhea. Eat foods like dry toast, crackers, rice, and pectin-rich fruits like bananas and apple sauce.

If diarrhea persists, adding in some beneficial bacteria or probiotic-rich foods or supplements (e.g., Florastor or Florastor Kids) may help replenish the natural microflora in your gut and keep your immune system strong. Studies have shown that probiotics can lessen the symptoms of IBS. Some of these foods are dairy-based (e.g., kefir, yogurt, and buttermilk) so be careful as they can aggravate diarrhea. Try nondairy probiotic foods, such as soy yogurt, miso, and tempeh (fermented soybeans). Add some soluble fiber such as oats, apples, oranges, and barley to aid in bulking up the stool.

Healing Hints

Colitis is an autoimmune, inflammatory bowel disease (IBD), which causes gas, bloating, and diarrhea. Its sister syndrome, ulcerative colitis, is similar except (as its name implies) it is accompanied by open sores in the colon. Eating a low-fat, bland diet with no alcohol or caffeine is the best way to minimize symptoms. Be sure to get enough calories and replenish fluids and electrolytes with broths, juices, or enhanced waters.

Crohn's Disease

Crohn's disease is unlike the other autoimmune inflammatory bowel diseases, as it's not confined to the bowel (large and small intestines); it can affect the mouth, skin, eyes, joints, and your concentration. Of the 1.4 million people in the United States who have IBD, half have Crohn's disease. Like other forms of IBD, the causes of Crohn's disease are a mystery, but it may be caused by the environment, your genetic makeup (20 to 25 percent of people have a close relative with it), or your immune system backfires by "turning on" without knowing how to shut off. The result is chronic diarrhea, cramps, abdominal pain, fever, rectal bleeding, and risk of cancer. Many people with Crohn's disease lose their appetite, lose weight, and are tired frequently. Children with Crohn's disease can have delayed growth and sexual maturation.

Specific foods will not cure Crohn's disease; however, fueling the body to give it energy and power is essential. Crohn's disease can rob the body of "The Big Three" macronutrients—carbs, protein, and fat—as well as the micronutrients—vitamins and minerals. People suffering from Crohn's disease must be extra vigilant about getting enough nutrition to maintain their health and heal their body. Being in the mood for food can be a challenge for people with Crohn's disease, so the diet should be flexible to accommodate flair-up times, as well as healthy, remission periods.

Balance eating with moderate fiber during periods of remission; during flair-ups, keep fiber low (as this can further irritate the colon). Choose from a variety of lean meat, skinless poultry, oily fish (e.g., salmon, tuna, halibut, barramundi, etc.), fruits, vegetables (starchy and nonstarchy), breads, cereals, olive oil, and canola oil. Avoid dairy products, if lactose intolerance is an issue (many people with IBDs are lactose intolerant); otherwise use low-fat varieties daily.

Gas It Up

Flatulence, the fancy word for "gas," is a normal bowel function. It can be caused by partially digested foods, carbohydrate by-products—think beans—and extra air taken in from the nose and mouth. Whatever the cause, medical professionals use gas release as an indicator of a healthy colon.

Gas-Forming Foods

Some foods pose more of a gas threat than others. Typically, gassy foods are carbohydrates that may be resistant to digestion in the upper, small intestine. Once these prebiotic foods reach the bacterial confines of the large intestine, they are feasted on by friendly microorganisms, and the gas ensues! Here is a list of classic gas-forming foods:

- Artichokes
- Beans (black, kidney, white, garbanzo, lima, navy, etc.)
- Cruciferous vegetables
- Garlic
- Dairy products (milk, yogurt, and cheese)
- Lentils (green, red, or yellow)
- Onions (including scallions, leeks)
- Potatoes (including sweet potatoes)
- Radishes
- Rutabagas
- Turnips
- Yeast in breads

Gas-Preventing Foods

Some herbs and spices are carminatives, which means they fend off gas production in the intestines. Sprinkle caraway, cinnamon, coriander, cumin, fennel, ginger, nutmeg, oregano, rosemary, saffron, thyme, and turmeric into your favorite dishes and leave the gas behind!

Good-for-the-Gut Recipes

Tasty foods can be good for your gut health, too. Here are a few from our kitchen to yours.

Gluten-Free Greek Salad

If you are lactose intolerant, you can always remove the cheese or add in soy cheese crumbles or tofu.

Yield:	Serving size:	Prep time:	Cook time:
2 servings	1½ cups	15 minutes	None
Each serving has:			
233 calories	15 g total fat	7 g saturated fat	0 g trans fat
33 mg cholesterol	805 mg sodium	19 g carbohydrates	7 g fiber
8 g sugars	9 g protein	23 percent iron	

Juice of 1 lemon

2 cloves garlic, minced

2 TB. extra-virgin olive oil

Pinch of oregano

Pinch of ground black pepper

1 head romaine lettuce, chopped

1 large cucumber, sliced

¼ cup black olives, pitted

½ cup small red onions, diced

1 cup green pepper, diced

1½ cups tomatoes, chopped

1 cup feta cheese or tofu, crumbled

1. To make the dressing, in a small bowl whisk together lemon juice, garlic, and oil. Stir in oregano and pepper to taste. Set aside.

2. When ready to serve, in a large bowl lightly toss lettuce with dressing. Divide lettuce among 4 bowls. Scatter cucumber, olives, onions, peppers, tomatoes, and cheese or tofu over the top of the greens. Serve and pass remaining dressing at the table.

Berry Oat Bake

This is a delicious high-soluble fiber treat to help combat IBS symptoms. Use any berry or fruit you desire.

Yield:	Serving size:	Prep time:	Cook time:
8 servings	½ cup	5 minutes	45 to 60 minutes

Each serving has:			
528 calories	17 g total fat	2 g saturated fat	0 g trans fat
0 mg cholesterol	5 mg sodium	92 g carbohydrates	13 g fiber
46 g sugars	9 g protein	16 percent iron	

1 cup raspberries	6 TB. canola oil
1 cup strawberries	2 TB. flaxseed, ground
1 cup fresh blueberries	2 tsp. cinnamon
2 tsp. sugar	3 tsp. maple syrup
¼ cup walnuts	½ cup white whole-wheat flour
2 cups oats	

1. Preheat oven to 375°F. Spread fresh berries in a baking dish. Sprinkle with sugar.

2. In a medium mixing bowl, combine walnuts, oats, flaxseed, cinnamon, maple syrup, and flour. Pour over berry mixture.

3. Cover tightly with sheet of foil and bake until fruit begins to bubble, about 30 minutes. Uncover and cook until golden brown, 20 to 30 minutes longer.

4. Scoop into bowls and serve warm.

Herb and Spice Rub

This rub can be a natural carminative (gas-preventer) to add to fish, chicken, or bean dishes. Use fresh or dried herbs and spices; add others to suit your tastes.

Yield:	Serving size:	Prep time:	Cook time:
3 rubs	2 TB.	5 minutes	None
Each serving has:			
77 calories	4 g total fat	0 g saturated fat	0 g trans fat
0 mg cholesterol	15 mg sodium	12 g carbohydrates	7 g fiber
0 g sugars	4 g protein	44 percent iron	

1 TB. coriander seed	1 TB. dried oregano
1 TB. cumin	1 TB. dried rosemary
1 TB. caraway seeds	A dash of curry powder

1. Combine coriander, cumin, caraway seeds, dried oregano, rosemary, and curry in a small bowl and blend together.

2. Store in an airtight container. It will last up to 6 months. To use, pat dry any lean meat, chicken breast, fish, or tofu and generously dab on the rub. Let the food sit for a few minutes, then grill, bake, or roast.

Essential Takeaways

- The digestive tract or gut is tied to the psyche. There is a brain-gut connection.
- Inflammatory bowel diseases include Crohn's, colitis, ulcerative colitis, celiac disease, and irritable bowel syndrome. Food can play a role in treating these diseases, depending upon the symptoms.
- Diarrhea should be treated with a bland, soluble-fiber diet with no dairy or spicy foods. Constipation may be alleviated with some fiber, too; however, some IBS-sufferers do not respond well to fiber, so listen to what your gut is telling you.
- Gas is a natural and healthy part of digestion. Eating fruits, vegetables, and starchy carbs can promote gas, while adding herbs and spices can decrease gas production.

chapter 24

It's All in Your Head

As we live longer and look for ways to enhance quality of life, it makes sense that we think about our noggins. It's not only our minds that need to remain sharp; we need to keep our vision, hearing, and mouth as healthy as possible, too. Healthful choices include eating foods with more potassium, antioxidants (carotenoids), vitamins, minerals, and omega-3 fats; and consuming less sodium, saturated fat, and cholesterol. All these can help keep your head on straight and fend off diseases and disorders in every part of your skull.

The world has two faces of malnutrition—according to the World Health Organization, one is hunger or nutrition deficiency and the other is dietary excess. Neither end of the spectrum is good for cognitive health or the other head-based senses.

This chapter delves into the optimal foods to keep everything in your head working well for life.

Brain Food

Although the brain constitutes only 2 percent of your total body weight, it uses a sizeable percentage of your body's oxygen supply and energy stores. Your brain uses 25 percent of the glucose (sugar) coursing through your entire body; if there's not enough glucose available, it goes into a state of hypoglycemia (low blood sugar), with symptoms of light-headedness, confusion, slow mental functioning, and lack of consciousness. Just like the heart, the brain requires special attention to diminish risk of stroke, dementia, and Alzheimer's disease.

Think Plants

The more fruits and vegetables you eat the better. The reasons for piling your plate with more plants and less red and processed meat, and salty and sugar-laden foods are very similar to why we do it for our hearts—to keep blood pressure, blood sugar levels, and your waistline in check. High blood pressure is the leading cause of stroke. Research shows that 80 percent of stroke risk is a result of high blood pressure (at or above 140/90). Strokes are caused by blood clots in the brain that come in contact with a clogged artery and cause a blockage. Lowering your blood pressure can lower your risk of stroke by 40 percent!

One study found that a Mediterranean-style diet, which emphasizes more whole grains, fruits, vegetables, nuts, olive oil, moderate alcohol and fish, and less red meat, refined grains (e.g., white flour products), and occasional sweets decreased the risk of stroke significantly in middle-aged women. Eating this type of plant-based diet was shown to positively affect blood pressure and promote weight loss, two results that are excellent for your brain's vascular health.

On top of preventing stroke, a Mediterranean-type diet can help fend off dementia (cognitive decline) or the more severe Alzheimer's disease (AD). Researchers anticipate that about 800 million people in the United States will have AD by the year 2030. As a potential preventive measure, experts recommend that we eat more plant-based foods, particularly colorful berries like blueberries and strawberries; balance fat intake with "good" unsaturated fats like olive oil and walnuts; and eat less animal products and saturated fat. Getting plenty of physical activity and mental stimulation helps, too!

Praise Potassium

Placing potassium center-stage in your eating life can reduce your risk of stroke, too. Potassium is an electrolyte that's important for optimal functioning of the brain and nerves. It's the twin sister of sodium, yet it functions completely different in your body. It helps lower and maintain good blood pressure levels by maintaining ideal fluid levels in and between the cells; plus, it works wonders for keeping bones strong and kidney stones at bay.

Healing
Hints
Nibbling on nuts can boost your potassium levels. An ounce of pistachios (49 nuts) has 300 milligrams of potassium; an ounce of almonds (23 nuts) has 210 milligrams. Coconut water is also high in potassium, and it's low in calories and fat-free.

Potassium is mainly found in fruits and vegetables; however fish, nuts, dairy products, and beans contain fair amounts of the mineral as well. Aim for at least 4,700 milligrams per day. It's not hard to get that amount with a plant-centric diet. For example, check out these whopping potassium levels, which will enable you to get your recommended daily dose:

- 1 medium baked potato = 1,080 milligrams

- 1 cup of tomato sauce = 940 milligrams

- 1 cup spinach = 840 milligrams

- 6 ounces salmon = 700 milligrams

- 4 ounces soybeans = 490 milligrams

- 6 ounces plain yogurt = 400 milligrams

- 4 ounces black beans = 370 milligrams

Eating for Vital Vision

Your eyes, although attached to your brain, have an independent lens into the world. Your eye lenses can get cloudy or obstructed with age causing a number of eye diseases that, if neglected, can greatly diminish your eyesight or even lead to blindness. Good nutrition, primarily from plant and fish food, has proven to be beneficial to eye health.

Aging Macula

As we age, our central vision, which is governed by the macula of the eye, can be destroyed through exposure to the sun's light, as well as strong blue light in the atmosphere. Typically diagnosed in people over age 65, age-related macular degeneration (AMD) is the most common cause of blindness. It's a debilitating eye disease in which you can no longer see the finer details of a face, a book, or a road sign.

AMD is caused by a combination of genetics and lifestyle factors. Age is the single biggest factor, followed by smoking, obesity, race (Caucasians are more prone than other races), family history (if you have a first-degree relative you are more prone), and being female (as women seem to get AMD more than men). The last 20 years of research in this area has shown that certain foods and nutrients can play a large role in fending off AMD. Let's take a look-see.

Food as Sunblock

Your eyes need sunblock, too—and that's where food comes in. One of the largest studies on eye health looked at the effects of high doses of antioxidant and zinc supplements on people with AMD. The study found that in people with moderate AMD, high doses of zinc oxide, copper (to balance out the zinc supplementation), and the antioxidants vitamin C, vitamin E, and beta-carotene (vitamin A) significantly reduced the risk for developing advanced AMD. In fact, high-potency antioxidant and/or zinc supplementation taken daily reduced the risk of advanced AMD by 25 percent! The antioxidant formulation is believed to reduce oxidative stress—the burden placed on cells by toxins, pollution, and unhealthy foods—in the eyes.

Colorful Eye Nutrients

Richly colored leafy greens like spinach, kale, turnips, as well as yellow corn and egg yolks—from hens that eat marigold petals and carotenoid-rich corn—contain two powerful carotenoids, lutein and zeaxanthin. Like fairy dust, these carotenoids deposit into the macula of your eyes and give them color (pigment). Macular pigment helps fend off AMD; it absorbs harmful wavelengths of light, thus reducing free-radical damage in the central retina. Eye health experts advise that you get at least 6 milligrams a day of these eye-salving nutrients; the average American adult gets a mere 2 to 4 milligrams of lutein and zeaxanthin a day from foods.

Create a visually stimulating plate, with the following carotenoid-rich foods:

Lutein and Zeaxanthin–Rich Foods for Eye Health	
Food	*Lutein+Zeaxanthin*
Beet greens, cooked, 1 cup	26.2 milligrams
Brussels sprouts, cooked, 1 cup	23.9 milligrams
Kale, cooked, 1 cup	23.7 milligrams
Spinach, cooked, 1 cup	20.3 milligrams

Food	Lutein+Zeaxanthin
Collard greens, cooked, 1 cup	14.6 milligrams
Turnip greens, cooked, 1 cup	12.1 milligrams

Source: Environmental Nutrition, May 2010, accessed at USDA National Nutrient Database Standard Reference, Release 22.

Healing Hints

Carotenoids are best absorbed in the presence of fat. Try sautéing dark, leafy greens in olive oil or tossing salads with oil-based dressings. The fat in egg yolks makes the lutein and zeaxanthin highly accessible to the eyes.

Fish Oil for the Eyes

Oily fish and seafood like salmon, mussels, sardines, shrimp, and prawns contain an arsenal of inflammation-fighting omega-3 fats. The two omega-3 fats, DHA and EPA, abundant in marine life, play a role in fending off inflammation in the eyes, which is linked to AMD. Plus, there are a lot of DHA stores in the retina of the eye.

When researchers followed people with risk for AMD, they found that those who ate fish and seafood regularly (thus, ate a lot of omega-3s) had a 30 percent lower chance of getting advanced AMD. Experts are looking at how 1,000 milligrams a day affects the progression of AMD. For now, aim to get at least 12 ounces of oily fish per week—that's two, 6-ounce servings twice a week.

Hear Me Now

Emerging research is revealing that certain vitamins, fats, and carbs may play a role in hearing loss. Making sound nutrition choices can play a role in maintaining optimal hearing for life.

Hearing Well with Folic Acid

More than 28 million Americans age 60 to 74 have hearing loss. Age-related hearing loss (ARHL), also known as prebycusis, is one of the most chronic conditions in older people. Nutrients can play a role in maintaining your auditory (hearing) system in working order. Lack of micronutrients (vitamin and minerals), such as folic acid, may hold an answer.

munch
on This
A study of 126 healthy Nigerian males and females over age 60 found that those with lower levels of folic acid in their blood had higher rates of hearing loss.

Save Hearing with Omega-3 Fats

Omega-3 fatty acids from fish may play a role in hearing loss, too. Results from a long-term study found that of the participants age 50 or above, those who ate two or more servings of fish per week showed a 42 percent lower risk of ARHL than those who only ate fish once or less per week. So on top of being healthy for your brain, heart, and eyes, omega-3s are good for your ears, too. So feel good about eating at least two servings of fish per week—your ears will thank you daily!

High-Fiber Noise

In the same study just mentioned, researchers looked at how participants' hearing responded to consumption of different kinds of carbs. They honed in on two components of carbohydrate eating: glycemic load (how much carbohydrate you eat at one time) and glycemic index (how much the carb-rich food increases blood sugar after eating it).

Participants who ate more highly refined carbohydrates and sugars—in other words, ate a high glycemic load and index diet (versus the high-fiber, lower glycemic load and index group) had a higher rate of hearing loss overall. The researchers concluded that blood sugar after eating (postprandial glycemia) might be a potential underlying biological mechanism in the development of ARHL. Choosing higher-fiber carbs, which tend to fill you up faster and keep your blood sugar from rising too high, may be a key to hearing health. So break out the whole-grain bread, whole-grain cereal, brown rice, and fruits and veggies to get more fiber for your ears today!

Beyond Brushing: Oral Health

The health of your teeth and gums is very important to your quality of life. The Centers for Disease Control and Prevention (CDC) reports that one third of all adults in the United States has untreated tooth decay; one in seven adults has gum disease; and 25 percent of adults have had associated facial pain in the past 6 months. And this all comes down to the quality of your diet and your oral health habits. As you know, brushing and flossing your teeth every day and getting regular dental exams and cleanings is important; however the nutrients you munch, bite, and chew every day can play a role in your oral health, too.

Feeding Dental Cavities

Dental cavities are a form of tooth decay. It's common in all age groups, particularly in children and adolescents. Sugar, particularly, sucrose—which is found in candy, cough drops, lollipops, suckers, etc.—can form a substance called glucan that aids bacteria in clinging to the surface of the tooth. Over time, these bacteria create acid that eat away at the enamel of the tooth and cause dental cavities.

Dental experts advise that children (and adults) avoid frequent consumption of juice or sugar-containing drinks. For infants and young children, avoid putting sugary drinks in a bottle or sippy cup, and discourage sleeping with a bottle. Offer nonsugary foods for snacks, limit sugary foods to once a day, and brush or rinse mouth shortly after the food is eaten. Overall, general good nutrition habits will keep teeth healthy and strong. Plant foods that are hard to chew, like apples, carrots, celery, and cucumbers, naturally clean the teeth.

Healing Hints	Since carbs, particularly refined sugars, create acid that can lead to dental cavities, eat protein and fat to lessen the acidic effect. Snack on a slice of low-fat cheese, skim milk, cottage cheese, and/or unsweetened yogurt.

Gum Disease

Inflammation in the mouth, specifically in the gums, is caused by a buildup of plaque. Eight percent of people in the United States have some form of periodontal disease or gum disease. The two common types are gingivitis and periodontitis. Gingivitis can lead to periodontitis if left untreated. The symptoms of gingivitis include swollen gums, bright red or purple gums (healthy gums are pink), gums that are tender or painful to touch, and gums that bleed with brushing and/or flossing. Halitosis (bad breath) can be associated with this inflammation of the gum tissue. Although the symptoms may seem to be localized in your mouth, research shows that gum disease can affect your heart health, as infections and bacteria can travel through the bloodstream and cause cardiac events.

Don't Forget to Floss

On top of brushing, flossing, and rinsing with hydrogen peroxide, good nutrition can come to the rescue for dental health. Calcium-rich foods may help to keep gum disease (a.k.a gingivitis) at bay. In a large national nutrition survey, which looked at calcium consumption and periodontal disease, researchers found that young men and women (20–39 years of age), as well as older men (40–59 years of age), who did not consume adequate amounts of calcium every day had higher rates of severe periodontal disease.

So to keep your teeth (and bones) healthy, aim for at least 2 to 3 servings of low-fat dairy products or calcium-fortified soy, rice, or nut milks and consume lots of calcium-rich veggies like broccoli, spinach, and kale daily. (Osteoporosis has been linked with tooth loss, a result of periodontal disease.)

Because gum disease is an inflammatory disease, eating anti-inflammatory foods can help, too. Follow a healthy pattern of eating that falls in line with the 2010 Dietary Guidelines for Americans. Also, drink plenty of water to rinse your mouth of potentially harmful bacteria before, during, and after you eat.

Head Strong Recipes

You can maintain brain, eye, ear, and mouth health with healthy and healing foods. Here are some fun recipes to keep your noodle strong for life.

Crunchy Carrot Crumble

This recipe can be made with string beans, sweet potatoes, broccoli, or cauliflower.

Yield:	Serving size:	Prep time:	Cook time:
8 servings	2 heaping TB.	5 minutes	30 minutes

Each serving has:			
184 calories	5 g total fat	1 g saturated fat	0 g trans fat
2 mg cholesterol	311 mg sodium	33 g carbohydrates	7 g fiber
10 g sugars	7 g protein	45 percent iron	

1 lb. carrots, peeled and thinly sliced	½ cup grated low-fat cheddar cheese
1 small yellow onion, peeled and finely chopped	⅛ tsp. smoked paprika (optional)
2 TB. olive oil	1 TB. chopped fresh parsley
2 TB. white whole-wheat flour	1 cup whole-grain or flax flakes, finely crushed
1 cup fat-free milk	

1. Preheat oven to 350°F. Steam carrots until brightly colored and tender (not mushy).

2. Place oil in skillet over medium heat and add onions, and sauté until clear.

3. Remove onions from heat, stir in flour, and cook for 1 minute. Gradually whisk in milk. Return the pan to the heat and stir until mixture is thickened and smooth, then remove from heat.

4. Stir in cheese until melted. Taste and season with salt and pepper, if desired.

5. Combine cooked carrots and parsley with cheese sauce and spoon into a baking dish.

6. Top mixture with crushed cereal flakes. Cook in oven for about 20 minutes or until golden brown on top. Serve warm.

Mozzarella Caprese Bites

These are a bite-size, tasty, and healthful start to a party or simple dinner.

Yield:	Serving size:	Prep time:	Cook time:
12 toasts	3 toasts	5 minutes	None

Each serving has:			
200 calories	10 g total fat	5 g saturated fat	0 g trans fat
18 mg cholesterol	304 mg sodium	16 g carbohydrates	2 g fiber
2 g sugars	11 g protein	5 percent iron	

1 cup cherry tomatoes, halved

1 cup fresh part-skim mozzarella cheese, diced

2 TB. fresh basil, chopped

2 TB. balsamic vinegar

1 TB. extra-virgin olive oil

¼ tsp. salt

Freshly ground black pepper

12 whole-grain toast rounds or pita chips

1. In a large bowl gently toss together cherry tomatoes, mozzarella cheese, basil, balsamic vinegar, olive oil, salt, and pepper.

2. Dollop a tablespoon of the mixture onto each of the toast rounds and serve.

Kale Fritters

This makes a great meal served with a dollop of light sour cream or plain yogurt. Delicious and high in the beneficial carotenoids, too!

Yield:	Serving size:	Prep time:	Cook time:
4 fritters	1 fritter	5 minutes	10 minutes

Each serving has:			
121 calories	9 g total fat	1 g saturated fat	0 g trans fat
53 mg cholesterol	106 mg sodium	8 g carbohydrates	1 g fiber
1 g sugars	4 g protein	6 percent iron	

2 cups kale, coarsely chopped

½ cup whole-grain breadcrumbs

1 large egg, beaten

Pinch of salt and ground black pepper to taste

2 TB. extra-virgin olive oil

1. Put freshly washed, still moist, kale in a large mixing bowl, coat with egg, and sprinkle with breadcrumbs. Use your hands to form small patties (about 2 tablespoons for each patty).

2. Heat oil in a skillet. Spoon patties into hot oil. Cook over a medium-high heat until golden brown on one side and very gently flip to cook on the other side.

3. Drain on paper towel to remove any excess oil. Add a touch more oil to the skillet, if needed, before making more fritters.

Essential Takeaways

- Your brain, eyes, ears, and mouth all thrive on good nutrition.
- Keeping your blood pressure in check can keep your brain healthy. Eat more potassium-rich fruits and vegetables and less sodium-laden processed foods.
- A plant-based diet along with fish and seafood can help keep the brain, eyes, ears, and mouth functioning well.

chapter 25

Nourishing Your Skin and Bones

Eating for youthful skin

Choosing bone-strengthening foods

Identifying foods for healthy joints

Making recipes for strong and supple skin, bones, and joints

Good skin is part genetic (look at your parents' skin) and part lifestyle, which means you have some control over your aging process. Skin protects your vital organs, bones, muscles, and ligaments; it helps regulate your body temperature; insulates your organs; and allows you to feel sensations. The skin is a vital part of the immune system. It readily adapts to its environment and is able to send off germs and harmful agents at a moment's notice. Dermatologists suggest that you feed your skin from the inside. That means getting plenty of antioxidants, B-vitamins, and minerals. All those nutrients play a role in skin health.

In this chapter, I explore the best foods for your skin and bones (and joints, too!).

Foods and Youthful Skin

The natural function of the skin is to slough off the old and bring in the new. Fortunately for us, skin's outer layer or epidermis sheds dead cells about every 27 days—new skin cells are put in their place. Typically, this is a seamless process, as the skin regenerates without you ever knowing it. (If skin is scaly, this may indicate an internal issue.) The second layer of skin, the dermis, consists of the strength-providing force called collagen and elastin, the part that gives your skin elasticity and bounce.

With age, the epidermis and the dermis layers become thinner (skin loses epidermal cells by 10 percent with every decade), plus the skin produces less collagen, and elastin fibers get tired and do not provide the same degree of elasticity. Thus, the smooth and thick skin of our youth slowly begins to thin, wrinkle, and sag as we age. To reduce wrinkles, protect your skin from the sun. The sun ages skin rapidly, but you may not see the effects until you are older. Ninety percent of the damage to skin is due to the sun's ultraviolet rays; the majority of photo (light) aging effects are believed to occur by age 20!

> **Healing Hints**
>
> Hone in on antioxidants in food (vitamin C–rich foods like citrus fruits and leafy greens, broccoli, and bell peppers) to help keep wrinkles at bay. They help fend off the free radicals produced from sunlight, smoke, and pollution, which can damage cells and breakdown elastin. Although there's no magic antiwrinkle pill (and food should come first), the American College of Dermatology recommends 500 to 1,000 milligrams of vitamin C each day.

Antioxidant Power for Skin

Some of the best foods for the rest of your body are also beneficial for skin health and keeping a youthful glow. Fruits, vegetables, nuts, seeds, and whole grains provide a whole host of antioxidants; the ones that have proven best for skin health are vitamins A, C, and E, and the mineral selenium.

Vitamin A (retinol) can relieve dry skin; this antioxidant is responsible for maintaining health and repair of skin. Topical creams that have vitamins A and C have shown to be effective in reducing fine lines and wrinkles on the face. Foods high in the carotenoid beta-carotene, a product of vitamin A, may play a role in preventing psoriasis—which can be an indicator of the arthritic condition, psoriatic arthritis. Beta-carotene–rich foods are sweet potatoes, carrots, kale, spinach, collard greens, and even fresh herbs like cilantro and thyme. In addition, tomato-based products, which are high in the carotenoid lycopene, have been shown to protect the skin against the sun's harmful UV rays.

Other foods that may keep the skin's elasticity in good shape are selenium-rich wheat germ, tuna, salmon, garlic, Brazil nuts, eggs, brown rice, and whole-wheat bread. Selenium is an antioxidant that's effective in keeping tissues pliable and reducing harmful oxidative stress.

B-Vitamins for Skin

You may have noticed the B-vitamin, biotin, in your favorite face cream or hand lotion. That's because biotin is a natural component of your skin, plus your nails and hair, too. If you are lacking this B-vitamin, you'll know it by getting dry skin—and possibly experiencing hair loss. Your body also makes its own supply of biotin, but you can also get it in foods like eggs, bananas, oats, and rice.

Another B-vitamin, niacin, which is a good anti-inflammatory nutrient, can fend off dry, itchy, and scaly skin. It's also used in a lot of topical creams because it's great for locking in moisture. Foods rich in niacin are chicken, fish, milk, eggs, avocados, dates, tomatoes, broccoli, and asparagus.

Skin-ny Fats

Healthy skin is yet another reason to eat oily fish, seeds, and vegetable oils regularly. Their essential fatty acids (EFA) or omega-3 fats can also fend off inflammation in skin, such as blemishes and blocked pores (e.g., white and/or black heads), dry, red, and scaly patches. Lack of EFAs in your diet can cause your skin to lose water, which leads to dry skin. Aim for at least 12 ounces of fatty fish per week and/or 2 tablespoons a day of flaxseed or chia seeds.

Optimize Bone Health

Besides supporting the structure of your body and enabling it to move, your bones incorporate many complex systems in which good nutrition plays a vital role. Bone health is contingent upon getting a good supply of calcium and phosphorus, two minerals that make up the rigid bone matrix. Bones are living, changing organs; they go through a process called "remodeling," which means that hormones and vitamins (mainly vitamin D) regularly signal a turnover of the old bone to be replaced with new bone tissue throughout your life. This allows for the normal growth and to repair any damaged bone due to stress from sports and regular high-impact activity (e.g., running). However, the primary reason for the remodeling is to keep calcium in balance.

Calcium in your bones and bloodstream is in constant flux—the bones release calcium from their stores as needed in the blood and take it from the blood, if needed. Thus, getting plenty of dietary calcium from food and, if necessary, from supplements is important. The average adult needs 1,000 milligrams of calcium; children need a bit more (1,200 milligrams) as their bones are rapidly growing. Good sources of calcium and phosphorus are low-fat dairy products (milk, cheese, and yogurt), leafy green veggies, fish with bones (e.g., sardines, salmon steak), and tofu.

> **Healing Hints**
>
> Want strong bones? Sip green tea. Green tea's emerald leaves contain plant-compounds called epigallocatechin (EGC) that can help your bones stay strong and solid. A study found EGC stimulated bone growth by 79 percent. This tea compound was also found to decrease resorption (the breakdown of bone) and increase bone formation.

Osteo-Friendly Foods

Osteoporosis is a disease in which the bones become weak due to gaps (holes) in the bone's architecture, leading to bone loss and dangerous fractures—breaks are most common in the hips, spine, and wrist.

Osteoporosis is the leading bone disease. The National Osteoporosis Foundation reports that 10 million Americans have it already, but another 34 million are at risk of getting it. It typically happens in older women—over 50 years old—as estrogen levels decline with age. Less estrogen sets off a cascade of bone destructive events. In a less estrogenic environment, the kidneys and intestines cut back on their absorption of calcium, and this signals the bone to slow down on construction of new bone and speed up demolition (or breakdown) of the bone you have. The results can be catastrophic to your health, with increased breaks, decreased mobility, and poor quality of life.

So what you do? Bone health experts tell us that focusing on bone nutrients—calcium, vitamin D, vitamin K, and protein—can help.

Vitamin D

This sunshine vitamin is a must for bone health. Vitamin D helps balance calcium and phosphorus in the blood and aids in the mineralization (getting calcium and phosphorus into the bone), growth, and remodeling of bones. Too little vitamin D can lead to thin, brittle, and weak bones, which are susceptible to breaks and osteoporosis. Vitamin D prevents the childhood weak bone disease called rickets and the milder adult version, osteomalacia, in which the bones become excessively soft.

Be sure to get enough vitamin D for optimal bone health. For children and adults that's at least 600 IU (although some experts recommend at least 1,000 IU per day); infants (0–12 months) can get by with 400 IU per day. Here are some natural ways to get vitamin D in your food. Remember exposure to the sun gives you vitamin D, too—so get at least 10 to 15 minutes a day of sunshine (before applying sunscreen).

Bone Up on Vitamin D	
Food	*Vitamin D Amount (IU)*
Cod liver oil, 1 TB.	1,360 IU
Mushrooms (exposed to sun), 3.5 oz.	400 IU
Milk, fortified, 1 qt.	400 IU
Salmon, cooked, 3.5 oz.	360 IU
Sardines, canned in oil, 1.75 oz.	250 IU
Tuna, canned in oil, 3.5 oz.	235 IU
Eel, cooked, 3.5 oz.	200 IU
Whole egg	20 IU

Source: National Institute of Health Office of Dietary Supplements, Dietary Supplement Fact Sheet: Vitamin D, Accessed on Dec 29, 2010.

Vitamin K

This fat-soluble vitamin is another nutrient that is vital for making dense, strong bones and fending off bone loss. Experts believe that a high level of vitamin K is needed in order for osteocalcin, the main protein in the bone matrix, to lay down enough bone. This is vital as we get older and breakdown is greater than bone formation. Studies back this up: in one study, women who took vitamin K–enhanced supplements (as well as calcium, vitamin D, and magnesium) had less bone loss than women who took only calcium, vitamin D, and magnesium supplements.

For bone health, supplemental vitamin K may work best due to the high quantities required. However, it can't hurt to boost your vitamin K levels with leafy greens like kale, spinach, collards, parsley, broccoli, and Brussels sprouts.

FOOD wise

Keep in mind that vitamin K can interfere with blood thinning medications like warfarin (Coumadin), so talk with your health-care provider before adding more vitamin K to your diet.

Bones on Base

Your bones thrive well in an environment that is balanced from a pH (acid-base) standpoint. Research has revealed that bones are more susceptible to fractures if your blood contains too much acid, meaning that the pH levels are low. Although the exact cause is unknown, many researchers believe that as we get older, our kidneys don't filter acid as well, thus our blood becomes more acidic. This also creates the potential for joint issues, such as *gout,* which is caused by high levels of uric acid in the bloodstream. A side effect of too much acid in the diet is losing lean body mass or muscle and bone loss.

Definition

Gout is a form of arthritis that strikes due to a high amount of purines, or acid, in the blood. It typically inflames the joint of the big toe. To relieve gout's painful effects, try eating cherries, blueberries, and strawberries, as studies have shown that they bring down inflammation and restore normal function again. The kicker is you have to eat half-pound of cherries to get relief!

Citrus or "acidic" fruits are not the culprits of low pH levels. Instead, experts contend that too much protein and grain (refined, processed) products lead to high acidity in the blood. Fruits and vegetables are more alkaline, or basic, in nature. Thus, eating a colorful cadre of these plants can neutralize the acid in your system. This is not to say you should not eat protein or grains; you need protein to fuel your muscles and keep your cells functioning properly, and whole grains are necessary for energy and proper bowel function, but balancing your plate with more veggies and fruits will maintain the pH equilibrium in your bloodstream. Bone health is another reason for loading your plate with more veggies and eating less protein and less starch!

Activity is good for your bones. Experts recommend at least 30 minutes of exercise per day (for weight loss get at least 60 to 90 minutes) of both weight bearing and strength training activity. Weight bearing activity is especially beneficial for bone health, as the weight on the bones signals bone-forming cells, osteocytes, to communicate the need for new bone tissue.

Choose a combination of weight bearing activity: low-impact (e.g., elliptical machine, stair-climber, and treadmill) and high-impact (e.g., dancing, aerobics, jogging, running, jumping rope, tennis). Nonweight bearing ventures are bicycling, yoga, pilates, free weights, and swimming.

Happy Joints

If your joints are happy, you don't even know they're there. Like the hinges on a door, if they squeak you have to oil them, but otherwise their beneficial function isn't fully realized. Your joints are the meeting place of two or more bones (such as your hip, knee, elbow, shoulder, and wrist) and arthritis, which is swelling of the joints, is the main cause of disability in people over age 55. Arthritic conditions have various causes, but they all cause discomfort—as they are inflammatory, with mild to severe pain. What you eat may or may not play a role in joint health, but if there is some food-based relief to these conditions, it's certainly worth exploring!

Osteoarthritis

This degenerative joint disease affects 27 million people in the United States. Osteoarthritis (OA) causes the joints to degrade and the cartilage to break down (causing bones to rub together). The pain associated with moving this joint may cause muscle and ligament loss surrounding the affected joint. OA can be caused by many factors, such as obesity, infection of the joint, diabetes, and/or abnormal anatomy during development.

Eating with osteoarthritis can be compromised, especially if the finger joints have developed nodes, or hard bony ball-like growths. Nodes make it difficult to articulate the fingers, thus holding utensils and serving food is a challenge. Anti-inflammatory foods can help keep the pain and swelling of OA at bay. A recent study found that nonstarchy veggies, garlic, and other alliums (e.g., onions) showed some improvement with hip OA. The researchers isolated a compound in alliums called diallyl disulphide, which is believed to be beneficial in fending off the degrading protein enzymes present with OA.

Rheumatoid Arthritis

This type of inflammatory joint disease is a chronic autoimmune disease, in which the body's immune system attacks the joints. Rheumatoid arthritis (RA) affects three times more women than men and about 1 percent of the global population overall. It can be very painful and causes extreme loss of mobility of the joints as well as disfigurement. It insidiously pervades the tiny joints of the hands, feet, and cervical spine (at the base of the neck). The suspected causes range from genes to infection to cigarette smoking, but whatever the cause, once its triggered, RA leads to a destructive course for the affected joints. Nutrition therapy along with physical and occupational therapies are necessary.

Decades of research has looked at how diet affects the inflammation associated with RA, and scientists have developed many theories on the topic. The types of diets that show some promise are low in saturated fat and red meat and high in fruits and vegetables; in other words, similar to the diet recommended for living a healthy life. They appear to help with alleviating pain, but not necessarily stiffness or physical function.

Some research suggests that food allergies are tied to RA. Studies have shown the gut of people with RA contain more antibodies to proteins from cow's milk, cereal, eggs, fish, and pork than people without RA. The immune complexes that are formed to combat potential allergens circulate throughout the body, and are believed to get lodged in the joints of people with RA. However, more research on this topic is needed. Based on this theory, experts believe that eliminating foods that cause the allergic response will help ease the symptoms of RA. You can always reintroduce that food back in later, if it wasn't the painful culprit. It's all about trial and error when it comes to eating with RA.

Another option for eating with RA is to go clean for a month with fruits, veggies, lean meats, and fish and see if that works. Research has shown that this type of eating improved symptoms of morning stiffness and pain, plus it got people back to their "normal" functioning lives, in which their joints were somewhat happy and moving! For more on RA and arthritis in general, take a look at www.arthritistoday.org.

Skin, Bones, and Joint Recipes

Your skin, bones, and joints can benefit from a bevy of whole foods. So incorporate some of these stick-to-your-bones recipes today!

Cauliflower with Garlicky Crust

You can use broccoli instead of cauliflower in this dish, which is a silky skin treat.

Yield:	Serving size:	Prep time:	Cook time:
4 servings	½ cup	5 minutes	15 minutes

Each serving has:			
312 calories	19 g total fat	3 g saturated fat	0 g trans fat
0 mg cholesterol	286 mg sodium	31 g carbohydrates	7 g fiber
7 g sugars	8 g protein	13 percent iron	

1 large cauliflower, cut into bite-size florets	5 TB. extra-virgin olive oil
1 cup whole-grain breadcrumbs	½ tsp. ground cayenne pepper
3 to 5 garlic cloves, thinly sliced or chopped	Pinch of salt

1. Steam the cauliflower in water until just tender (about 8 minutes). Drain and let cool.

2. Heat 4 tablespoons of olive oil in a pan, add breadcrumbs, and cook over medium heat, tossing until browned and crisp.

3. Add garlic to breadcrumbs, stir a few times, then remove from the pan and set aside.

4. Heat remaining oil in the pan, add cauliflower, breaking it up a little as it lightly browns in the oil; do not overcook it.

5. Add garlic breadcrumb mixture to the pan and cook, stirring, until well combined, with some of the cauliflower still holding its shape. Season and serve warm.

Asparagus, Onions, and Mushroom Roast

This is a fun vegetable medley that goes well with lean meat, fish, or tofu. Feel free to throw in your favorite veggies.

Yield:	Serving size:	Prep time:	Cook time:
4 servings	½ cup	5 minutes	20 minutes

Each serving has:			
85 calories	7 g total fat	1 g saturated fat	0 g trans fat
0 mg cholesterol	28 mg sodium	5 g carbohydrates	2 g fiber
2 g sugars	2 g protein	7 percent iron	

1½ cups asparagus spears	2 TB. extra-virgin olive oil
1 small onion, quartered	1 small handful of fresh basil leaves
2 cups mushrooms, chopped	Salt and ground black pepper

1. Preheat the oven to 375°F. Put asparagus, onions, and mushrooms in a roasting pan and drizzle with olive oil. Sprinkle basil over veggies and season with salt and ground pepper. Stir to coat with oil.

2. Roast in the oven for 20 minutes, stir, and put back into the oven for 10 more minutes, or until veggies are golden brown and tender. Serve immediately.

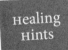

Healing Hints

Use mushrooms that contain vitamin D for that extra bone-strengthening boost.

Essential Takeaways

- Eating well can keep your skin, bones, and joints strong and healthy for life.
- Calcium is a big bone builder; choose low-fat dairy, leafy greens, and fish with bones to get your daily dose.
- Vitamin D can help your bones stay strong, but too much sunlight will damage skin, so choose foods high in vitamin D, such as fortified milk, fish, mushrooms, and eggs.
- Fruits and vegetables can do wonders for your skin, bones, and joints; eat a wide variety every day.

chapter 26

Sex and Conception Connection

Sexual healing for men and women

Balancing your hormones

Eating foods for fertility

Following pregnancy eating protocol

Cooking up some have-more-fun-in-bed recipes

Let's face it, sex is everywhere, and it sells; but are people really doing it? Intercourse is the most primal act there is, as it's essential for procreation; however, sexuality ebbs and flows throughout an adult's life. Many factors affect whether sex takes priority or a back seat. Age, stress level, weight gain, and health issues all affect the frequency and quality of your sex life.

Statistics reveal that 40 percent of women have had sexual problems; in men it occurs in about 5 percent of 40 year olds and 15 to 25 percent of men over 60 years. Sexual issues can lead to depression, anxiety, and broken relationships. Lack of arousal for both men and women is one of the biggest sex squelchers. In men it's called erectile dysfunction (ED); in women it's called sexual arousal disorder; they are both bona fide psychological disorders. The reason for the malfunctioning turn-on buttons is complex; however, good nutrition—or lack of it—can play a vital role.

In this chapter, I explore how food can help or hinder your sexual and reproductive life. Experts agree that a satisfying sex life is important to overall quality of life.

Erectile Dysfunction

The reality is that as we get older, sexual activity drops, according to sex authorities at The Kinsey Institute. Research shows that people in their 20s have sex about 112 times per year, whereas frequency for people in their 30s and 40s drops to 86 and 69 times per year, respectively. The reasons for the sex decline may be embedded in the fact that sexual dysfunction goes up; in men the rate of ED, the inability of the penis to become erect to perform sex, rises with age.

A large study found that men in their 40s had a 40 percent rate of ED, and once they hit their 70s the rate shot up to 70 percent. Coupled with this, the actual desire for sex declines during midlife for men (and women) with each passing birthday. A large national study showed that men ages 50 to 59 years were three times more likely to have low sexual desire and ED compared with teens and 20-somethings.

Healing Hints	Erectile dysfunction does not exist as a stand-alone problem; it's been linked to high blood pressure, diabetes, and heart disease. So replace saturated fat from red meat and full-fat dairy with unsaturated fat from fish, olive oil, avocados, and seeds, and nuts like flaxseed, chia seeds, pistachios, and walnuts. Also lay off the salt shaker, and add more veggies and fruits to your day. All those healthy choices can help bring on natural erections that help you say goodbye to Viagra!

Eating with ED

The best remedies for ED are healthful foods and an active lifestyle. Research shows that ED was more likely to occur among men in poor physical and emotional health (depression and anxiety disorders are linked to ED). Diabetes, high blood pressure, and high cholesterol levels affect vascular health, common problems in men with ED. So follow a heart-healthy diet (see Chapter 20) and blood sugar–friendly diet (see Chapter 21) to bring excitement back to your sex life!

Hypertension and ED

Not only is maintaining normal blood pressure good for your heart, but a man's sexual arousal relies on it. If your blood pressure is 140/90 or higher, your chances for getting ED go up. One study found that 45 percent of men with high blood pressure had ED; and they didn't just have it, they had a severe degree of ED.

Erections depend on the intricate interplay of blood vessels servicing the penis and hormones during arousal. High blood pressure decreases the amount of blood flow to the penis by not allowing blood vessels to dilate (widen) or the smooth muscles of the penis to relax and allow blood in. The hormonal whammy is that men with high blood pressure typically have low levels of testosterone, the male hormone that facilitates healthy erections. So keeping an eye on blood pressure is important for a healthy sex life.

With statistics revealing that blood pressure has a natural tendency to increase with age (as does ED), monitoring what you eat, your weight, alcohol intake, and activity level can help. Follow a heart-healthy diet by eating more whole foods, such as leafy greens, orange, yellow, purple, and/ or red vegetables, as well as low-fat dairy products, whole grains, less red meat, and more plant-based proteins.

Blood pressure medications such as diuretics and beta-blockers can cause less blood flow to the penis and interfere with erections as well. They can also cause nerve impulses to be less strong, making it more challenging for men to have an erection. Beta-blockers might also cause a depressive state of mind, which can squelch an amorous mood and lead to ED. Aim to get off your blood pressure medication by making healthful eating and regular exercise your number one blood pressure regulator!

> **Food wise**
>
> Although an alcoholic drink or two a day can be good for heart health, drinking too much alcohol can cause blood pressure to soar and lead to ED. To avoid dampening the mood in the bedroom, monitor how much you drink, alternate alcohol with water, or abstain from alcohol prior to sex.

Popular prescription medications like Viagra and Cialis can have side effects and do not cure ED or lack of sexual desire. Plus, they may interfere with other medications, so talk with your health-care provider before taking these medications.

Sexual Arousal Disorder

For women, getting "in the mood" can sometimes be a challenge, too. Sexual arousal disorder is just one form of female sexual dysfunction (FSD). About 40 million women in the United States have FSD; of that several million suffer from lack of sexual arousal. Just like ED in men, the turn-on factor for females is a complex phenomenon. A sexual arousal disorder rears its head in many ways, from vaginal dryness or lack of lubrication to lack of clitoral swelling called tumescence (which is equal to an erection of the male's penis) to lack of sensation in the nipples of the breasts and genitals, to difficulty reaching climax (also called orgasmic disorder).

The reasons for a woman's cold response in the bedroom are varied. However, a woman's libido or sex drive is not only about arousal. Physical and mental factors like depression, anger, resentment, or relationship issues, as well as hormonal imbalances, poor blood flow to the genitals, and nerve damage can come into play. Sex therapy entails professional psychological and physical therapy, such as doing pelvic floor exercises, which can enhance arousal and put women in touch with their bodies.

Nourishing the Female Libido

There's no doubt that women require special tender love and care when it comes to igniting a sexual spark. With hormonal changes (e.g., after giving birth or during and after menopause) and the dynamic nature of the vagina during certain times in a woman's monthly cycle, arousal may be compromised. Even levels of the male hormone testosterone affect sexual function in women. During the month, as the female cycle ebbs and flows, testosterone levels do the same, dictating sexual desire. As in men, high testosterone levels peak sexual interest and lead to optimal arousal in women.

Being properly nourished can affect the delicate balance of hormones in a female's body. If a woman is too thin or obese, her estrogen levels can be thrown off, causing hormonal imbalances like amenorrhea, absence of the menstrual cycle, heavy bleeding during menstruation, or early menopause—all of which can affect sexual arousal. If you don't have a menstrual cycle, you also miss out on the natural libido lift that occurs a few days before ovulation, when the ovary releases an egg to be fertilized.

Eating for Your Libido

Here are some eating tips to lift your libido and create A+ arousal:

- Eat enough calories, but not too much. Maintaining a healthy body weight with three square meals a day, plus two snacks, should ensure enough fuel for your sexual desire.

- Avoid skipping meals or overeating at one time in the day. Get a steady flow of calories throughout the day. Hunger or fullness can squelch the sexual flame fast.

- Eat enough fat; going fat-free is a hormonal nightmare. Hormones need fat to function. Balance your hormones with low-fat dairy products, nuts, seeds, olive oil, and avocados.

- Fuel up on high-fiber veggies, fruits, and some whole grains every day. Your vascular health will benefit—and that promotes good blood flow down there!

- Avoid drinking too much alcohol, as this can depress your mood and sedate you—and you'll miss out on the moment completely. Don't drink more than one alcoholic beverage a day!

Taking a Closer Look at Aphrodisiacs

Food has a long association with sexual stimulation and arousal. The ancient Greek myths tell us that the gods considered certain foods to be natural aphrodisiacs, or substances that increase sexual desire. Foods long thought to stimulate passion run the gamut from fruits like cherries, bananas, strawberries, and tomatoes to vegetables like artichokes, asparagus, and arugula, as well as truffles, oysters, and dark chocolate. Herbs and spices believed to ignite the sexual flame include saffron, ginkgo biloba, and ginseng.

But before you run out and buy any of these foods to give you a boost in the bedroom, stop to read this: a recent research review that looked at natural aphrodisiacs found that the science is lacking to back any of these foods as genuine remedies for female or male sexual dysfunction. So eat and enjoy—and if any of these foods stimulate anything besides your taste buds, consider yourself lucky!

Food and Fertility

One out of every six couples experience *infertility*. Conceiving a baby relies on a delicate system of checks and balances including the intricate interplay of hormones, the quality of sperm and egg, the timing and presence of ovulation, a healthy body weight, and fitness level. The reasons for infertility vary; however, ovulatory disorders in women are present in more than 25 percent of infertile females.

Definition

Infertility is the attempt to conceive for a least one year (or six months for women over 35) without success; it's one of the most prevalent chronic health disorders involving young adults today.

In men, ED from diabetes or related conditions, as well as endurance sports, such as long distance running, may diminish sexual encounters and/or affect sperm count and quality. Research has identified omega-3 fats as a nutrient that is high in the sperm of fertile men, but lacking in infertile men. So that means oily fish, flaxseed, and possibly omega-3 supplementation may play a role in male fertility.

Although everyone has different dietary needs when it comes to conception, certain foods may come into play in preventing infertility—and magically promote conception.

Studies have shown that relatively simple changes in diet and lifestyle can have a profound effect on fertility. A large study of healthy women who were trying to get pregnant over an eight-year period identified a "fertility eating pattern" to prevent ovulatory disorders in women, as well as lifestyle factors like physical activity that can play a large role in fertility.

As we point out again and again in this book, just as it's your total diet and nutrients working together synergistically that play a role in overall health, the same is true for fertility. Eating a variety of nutrient-rich whole foods the majority of the time is your best bet for conception. The dietary pattern for fertility that researchers found to work includes more monounsaturated fatty acids (MUFAs), such as avocado, olive oil, and nuts instead of trans fatty acids found in partially hydrogenated vegetable oil (found primarily in store-bought baked goods); vegetable proteins rather than animal proteins (less red meat and more beans, legumes, and hummus); high-fiber breads, cereals, and pastas; dairy products with some fat versus fat-free varieties (the fat is beneficial for ovulation and fertility); and iron from plants like leafy greens, cereals, and beans. They concluded that women who combined this pattern of eating with regular physical activity and weight control had a 69 percent lower risk of ovulation problems that cause infertility.

Polycystic Ovarian Syndrome

Healthy reproduction is closely tied to body weight and nutritional status. Overweight and obese women can have problems ovulating and so are more likely to experience irregular menstrual cycles. Half of young women who are overweight or obese with menstrual irregularities are diagnosed with polycystic ovarian syndrome (PCOS), a hormonal disorder characterized by large cysts around the outer edge of each ovary. PCOS is considered the most common cause of female infertility.

Females with PCOS have elevated levels of male hormones called androgens. The other defining feature of this disorder is excess facial and body hair—its medical term is hirsutism. Plus, some women lose hair on their head called androgenic alopecia. The symptoms of PCOS are very individual and it may not be diagnosed until a woman tries to conceive a child.

Eating with PCOS

Extremes are not good for fertility—being underweight or overweight can affect ovulation, which in turn can cause infertility. When obesity is coupled with PCOS in women, the physiological phenomenon of insulin resistance occurs, in which the cells of the body are no longer as sensitive to insulin, thus resistant to it. This can lead to type 2 diabetes in women with PCOS.

Studies show that women with PCOS typically binge eat. They have cravings for carbohydrate-rich foods (e.g., cookies, cake, and candy). To avoid surges in blood sugar and insulin levels, the recommendation is high-fiber whole grains or "slow carbs," which take longer to digest versus the high sugar, more refined carbohydrates or "fast carbs" like regular soda, white bread, and potatoes. Because muscle cells utilize insulin better with activity, experts recommend some type of movement daily.

> **Food Wise**
>
> Because women with PCOS can have low-grade inflammation, they should focus on eating small meals with healthful, inflammation-fighting foods. Aim for the best-quality whole foods, such as wild salmon, halibut, or tuna; low-fat dairy foods; high-fiber cereal and breads; plenty of colorful fruits and veggies; and "good" fats like extra-virgin olive oil, nuts, seeds, and avocados; and plant proteins like beans, peas, lentils, tofu, tempeh, and quinoa.

Experts agree that women with PCOS who stop bingeing regulate their menstrual cycles better—and lose weight. It's not just the number on the scale, but your body composition—lean tissue like muscle, bone, and organs versus fat tissue—that counts. Fertility doctors recommend that women with PCOS who are trying to conceive wear adjustable weight vests, which help increase muscle mass, burn more calories, lose weight, and may improve chances of conception.

Weight Gain Guidelines for Moms

Pregnancy is a unique metabolic state in which gestational weight gain encompasses a lot more than just pounds on the scale. It also includes the "products of conception," such as the fetus and placenta, the mother's fat stores, blood volume (which increases greatly), and uterine and breast tissue. Thus, the ultimate challenge is balancing the amount of weight gain needed to optimize the health of the baby without jeopardizing the health of the mother both in the long and short term.

Pregnancy is certainly not the time to diet or restrict calories. Some women experience an unhealthy obsession with weight gain during pregnancy called *pregorexia,* a form of disordered eating some women experience as their familiar body size and shape changes due to pregnancy. If this is an issue, professional help or support is essential.

On the other side of the spectrum, *pregobesity*, or excessive weight gain during pregnancy, is a more prevalent problem. Although you are technically eating for two or maybe more—when you are pregnant, although your calorie needs during pregnancy go up, they are not much more than what you usually need in a day.

Munch on This

The Institute of Medicine (IOM) has guidelines for weight gain during pregnancy, but many pregnant women don't adhere to them. The IOM guidelines for weight gain during pregnancy were revised in 2009 and are based on pre-pregnancy body mass index (BMI) To figure out your BMI go to: www.nhlbisupport.com/bmi/.

Not gaining enough weight can lead to a number of complications including low birth weight, preterm delivery, and infant mortality; gaining too much weight may lead to gestational diabetes or high blood sugars during pregnancy, which must be controlled with a tailored eating plan from a registered dietitian and/or insulin shots prescribed by your health-care provider. Other complications include a big baby at birth, a difficult labor and delivery, and excessive weight to lose after your baby is born.

About 75 percent of women who deliver at term have appropriate weight gain. If you eat normally, listen to your body cues for hunger and fullness, and get regular physical activity (if medically acceptable), you and your baby are likely to have a healthy weight.

Appropriate Weigh-Ins for Expectant Mothers

Pre-Pregnancy Body Mass Index	Recommended Weight Gain
Low (<18.5 kg/m^2)	28–40 pounds
Normal (18.5–24.9 kg/m^2)	25–35 pounds
High (25.0–29.0 kg/m^2)	15–25 pounds
Obese women (> 30 kg/m^2)	11–20 pounds

Sources: Institute of Medicine. Weight Gain During Pregnancy: Reexamining the Guidelines. *Washington, D.C.: National Academy Press; 2009.*

Pregnant with multiples? The IOM advises that those beginning their pregnancy with a normal BMI gain 37 to 54 pounds; those with an overweight BMI gain 31 to 50 pounds; and obese BMI gain 25 to 42 pounds.

According to the IOM, weight gain during the first trimester of pregnancy is a concern. Some women may not gain anything or lose weight due to nausea or vomiting, but others may use their pregnancy as a license to eat anything. With that in mind, the advisable weight gain range in the first trimester is 1.1 to 4.4 pounds.

Keep in mind: you only need an extra 300 calories a day during the second and third trimester (during breast feeding it's an extra 500 calories a day). So what does that 300 calories look like? It's a regular yogurt with a large piece of fruit; two slices of whole-grain toast with a tablespoon of almond butter; or a cup of 1 percent milk and an ounce of whole-grain cereal. So it's not that much more! For more information on pregnancy and weight gain, visit the IOM website at www.iom.edu/pregnancyweightgain.

Have-More-Fun-in-Bed Recipes

Food can be fun and exciting—especially after having some fun in the bedroom. Take time to ignite your passion for food and quite possibly your amorous appetite will become ablaze!

Soybean and Red Pepper Salsa

The crunch of the soybeans and the crisp red peppers give this salsa a delicious and clean flavor. Enjoy it as a side to chicken, fish, or tossed into a salad.

Yield:	Serving size:	Prep time:	Cook time:
2 servings	½ cup	10 minutes	None
Each serving has:			
275 calories	15 g total fat	3 g saturated fat	0 g trans fat
8 mg cholesterol	147 mg sodium	17 g carbohydrates	5 g fiber
5 g sugars	19 g protein	43 percent iron	

1 cup soybeans (edamame), frozen, shelled

½ red bell pepper, chopped

1 shallot, minced

2 TB. feta or goat cheese, crumbled

1 TB. cilantro, chopped

1 TB. extra-virgin olive oil

1 TB. balsamic vinegar

1 tsp. Dijon mustard

Pinch of salt and pepper

1. Defrost edamame on the countertop for an hour or in the microwave on high for 90 seconds.

2. In a large bowl toss together edamame, red pepper, shallot, feta cheese, and cilantro.

3. In a small bowl whisk together olive oil, vinegar, and mustard and pour on top of vegetable cheese mixture. Toss to coat and add salt and pepper as desired.

4. Serve with whole-grain pita chips or top fish, chicken, or pork chops.

Artichoke Purée

This simple dish is fun as a dip, a spread on a whole-grain wrap, or added to tomato soup for added flavor. The optional fresh rosemary gives this purée a wonderful aromatic essence.

Yield:	Serving size:	Prep time:	Cook time:
8 servings	2 tablespoons	5 minutes	None

Each serving has:			
57 calories	0 g total fat	0 g saturated fat	0 g trans fat
0 mg cholesterol	130 mg sodium	13 g carbohydrates	6 g fiber
1 g sugars	4 g protein	9 percent iron	

2 cups artichoke hearts, marinated

1 tsp. curry powder

2 garlic cloves, peeled

2 sprigs of fresh rosemary (optional)

Pinch of salt and pepper

1. Drain artichokes in a colander to remove excess oil.

2. Put artichokes, cloves, and rosemary in a food processor and purée.

3. Taste and add a dash of salt and pepper if needed.

Creamy Curry Salmon Salad

This is perfect in a whole-grain pita bread, with crackers or on a bed of mixed greens.

Yield:	Serving size:	Prep time:	Cook time:
2 servings	¾ cup	5 minutes	None

Each serving has:			
305 calories	16 g total fat	2 g saturated fat	0 g trans fat
94 mg cholesterol	244 mg sodium	4 g carbohydrates	1 g fiber
1 g sugars	35 g protein	12 percent iron	

12 oz. wild salmon, flaked and mashed	1 medium scallion, diced
2 TB. low-fat mayonnaise or nayonaise	½ cup cherry tomatoes, diced
	2 tsp. curry powder
	1 tsp. fresh dill

1. Add salmon, mayonnaise, scallion, tomatoes, and curry powder into a mixing bowl and stir just until combined.

2. Serve with whole-grain pita bread or on a bed of mixed greens.

Munch on This

Salmon in a can or pouch works well for this recipe because it's already flaked and mashed up.

Nayonaise is an egg-free, dairy-free alterative to mayonnaise. Use it anywhere you'd use mayo.

Essential Takeaways

- Sexual health is a big part of overall health.

- Sexual dysfunction in men is called erectile dysfunction (ED); in women it's female sexual dysfunction (FSD).

- Because ED can be linked to heart disease, diabetes, and high blood pressure, eating low-fat dairy, plenty of plant proteins, and less saturated fat can help fend off ED.

- Physical activity can help both men and women in the bedroom, as it can fend off depression and make you more attuned to your body.

- Infertility is a big issue among married couples. Improving eating patterns and physical activity can help both men and women.

- Polycystic ovarian syndrome (PCOS) is the biggest reason for infertility in women. The right food, fitness, and support can play a big role in dealing with this hormonal disorder.

- Pregnancy is a unique metabolic state in which weight gain is inevitable; however, gaining the right amount is important for the health of the mother and growing baby.

chapter 27

Mood Matters

Making the food and mood connection

Soothing common mood disorders

Alleviating mood symptoms

Your mood determines a lot in life; it's your view of the world and a portal to the whims of your food cravings. From an emotional standpoint, moods can be happy and joyful or sad and angry—however, in a healthy mind moods change. Like a mood ring that turns colors, your state of mind or mood can change with the weather—and last for fleeting moments or days. However, when people get stuck in a mood rut, they're typically not in a good and healthy mood. Over 20 million adults in the United States have mood disorders or disturbances that have a negative impact on their health.

The food you choose to eat—or not eat—can be a direct reflection of your mood. Some people with mood disorders, such as major depression and bipolar disorder have intense cravings for refined carbs (e.g., candy, cookies, fried foods, etc.) and others lose their appetite altogether. In this chapter, I discuss the gamut of moods and point out healthful foods that can heal mental illness and help change the forecast in the mind to bright and sunny!

Mood and Health

Your everyday moods can affect your health and your health can affect your moods. Studies show that a positive frame of mind can reduce risk of heart disease and boost immunity. A positive outlook has been linked with lowering stress hormones and keeping blood pressure, heart rate, and inflammatory markers down, which are all signs of good health.

In the face of illnesses like the flu or the common cold, studies show that those with positive emotions like happiness and pleasure had fewer upper respiratory infections compared to those with negative emotions like anxiety, hostility, and/or depression.

Food and Depression

Feeling blue for a day or two is nothing to be concerned about, but when these feelings last for a long time and escalate to feelings of helplessness, disordered eating, loss of pleasure in everyday life, restlessness, and/or anxiety, this can be full-blown depression, which requires professional help. The good news is depression is highly treatable, especially if caught early. Whether the depression causes the sufferer to overeat or not eat enough, treating the underlying depression and incorporating nutrient-rich foods as part of the treatment plan may help.

Let's look at some key terms for mood disturbances:

- **Mood disorders** (used to be called "affective disorders")   A group of distinct disturbances in a person's mood or behavior; includes major depression, bipolar disorder, and anxiety disorder.

- **Major depression**   A mood disorder characterized by chronic sadness, feelings of hopelessness, overeating, or appetite loss.

- **Bipolar disorder**   A mood disorder in which the person swings between mania and depression.

- **Anxiety disorder**   A group of emotional disturbances characterized by fear and anxiety; for example, generalized anxiety disorder is chronic worrying for six months or more.

Depression and Disordered Eating

Major depression is the leading cause of disability in the United States for people ages 15 to 44 years. There is a direct link between depression and eating disorders; research shows that half of people diagnosed with binge eating disorder (BED) have depression. Depression can be so pronounced in people with anorexia nervosa (AN); people with this eating disorder are

50 times more likely to commit suicide. (See Chapter 2 for details on these disorder.) Binge eating is also associated with night-eating disorder (see Chapter 19).

Treating people with both depression and an eating disorder is tricky. Antidepressant medication has been shown to help with disordered eating, particularly for AN; for BED, the anticonvulsant medication, Topomax, has shown some benefit, but it may only be temporary. Eating disorders may require a type of psychotherapy called cognitive behavioral therapy (CBT), as studies have shown that CBT helps alleviate the disordered eating and the associated depression, too. So a combination of nutrition, psychological, and medical therapies is the most effective.

Winter Blues

Seasonal affective disorder (SAD), or winter blues, can affect sleep patterns and make waking up difficult. It leads to a lack of energy, difficulty concentrating, and cravings for high carbohydrate and fatty foods, which can cause weight gain. Because it gets darker earlier in the winter and sunlight is covered by clouds in the northern climates during winter months, light therapy with a light box is prescribed. It helps increase levels of the hormone melatonin, which can boost appetite, decrease cravings, and regulate mood.

Mediterranean Diet and Depression

Nutrition offers an inexpensive, side-effect free adjunct therapy for depression. Research has shown that incorporating Mediterranean-type foods (plant foods such as vegetables, fruits, nuts, whole-grain cereals, beans, and legumes; as well as fish) into the diets of people with depression works. A large study found that healthy people who ate the most fruits, nuts, and beneficial monounsaturated fats experienced lower rates of depressive disorders.

Mood Lifting B-Vitamins

One of the components of the Mediterranean diet that is lacking in the refined Western diet is B-vitamins, primarily B_1, B_2, B_{12}, B_6, and folic acid (B_9). Experts believe that B-vitamins are powerful players in fending off depression in people of all ages. Through a complex metabolic process, B-vitamins—specifically B_{12} and B_6—help balance the levels of homocysteine (an amino acid that is linked to heart disease) in the bloodstream. Too much homocysteine throws off mood regulators in the brain, and depression can ensue! So not eating enough B-vitamins—specifically folic acid, B_{12}, and B_6—has been shown to have a negative effect on your mood.

Folic Acid Defense

A folic acid deficiency can thwart the production of the feel-good brain cell transmitters serotonin, dopamine, and norepinephrine. Studies have shown that low levels of folic acid in men and women leads to depression. Plus, people with low levels of folic acid do not respond to antidepressant medications as well.

> **Food wise**
>
> Smoking can deplete folic acid levels. One study found that men who smoke and suffer from depression are better able to fend off depressive symptoms by boosting folic acid intake. Quitting smoking helps, too!

Dietary folic acid (folate) is found in leafy greens, beans, dried peas, legumes, and nuts. Of course, if you have a deficiency, you can always take a supplement to boost levels—and your mood at the same time! Pregnant women should take prenatal vitamins, which contain folic acid and can reduce this risk of birth defects. (Men should not take more than the recommended amount of folic acid, as high doses may be linked to prostate cancer.)

> **Healing Hints**
>
> Not only will whole grains give you depression-defending B-vitamins, but their high-fiber content can help alleviate constipation, which can be a side-effect of antidepressant medications. Aim for three, 1-ounce servings daily.

To up your mood with B-vitamins choose whole-grain breads, cereals, and pastas over the white, refined flour products. (In the ingredient statement on the package, look for the word *whole* before the grain to make sure the B-vitamins have not be stripped away during processing.) Other foods that contain B-vitamins are turkey, tuna, lentils, beans, tempeh, and fortified nutritional yeast.

Omega-3 Fats and Depression

Some omega-3 fatty acids may do wonders for boosting mental health. In particular, alpha-linolenic acid (ALA)—found in flaxseed, chia seeds, and walnuts; and docosahexaenoic acid (DHA) and eicosapentaenoic acid (EPA)—found in oily fish like salmon, halibut, tuna, and sardines—have been shown to help with depression. Studies have shown that deficiency of omega-3 fats has been linked to higher levels of aggression, stress, and depression. Research tells us that omega-3 fat's anti-inflammatory nature fends off the action of proinflammatory bodies in the brain that suppress the feel-good messengers (neurotransmitters). Omega-3 fats have been found to be particularly protective against depression in women.

Try these simple ways to get more omega-3 fats in your diet:

- Make fish tacos at least one night a week and salmon salad another day. (See recipes in Chapters 10 and 26.)

- Sprinkle a tablespoon of ground flaxseed into pancake batter, banana bread, on yogurt, or into chili. (Aim for 2 tablespoons a day.)

- Toss an ounce of walnuts (7 whole or 14 halves) into oatmeal, meatloaf, and roasted veggie dishes.

- Purée walnuts into basil pesto or other dips and sauces.

- Mix some ground chia seeds into quick breads, puddings, and cakes.

Eating Alone and Depression

People who eat alone are less happy than people who eat in a community or social setting. It makes sense because eating alone is isolating and can contribute to overeating, and this sets up a vicious cycle of depression. A recent study of older caregivers (age 50 +) found that the ones with depressive symptoms had a poorer appetite and were at a higher risk of malnutrition (due to eating imbalanced meals), however they were overweight! The real kicker is that a quarter of them ate meals alone, which is not only no fun, but can lead to depression.

Connectedness with others or a healthy social network cannot only add years to your life, but can make you happier.

In his book, *The Blue Zones: Lessons for Living Longer from the People Who've Lived the Longest* (National Geography Society, 2010), Dan Buettner describes five zones in the world where people live longer (over 100 years) and depression is virtually nonexistent due to the importance of a social community, mindful eating, and a healthy outlook on life. We can all learn a lesson from these parts of the world. Here are five ways to enjoy meals mindfully with others and be happy today:

- Make family meal time sacred. Cook with your family every night (or most nights) and sit, enjoy, and linger over the meal.

- Use your appetite as your barometer of eating pleasure; give your brain time to register fullness (at least 20 minutes) and your palate time to enjoy the food.

- Set up a weekly date with your spouse or partner to eat in each other's company. To enjoy the food, conversation, and connectedness of the moment without other distractions.

- Host a hands-on cooking class or party in your home once a month and enjoy the preparation, eating, and even the clean-up with your community of friends.

- At lunchtime, when it can be tempting to eat at your desk or go off alone to dine out, make plans with co-workers or friends around your office to connect over a meal.

Anxiety Disorder and Eating

About 40 million Americans are walking around with an anxiety disorder—whether it's panic disorder, obsessive-compulsive disorder, post-traumatic stress disorder, generalized anxiety, and/or phobias. Anxiety can grip you in the gut and take hold, and it's frequently tied to depression and/or drugs or alcohol abuse. People with anxiety often obsess about food in general or certain foods, particularly carbohydrates like bread, pasta, rice, and crackers.

Treatment for anxiety disorder coupled with an eating disorder can involve medication, nutrition therapy with a registered dietitian, and a CBT-trained psychologist. The good news with some forms of anxiety is that early diagnosis can lead to big results.

Food wise

Natural herbal remedies like kava and St. John's wort promise to end some depression and anxiety disorders, but their effectiveness is inconclusive. Your best bet is moving your body regularly, getting a good night's sleep, and cutting back on the caffeine.

Caffeine Connection

There's no proof that caffeine causes anxiety, but because it is a stimulant, it may magnify the symptoms of anxiety. Experts advise cutting back on the java as part of treatment for people who suffer from anxiety. Because caffeine can interrupt sleep, and getting a good night's sleep is necessary for good health, everyone should avoid drinking caffeine too close to bedtime.

Premenstrual Syndrome

There's no doubt that the hormonal changes that women go through during their menstrual cycle can be challenging. A week before their period women typically experience a cluster of mood-altering symptoms that are appropriately called premenstrual syndrome (PMS). Many women experience physical changes in their bodies like bloating and breast tenderness, but the actual diagnosis of PMS requires more severe symptoms that interfere with your daily life. Although statistics show that only about 2 to 5 percent of females have actual PMS, some research estimates show that 25 percent need some form of treatment for symptoms.

Of all the symptoms—and there are about 150—that women can have during or just prior to their period, three stand out as the diagnostic tell-tales of PMS: irritability, tension, and dysphoria (unhappiness or anxiety). A more severe type of PMS is called premenstrual dysphoric disorder (PMDD), which has a lot of symptoms as depression, such as feelings of hopelessness, guilt, and loss of control.

Food and Your Cycle

Food can be a factor in PMS. Hormone surges in the body during this time can make women feel ravenous the week before their period. Good nutrition can help keep hormones and your mood steady. Upping minerals like calcium carbonate (1,000–1,200 milligrams/day) can help regulate cravings, so be sure to eat at least two to three servings of low-fat dairy products, leafy greens, and tofu. Adding more vitamin B$_6$ to your diet has shown to alleviate symptoms of depression. Foods like whole grains, fruits, veggies, and nuts contain B$_6$.

Eat whole foods like veggies, fruits, and lean protein; and consuming less refined sugar and sodium, as too much processed and salt-laden foods can make you bloated and uncomfortable. Lastly, cut back on the caffeine (and that means chocolate, too!) as this will only feed into lack of sleep, food cravings, and irritability.

Healing Hints	When stress, PMS, anxiety, or depression hit, don't reach for the refined carbs. Eating them will only make you want more, sucking you into the dreaded craving cycle. Instead have some protein like a handful of nuts, a tablespoon of almond butter on whole-grain toast, and/or $\frac{1}{2}$ cup of low-fat cottage cheese and a brown rice cake.

Also, increase your activity levels at this time of the month. Regular physical activity can do wonders for relieving stress and elevating your mood. Combine both cardio work and strength-training to build muscle and efficiently burn calories.

Chronic Fatigue Syndrome

People suffering from chronic fatigue syndrome (CFS) often feel exhausted even though they haven't exerted themselves, or wake up feeling not rested, or have joint or muscle pain for no reason. Although the cause for CFS is unknown, about 1 million people in America have it. It's an adult affliction that rears up in the 40s and 50s, and it causes mood disturbances like depression. While CFS can be disabling and extremely painful for some, in others the symptoms are more tolerable.

People with CFS can compensate for their symptoms by living a healthier life—less smoking, drinking, and keeping weight down. Replace saturated fat with mood-boosting omega-3 fats and get plenty of B-vitamins for energy and to boost your immune system.

Keeping your eating balanced and consistent from day to day will help keep blood sugar regulated and avoid energy-draining highs and lows. Be sure to include high-fiber carbs, whole grains, fruits, and veggies instead of energy-sapping refined, processed white flour foods. Try to get regular physical activity: studies have shown that light aerobic exercise such as walking, swimming, or bicycling can help people with CFS feel better and have more energy.

Essential Takeaways

- Eating well and exercising can boost mood and health at the same time.
- Depression is a serious mood disorder with symptoms such as hopelessness, disordered eating, and lack of pleasure in life. Omega-3 fats, B-vitamins, and whole foods can help.
- Anxiety disorder is excessive fear and worry; it causes sleep disturbances, malnutrition, and eating disorders. Avoid caffeine, alcohol, and eat balanced meals and snacks.
- Premenstrual syndrome (PMS) is a painful and discomforting time of month for women. Focus on foods like calcium, whole grains, beans, and nuts; and get regular physical activity.
- Chronic fatigue syndrome is extreme tiredness for no reason, plus painful joints and muscles. Fuel your body with a steady stream of high-fiber carbs, lean protein, and "good" fats.

Glossary

allergic reactions   The body's response to the immune system's release of chemicals; symptoms range from hives, rash, wheezing, trouble breathing, and eventual death.

anaphylaxis   A potentially fatal allergic reaction that progresses quickly from a rash, wheezing, and swollen lips to a drop in blood pressure and loss of consciousness.

anthocyanins   Water-soluble pigments that appear blue, red, or purple in fruits and vegetables and have been found to prevent chronic diseases.

anxiety disorder   A group of emotional disturbances characterized by fear and anxiety.

artificially acquired immunity   Temporary protection against disease or illness by vaccinations, in which the body is given a small dose of the disease to the immune system to build antibodies.

autoimmune disease   Occurs when the body's immune system attacks itself causing illness and diseases.

bipolar disorder   A mood disorder in which individuals swing between mania and depression.

circadian rhythm   Your inner timekeeper based on the light and darkness in a 24-hour period.

conventional foods   Foods produced with synthetic chemicals, irradiation, and in the presence of sludge or toxic waste.

dehydration   Extreme loss of body water; typically noticeable when 2 percent of the body's normal body water is lost. Symptoms include headache, dizziness, and fatigue.

diet   All of the food and beverages regularly consumed.

Dietary Guidelines for Americans   Nutrition recommendations to promote health and prevent chronic diseases.

dietary reference intake (DRI)   Nutrition recommendations in the United States and Canada developed by the Institute of Medicine, used to create the USDA Dietary Guidelines for Americans.

empty-calorie food   Contains more calories than nutrients; examples include candy, cookies, white bread, fried foods, and alcoholic beverages.

evolutionary eating   Gradual, slow changes in food choices and eating habits that are good for overall health.

fat-soluble vitamins   Vitamins that can be stored for long periods of time in the body and do not need to be replenished as frequently.

food allergens   Proteins in certain foods that the immune system attacks.

food guide pyramid   A visual guideline that depicts how many daily servings you should eat from each of the food groups.

garam masala   A popular blend of aromatic ground spices used in Indian and south Asian cooking.

ghrelin   The only known hormone in humans that stimulates appetites and cravings for certain foods.

glucose   Sugar and starches that give the brain and body energy and growth.

goitrogens   Foods that may block the thyroid from getting enough iodine, the mineral needed for proper thyroid function.

heat stress   Exposure to extreme hot temperatures, which can lead to dizziness, fatigue, nausea, muscle cramps, and death.

hidden hunger   The chronic lack of vitamins and minerals that often has no visible warning signs.

histamine   One of the chemicals released in the body that causes an allergic reaction.

hydration   The state of having optimal levels of water in the body to maintain normal metabolism, body temperature, and organ function.

innate immunity   The body's natural resistance to disease and infection; it's a fast-response defense against general infections and typically offers short-term protection.

insulin   The hormone that enables glucose to get into the body's cells for energy.

insulin resistance   Occurs when the body's cells can no longer use insulin effectively (resists it), thus preventing glucose from entering the cells.

insulin sensitivity   The body's ability to use insulin; the higher the sensitivity the better.

internal cues   Your body's natural feelings of hunger (i.e., stomach grumbling, light-headedness) and fullness (i.e., bloating, discomfort).

lipids   Fats, oils, waxes, and related compounds found in foods and the human body.

major depression   A mood disorder characterized by chronic sadness, feelings of hopelessness, overeating, or appetite loss.

mindful eating   Consciously choosing to eat food that is both pleasing and nourishing to your body to use all of your senses to explore, savor, and taste.

mindless eating   Unconscious decision-making about what and how much we eat.

minerals   Support chemical reactions in the body for proper functioning of organs, bones, and hormones.

mood disorders   A group of distinct disturbances in a person's mood or behavior; includes major depression, bipolar disorder, and anxiety disorder.

MyPyramid food guidance system   A system of healthy eating that provides motivational tools, personalized eating plans, and a physical activity component for every American age 2 and older.

nutrient   A chemical substance in foods; nutrients provide energy, growth, enable repair of cells, and regulate body processes.

nutrient-dense foods   Foods that provide a lot of vitamins, minerals, and fiber with relatively few calories.

organic   A designation used by the U.S. Department of Agriculture's National Organic Program to certify food that is produced without synthetic chemicals or fertilizers, genetic engineering, radiation, or sewage sludge.

oxygen radical absorbance capacity (ORAC) scale   Used in laboratories to determine the antioxidant capacity of certain foods.

probiotics   Live microorganisms that, when administered in adequate amounts, confer a health benefit on the host.

processed foods   Foods altered from their natural state and that typically contain a lot of sugar, salt, and fat.

recombinant bovine somatotropin (RBST)   An artificial growth hormone injected in dairy cows to increase milk production.

saturated fats   The unhealthy fats; solid fats, such as butter, bacon, cheese, and marbling in meat.

self-regulation   The body's ability to know when to start eating and when to stop.

sleep hygiene   Healthy bedtime practices that help ensure a good night's sleep.

thermic effect of food   The extra energy or calories it takes your body to chew, bite, swallow, and process (move, digest, and store) nutrients.

thyroid gland   Controls metabolism and hormone levels in your body.

total diet   Overall pattern of eating over the course of a few days to a week.

trans fats   Partially hydrogenated vegetable oils found in store-bought baked goods.

unsaturated fats   The heart-healthy fats; typically liquid fats, such as vegetable oils; they are also found in avocados, nuts, seeds, dark leafy greens (e.g., broccoli, cabbage, and spinach), and fish oil.

vitamins   Natural compounds in animals and plants that the body requires for overall health and vitality.

water intoxication   A dangerous, life-threatening condition caused by drinking too much water; it can lead to loss of electrolytes, abnormal brain function, and possible death.

water-soluble vitamins   Vitamins that dissolve easily in water and are eliminated from the body quickly; they must be replenished regularly.

Food and Beverage Log

Use the following log to keep track of your daily food and beverage intake.

Day/Date: _____

Time	Meal	All Food & Drinks Consumed	Hunger Rating (on a scale of 1–10, 1 = starving; 10 = not hungry)
_____	_____	_____	_____
_____	_____	_____	_____
_____	_____	_____	_____
_____	_____	_____	_____
_____	_____	_____	_____
_____	_____	_____	_____
_____	_____	_____	_____
_____	_____	_____	_____
_____	_____	_____	_____
_____	_____	_____	_____
_____	_____	_____	_____
_____	_____	_____	_____
_____	_____	_____	_____
_____	_____	_____	_____
_____	_____	_____	_____
_____	_____	_____	_____
_____	_____	_____	_____
_____	_____	_____	_____
_____	_____	_____	_____
_____	_____	_____	_____
_____	_____	_____	_____
_____	_____	_____	_____

Resources

Websites

American Dietetic Association
www.eatright.org

American Heart Association
www.americanheart.org

Dietary Guidelines for Americans 2010
www.dietaryguidelines.gov

CDC Division of Nutrition, Physical Activity & Obesity
www.cdc.gov/nccdphp/dnpa

Center for Science in the Public Interest
www.cspi.net

USDA National Agricultural Library Food and Nutrition Information
fnic.nal.usda.gov

International Food Information Council (IFIC) Foundation
www.ific.org

Nutrition.gov
www.nutrition.gov

USDA Food Guide System
www.mypyramid.gov

Nutrient-Rich Coalition
www.nutrientrichfoods.org

The Food Allergy and Anaphylaxis Network
www.foodallergy.org

Environmental Working Group
www.ewg.org

National Institutes of Health (NIH) Office of Dietary Supplements (ODS)
ods.od.nih.gov

International Tree Nut Council
www.nuthealth.org

California Walnuts
www.walnuts.org

California Avocado Commission
www.avocado.org

US Highbush Blueberry Council
www.blueberry.org

The Cranberry Institute
www.cranberryinstitute.org

The Whole Grains Council
www.wholegrainscouncil.com

National Heart, Lung and Blood Institute
www.nhlbi.nih.gov

USDA National Nutrition Database
www.nal.usda.gov/fnic/foodcomp/search

Books

Albers, Susan, Ph.D. *Eat, Drink, and Be Mindful.* Oakland: New Harbinger Publications, Inc. 2008.

Case, Shelley, B.Sc., R.D. *Gluten-Free Diet.* Canada: Case Nutrition Consulting, Inc. 2008.

Craighead, Linda W., Ph.D. *The Appetite Awareness Workbook.* Oakland: New Harbinger Publications, Inc. 2006.

Geagan, Kate, M.S., R.D. *Go Green, Get Lean.* New York City: Rodale, 2009.

Grotto, David, R.D., L.D.N. *101 Optimal Life Foods.* New York City: Bantam Dell, 2009.

Jackson Blatner, Dawn, R.D., L.D.N. *The Flexitarian Diet.* New York City: McGraw-Hill, 2008.

Scarlata, Kate, R.D., L.D.N. *The Complete Idiot's Guide to Eating Well with IBS.* Indianapolis: Alpha Books, 2010.

Taub-Dix, Bonnie, R.D., L.D.N. *Read It Before You Eat It.* New York City: Penguin Group, 2010.

Tessmer, Kimberly A., R.D., L.D., and Chef Stephanie Green, R.D. *The Complete Idiot's Guide to The Mediterranean Diet.* Indianapolis: Alpha Books, 2010.

Wansink, Brian, Ph.D. *Mindless Eating: Why We Eat More Than We Think.* New York City: Bantam Dell, 2006.

Young, Lisa R., Ph.D., R.D. *The Portion Teller Plan.* New York City: Morgan Road Books, 2005.

index